BMA

Essentials of Pediatric Neuroanesthesia

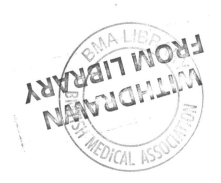
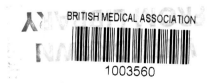

Essentials of Pediatric Neuroanesthesia

Edited by

Sulpicio G. Soriano
Boston Children's Hospital and Harvard Medical School

Craig D. McClain
Boston Children's Hospital and Harvard Medical School

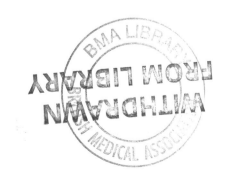

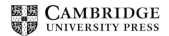

CAMBRIDGE
UNIVERSITY PRESS

CAMBRIDGE
UNIVERSITY PRESS

University Printing House, Cambridge CB2 8BS, United Kingdom

One Liberty Plaza, 20th Floor, New York, NY 10006, USA

477 Williamstown Road, Port Melbourne, VIC 3207, Australia

314–321, 3rd Floor, Plot 3, Splendor Forum, Jasola District Centre, New Delhi – 110025, India

79 Anson Road, #06–04/06, Singapore 079906

Cambridge University Press is part of the University of Cambridge.

It furthers the University's mission by disseminating knowledge in the pursuit of education, learning, and research at the highest international levels of excellence.

www.cambridge.org
Information on this title: www.cambridge.org/9781316608876
DOI: 10.1017/9781316652947

© Cambridge University Press 2019

First published 2019

Printed in the United Kingdom by TJ International Ltd Padstow Cornwall

A catalogue record for this publication is available from the British Library.

Library of Congress Cataloging-in-Publication data
Names: Soriano, Sulpicio, editor. | McClain, Craig (Craig D.), editor.
Title: Essentials of pediatric neuroanesthesia / edited by Sulpicio Soriano, Craig McClain.
Description: Cambridge, United Kingdom ; New York, NY : Cambridge University Press, 2019. | Includes bibliographical references and index.
Identifiers: LCCN 2018028364 | ISBN 9781316608876
Subjects: | MESH: Anesthesia | Neurosurgical Procedures | Nervous System Diseases – surgery | Child
Classification: LCC RD139 | NLM WO 440 | DDC 617.9/6083–dc23
LC record available at https://lccn.loc.gov/2018028364

ISBN 978-1-316-60887-6 Paperback

This book is dedicated to my family (Carmen A. Perez, Richard, Steven, Laura, Teresa, Sara, Kristen, Isa, Koa and Leo Soriano) and mentors (Babu V. Koka and Gerald A. Gronert) who have blessed me with unwavering support and guidance.

SGS

I would like to dedicate this work to the three groups of people that I will forever be indebted to for anything good I've been able to do in my life. First and foremost, I want to thank my family—Natalie, Isla, Callum, and Finlay as well as the extended McClains, Murphys, and Vuyks. Thanks for your continued support, patience, and understanding. I am an incredibly lucky man to have you all in my life, and I love you all so very much. Second, I'd like to thank my mentors throughout my training and practice who have tried to teach me how to be a good and caring doctor. A complete list is impossible, but I'd like to single out Terry Yemen, Keith Littlewood, Sol Soriano, Mike McManus, and Bob Holzman as folks that I find myself quoting and emulating on a daily basis. Finally, and most importantly to this book, I'd like to thank the patients and families that have allowed me to participate in their care and hopefully help them as they negotiate often Promethean tasks. I am humbled on a daily basis by the grace with which they go about their lives during times that are often unfathomably difficult. Thank you.

CDM

Contents

Contributors

Hubert A. Benzon
Ann and Robert H. Lurie Children's Hospital of Chicago and Northwestern University Feinberg School of Medicine, Chicago, IL, USA

Ken M. Brady
Ann and Robert H. Lurie Children's Hospital of Chicago and Northwestern University Feinberg School of Medicine, Chicago, IL, USA

Eric Darrow
Cook Children's Hospital, Fort Worth, TX, USA

Rebecca Dube
Hospital for Sick Children and University of Toronto School of Medicine, Toronto, Canada

Thejovathi Edala
Arkansas Children's Hospital and University of Arkansas for Medical Sciences, Little Rock, AR, USA

Thomas O. Erb
University Children's Hospital and University of Basel, Basel, Switzerland

David Faraoni
Hospital for Sick Children and University of Toronto School of Medicine, Toronto, Canada

Audrice Francois
Stritch School of Medicine of Loyola University Chicago, Chicago, IL, USA

Susan M. Goobie
Boston Children's Hospital and Harvard Medical School, Boston, MA, USA

Indu Kapoor
All India Institute of Medical Sciences (AIIMS), New Delhi, India

Babu V. Koka
Boston Children's Hospital and Harvard Medical School, Boston, MA, USA

Rahul Koka
Johns Hopkins Children's Center and Johns Hopkins University, Baltimore, MD, USA

Mary Landrigan-Ossar
Boston Children's Hospital and Harvard Medical School, Boston, MA, USA

Jennifer K. Lee
Johns Hopkins Children's Center and Johns Hopkins University, Baltimore, MD, USA

David Levin
Hospital for Sick Children and University of Toronto School of Medicine, Toronto, Canada

Elaina E. Lin
Children's Hospital of Philadelphia and Perelman School of Medicine at the University of Pennsylvania, Philadelphia, PA, USA

Charu Mahajan
All India Institute of Medical Sciences (AIIMS), New Delhi, India

Jason T. Maynes
Hospital for Sick Children and University of Toronto School of Medicine, Toronto, Canada

John McAuliffe
Cincinnati Children's Hospital Medical Center and University of Cincinnati College of Medicine, Cincinnati, OH, USA

Mary Ellen McCann
Boston Children's Hospital and Harvard Medical School, Boston, MA, USA

Craig D. McClain
Boston Children's Hospital and Harvard Medical School, Boston, MA, USA

Michael L. McManus
Boston Children's Hospital and Harvard Medical School, Boston, MA, USA

Douglas Hale McMichael
Ann and Robert H. Lurie Children's Hospital of Chicago and Northwestern University Feinberg School of Medicine, Chicago, IL, USA

Petra M. Meier
Boston Children's Hospital and Harvard Medical School, Boston, MA, USA

Hemanshu Prabhakar
All India Institute of Medical Sciences (AIIMS), New Delhi, India

Laura C. Rhee
Boston Children's Hospital and Harvard Medical School, Boston, MA, USA

Ravi Shah
Ann and Robert H. Lurie Children's Hospital of Chicago and Northwestern University Feinberg School of Medicine, Chicago, IL, USA

Sulpicio G. Soriano
Boston Children's Hospital and Harvard Medical School, Boston, MA, USA

Paul A. Stricker
Children's Hospital of Philadelphia and Perelman School of Medicine at the University of Pennsylvania, Philadelphia, PA, USA

Santhanam Suresh
Ann and Robert H. Lurie Children's Hospital of Chicago and Northwestern University Feinberg School of Medicine, Chicago, IL, USA

Robert C. Tasker
Boston Children's Hospital and Harvard Medical School, Boston, MA, USA

Kha M. Tran
Children's Hospital of Philadelphia and Perelman School of Medicine at the University of Pennsylvania, Philadelphia, PA, USA

Cynthia Tung
Boston Children's Hospital and Harvard Medical School, Boston, MA, USA

Monica S. Vavilala
Harborview Medical Center and University of Washington, Seattle, WA, USA

Frederick Vonberg
Boston Children's Hospital and Harvard Medical School, Boston, MA, USA

Lazslo Vutskits
University Hospital Geneva and University of Geneva, Geneva, Switzerland

Jue Wang
Boston Children's Hospital and Harvard Medical School, Boston, MA, USA

Preface

This book was written to provide practical recommendations for the perioperative management of neurosurgical procedures in pediatric patients. The constant evolution in the care of infants and children with neurosurgical conditions and the recognition of age-related differences in the surgical lesions, anatomy, and physiological responses to surgery and anesthesia have fueled pediatric subspecialization by our colleagues in neurosurgery and critical care. The guidance prescribed by these chapters is founded on anatomy, physiology, and pharmacology unique to the infant and child and is based on the expertise and experience of international authorities on the care of pediatric neurosurgical patients. This approach ensures that best practices in pediatric neuroanesthesia are part of the repertoire and skill set of the reader as technological innovations in neurosurgery and interventional neuroradiology emerge.

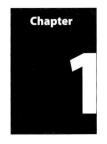

Developmental Approach to the Pediatric Neurosurgical Patient

Jue Wang and Sulpicio G. Soriano

Introduction

The anesthetic management of infants and children undergoing neurosurgical procedures should be based on the developmental stage of the patient. The evolving maturational changes of the various organ systems have a significant impact of the drugs and techniques used for the safe conduct of anesthesia. Subspecialty training in pediatric neurosurgery has driven advances in intracranial surgery in infants and children, prompting calls for similarly trained anesthesiologists and intensivists for the management of these infants and children.[1] Age-dependent differences in cranial bone development, cerebrovascular physiology, and neurologic lesions distinguish neonates, infants, and children from their adult counterparts. In particular, the central nervous system (CNS) undergoes a tremendous amount of structural and physiological change during the first two years of life. Neurosurgical lesions and associated surgery in this vulnerable age group have been linked to increased mortality and decreased academic achievement scores at adolescence.[2] Furthermore, outcome studies reveal increased perioperative morbidity, mortality, and cognitive deficits in this patient population.[3–5] This chapter highlights these age-dependent differences and their effect on the anesthetic management of the pediatric neurosurgical patient.

Developmental Aspects

Central Nervous System

The CNS develops early in gestation and is orchestrated by a combination of transcriptional and mechanical factors.[6] A basic understanding of normal and abnormal development of the CNS is essential for comprehending the pathology of congenital lesions of the CNS.[7]

The primitive CNS is derived from the neural plate, which folds and fuses dorsally. Primary neurulation occurs when the neural plate folds to form the neural tube. The walls of the neural tube give rise to the brain and spinal cord, while the canal develops into the ventricles and central canal of the brain and spinal cord, respectively. Fusion of the cranial neural folds and closure of the cranial neuropore, which give rise to the forebrain, midbrain, and hindbrain, arise from these structures. Failure of the anterior neuropore to close by 24 days results in anencephaly. Secondary neurulation ensues when the neuroepithelium caudal to the posterior neuropore closes. Derangements in this progression can lead to spinal dysraphism (spinal bifida, myelomeningocele, and tethered cord).

After birth, the CNS is essentially fully developed, with some fine tuning that occurs between the neonatal and toddler periods.[8] Cerebral blood flow (CBF) varies with the age of the patient, which peaks between 2 and 4 years and settles to adult levels at 7–8 years.[9] Prematurity, traumatic brain injury, neurovascular anomalies, hypoxic brain injuries, intracranial hemorrhage, inflammatory processes, and congenital heart defects have an impact on cerebral hemodynamics. Although the theoretical autoregulatory range of blood pressure in infants is lower than in adults due to the relatively low cerebral metabolic requirements and blood pressure during infancy, recent evidence demonstrates heterogeneity of the lower limits of autoregulation in pediatric pateints.[10] Although cerebral autoregulation is intact in healthy full-term neonates,[8] it may be absent in critically ill premature neonates.[11] CBF pressure-passivity is common in premature neonates with low gestational age and birth weight and systemic hypotension. Systolic arterial blood pressure is a poor surrogate of cerebral perfusion pressure in these patients, and the diastolic closing pressure may be a better measure of cerebral perfusion in this population.[12] Extremes in blood pressure can lead to cerebral ischemia and intraventricular hemorrhage and dictate rigorous control of hemodynamics in this vulnerable population.

Children have high cerebral metabolic requirement for oxygen and glucose ($CMRO_2$ and CMRGlu) relative to adult values ($CMRO_2$ 5.8 vs. 3.5 mL/100g/m and CMRGlu 6.8 vs. 5.5 mL/100g/m, respectively).[13] At birth, CMRGlu is approximately 13–25 µmol/100g/min and rises to 49–65 µmol/100g/min at 3–4 years. It remains at this rate until 9 years and subsequently settles at 19–33 µmol/100g/m.[14] These ontological changes in $CRMO_2$ and CMRGlu are reflected in CBF values derived from brain perfusion computed tomographic (CT) scans.[9] Cerebrovascular reactivity to carbon dioxide appears to be normal in newborns, but may be deranged in the setting of perinatal asphyxia.[15] Inspired concentrations of oxygen (FIO_2) have an impact on CBF. Decreasing FIO_2 from 1.0 to 0.21 decreases CBF by 33%.[16] Premature neonates are also vulnerable to the detrimental effects of high FIO_2 due to liberation of reactive oxygen species leading to bronchopulmonary dysplasia and retinopathy of prematurity.[17]

Neonates and infants initially have compliant intracranial space due to several open fontanelles, which close in sequence from 4 months to 1 year. Therefore, gradual increases in intracranial mass due to tumor, chronic hydrocephalus, and hemorrhage are undetectable due to compensatory distension of the fontanelles and widening of the cranial sutures. However, given the diminutive neonate and infant intracranial volume, acute increases in cranial content due to blood or cerebrospinal fluid often result in life-threatening intracranial hypertension.[18]

Cardiac System, Including Transitional Circulation

The cardiac system is an integral component of neurovascular development, and factors that affect changes in the growth and development of the heart, including the changes during transitional circulation from intrauterine to extrauterine conditions, will also affect the brain and CNS. The neonatal myocardium is immature and incompletely developed with fewer muscle cells and more connective tissue compared to adults, which results in poor ventricular compliance and limited response to increasing preload to augment cardiac output. The high metabolic rate of neonates requires a proportional increase in cardiac output. Furthermore, the neonatal heart functions at close to its maximal rate and stroke volume just to meet basic oxygen demand. This makes the immature myocardium very susceptible to hypocalcemia, which

is exacerbated by increased citrate from administration of blood products and albumin, as well as increased sensitivity to volatile anesthetics and calcium channel blockers.

Pediatric Airway

Anatomic differences between the pediatric and adult airway are primarily due to the size and orientation of the upper airway, larynx, and trachea. Neonates and infants have the greatest differences from adults in this respect, with the configuration of the larynx becoming similar to that of adults after the second year of life. An infant's larynx is funnel shaped and narrowest at the level of the cricoid, thus making this region the smallest cross-sectional area in the infant airway. This places the infant at risk for life-threatening subglottic obstruction secondary to mucosal swelling after prolonged intubation with a tight-fitting endotracheal tube. An endotracheal tube can also migrate into a mainstem bronchus if the infant's head is flexed for a suboccipital approach to the posterior fossa or the cervical spine. Therefore, the anesthesiologist should auscultate both lung fields to rule out inadvertent intubation of a mainstem bronchus after the patient is positioned for the surgical procedure.

Renal and Hepatic System

Renal blood flow doubles during the first 2 weeks of postnatal life, when adjusted for body surface area, and continues to increase until it reaches adult values by 2 years. The glomerular filtration rate (GFR) also doubles over the first 2 weeks of life and continues to increase until 1 to 2 years. As a result, neonates are much less able to conserve or excrete water compared to older children and adults; thus meticulous attention must be paid to fluid management during long cases and cases with significant blood loss or fluid shifts. In addition, neonates are also inefficient at excreting potassium, and the normal range of potassium may be higher in neonates and children compared to adults. Neonates in particular maintain a slightly acidotic pH (7.37) and have lower plasma bicarbonate concentrations (22 mEq/L) compared to older children and adults (pH 7.39 and bicarbonate 22 mEq/L). Thus, while neonates are able to maintain acid-base homeostasis, they are less able to buffer larger acid loads.

At birth the liver is structurally and functionally immature, with the neonatal liver containing 20%

fewer hepatocytes, which are each only half the size of adult hepatocytes; the liver is even more underdeveloped in preterm infants. Due to the relative immaturity of the neonatal liver, drug metabolism and excretion as well as glucose management can be significantly affected. A dextrose-containing intravenous fluid may be used for maintenance in long cases with neonates given the immature liver's limited ability to store and utilize glycogen.

Hepatic drug metabolic activity appears as early as 9 to 22 weeks. Drug metabolism by the liver usually involves enzymatic conversion of medications from a lipid soluble (less polar) state into a more water-soluble (more polar) state. Phase I reactions transform drugs via oxidation, reduction, or hydrolysis. The cytochrome P450 (CYP) enzyme system provides most of the phase I drug metabolism for less polar (lipophilic) compounds. Neonates have a reduced total quantity of CYP enzymes, with activity 50% of adult values. This reduction in CYP decreases clearance for many drugs, including theophylline, caffeine, diazepam, phenytoin, and phenobarbital.

Phase II reactions transform drugs via conjugation reactions such as sulfation, acetylation, and glycuronidation. Activity of uridine diphosphoglucuronosyltransferases (UGT), which is responsible for glucuronidation of bilirubin and many medications like morphine, acetaminophen, dexmedetomidine, and lorazepam, is limited immediately after birth and different isoforms mature at different rates with growth and development, but in general adult activity levels are reached by 8 to 18 months of age.

The immature liver also has a limited capacity for protein synthesis, which decreases the proportion of drugs bound to proteins in circulation and increases the amount of free drug. Acidic drugs (e.g., diazepam) mainly bind to albumin, while basic drugs (e.g., amide local anesthetic drugs) bind to globulins, lipoproteins, and glycoproteins. Due to decreased synthesis of all proteins, both basic and acidic drugs can have significantly greater effects in neonates than adults.

In addition to differences in hepatic enzymatic activity, hepatic blood flow and body composition also significantly affect enzymatic drug degradation. As neonates mature, a larger proportion of the cardiac output is delivered to the liver, thus increasing drug delivery and subsequent degradation.

In general, the half-lives of medications that are cleared by the liver are increased in neonates, decreased in children 4 to 10 years of age, and reach adult levels in adolescence. Preterm and term infants have proportionally more water than older children and adults, which increases the volume of distribution of water-soluble drugs. However, neonates oftentimes are more sensitive to the neurologic, respiratory, and cardiovascular effects of many medications, and a lower dose may be needed to achieve the desired effect. Preterm infants are particularly susceptible to anesthetic medication and may require even smaller blood concentrations to achieve the desired effect.[19] Due to the complexity of differences in enzymatic activity, circulatory volume, and variable neurologic and hemodynamic responses to anesthetic medications, it is important to titrate the dose of all medications to the desired response to all preterm and term infants.

Preoperative Assessment and Planning

Neonates and infants have the highest risk for perioperative respiratory and cardiovascular morbidity and mortality of any age group.[20,21] They are particularly sensitive to the depressant effects of general anesthesia and the physiological stress of surgery. Therefore, a thorough review of the patient's history can reveal conditions that may require further evaluation and be optimized before surgery (Table 1.1). An echocardiogram and consultation by a pediatric cardiologist may be needed to optimize cardiac function prior to surgery. The neonatal respiratory system may be challenging due to the diminutive size of the airway, neonatal pulmonary physiology, craniofacial anomalies, laryngotracheal lesions, and acute (hyaline membrane disease, retained amniotic fluid) or chronic (bronchopulmonary dysplasia) disease. These conditions are in a state of flux as the patient matures.

Preoperative fasting guidelines have evolved and are frequently dictated by regional practices.[22] The purpose of limiting oral intake is to minimize the risk of aspiration of gastric contents on induction. However, prolonged fasting periods and vomiting may induce hypovolemia and hypoglycemia, which can exacerbate hemodynamic and metabolic instability under anesthesia.

Table 1.1 Coexisting Conditions That Impact Anesthetic Management

Condition	Anesthetic Implications
Congenital heart disease	Hypoxia
	Arrhythmias
	Cardiovascular instability
	Paradoxical air emboli
Prematurity	Postoperative apnea
Gastrointestinal reflux	Aspiration pneumonia
Upper respiratory tract infection	Laryngospasm, bronchospasm hypoxia, pneumonia
Craniofacial abnormality	Difficult tracheal intubation
Denervation injuries	Hyperkalemia after succinylcholine
	Resistance to non-depolarizing muscle relaxants
	Abnormal response to nerve stimulation
Epilepsy	Hepatic and hematological abnormalities
	Increased metabolism of anesthetic agents
	Ketogenic diet
Arteriovenous malformation	Congestive heart failure
Neuromuscular disease	Malignant hyperthermia
	Respiratory failure
	Sudden cardiac death
Chiari malformation	Apnea
	Aspiration pneumonia
Hypothalamic/ pituitary lesions	Diabetes insipidus
	Hypothyroidism
	Adrenal insufficiency

Intraoperative Management

Induction of Anesthesia

A smooth transition into the operating suite depends on the level of anxiety and the cognitive development and age of the child.[23]

Induction of anesthesia should be dictated by the patient's developmental stage, comorbidities, and neurologic status. Children between the ages of 9–12

months and 6 years may have separation anxiety. Midazolam, administered orally or intravenously, is effective in relieving anxiety and producing amnesia. Parental presence during induction of anesthesia is common in pediatric operating rooms and requires full engagement of the surgical team. If the patient does not have intravenous access, anesthesia can be induced with sevoflurane, nitrous oxide, and oxygen by mask. However, intracranial hypertension may be exacerbated if the airway becomes obstructed during induction. Maintenance of a patent airway with mild hyperventilation will alleviate this problem. In patients with intravenous access, anesthesia can be induced with a propofol. It should be noted that significant hypotension and possible cerebral ischemia might occur after an induction dose of propofol,[24] due to the lack of surgical stimulation or in the setting of hypovolemia. This can be minimized by reducing the dose of propofol and adjuvant opioids for induction and an intravenous fluid bolus. Some patients presenting for neurosurgical procedures may be at particular risk for aspiration of gastric contents, and a rapid-sequence induction of anesthesia with succinylcholine is required to expeditiously intubate the trachea. Contraindications to the use of succinylcholine include malignant hyperthermia susceptibility, muscular dystrophies, and recent denervation injuries.

Airway Management

Since the head and airway are inaccessible to the anesthesiologist during most neurosurgical procedures, tracheal intubation requires careful planning. Orotracheal intubation is acceptable for most neurosurgical procedures, especially for surgical approaches to the supratentorial area and when transsphenoidal exposure is planned. However, patients in the prone position are at increased risk for kinking of the orotracheal tube and macroglosia due direct pressure injury to the tongue. Nasotracheal tubes are best suited for these situations because they are easily secured and less likely to be kinked or dislodged during long procedures.

Vascular Access and Positioning

Given the diminutive size of pediatric patients and limited access, the patient should be positioned with all vascular access, monitors, and endotracheal tube secured prior to the start of surgery. Large peripheral venous cannulae are sufficient for most craniotomies.

Central venous cannulation may be necessary. Femoral vein catheterization avoids the risk of pneumothorax and does not interfere with cerebral venous return. Furthermore, femoral catheters are easily accessible. The routine use of central venous catheters was not effective in reducing hypotension in craniofacial surgeries in pediatric patients.[25] Given the small caliber of an infant cerebral venous catheter, its use as a conduit for aspiration of venous air embolism (VAE) is questionable.[26] Placement of peripherally inserted central catheter (PICC) through the cephalic, basilica, or brachial veins and advanced to the distal superior vena cava under ultrasound guidance has the advantage of being a noninvasive and long-term access to the central circulation.[27] Cannulation of the radial artery provides direct blood pressure monitoring and sampling for blood gas analysis. The dorsalis pedis and posterior tibial artery are more accessible should attempts at radial artery cannulation fail.

Patient positioning requires careful preoperative planning to allow adequate access to the patient for both the neurosurgeon and anesthesiologist. Children have relatively thin skulls and are at risk for depressed skull fractures and perforation of underlying blood vessels with cranial fixation devices.[28,29] Should a depressed skull fracture or intracranial hemorrhage be suspected, urgent imaging with CT or magnetic resonance imaging (MRI) scanning can detect the extent and location of the injury and prompt immediate evacuation of the hematoma.[30] Modifications of these standard fixation devices and headrests should be utilized to minimize this preventable and potentially lethal complication.[31]

Surgical positioning affects the physiologic status of the patient (Table 1.2). The prone position can increase intra-abdominal pressure and lead to impaired ventilation, venocaval compression, and bleeding due to increased epidural venous pressure. Soft rolls are generally used to elevate and support the lateral chest wall and hips in order to minimize abdominal and thoracic pressure. Neurosurgical procedures performed with the head slightly elevated facilitate venous and cerebrospinal fluid (CSF) drainage from the surgical site. However, this increases the likelihood of VAE. Significant rotation of the head can also impede venous return via compression of the jugular veins and can lead to impaired cerebral perfusion, increased intracranial pressure (ICP), and venous bleeding. Vigilant assessment of the airway is critical in prone patients throughout the case because

Table 1.2 Physiologic Effects of Patient Positioning

Position	Physiological Effect
Head up/ sitting	Increased cerebral venous drainage
	Decreased cerebral blood flow
	Increased venous pooling in lower extremities
	Postural hypotension
Head down	Increased cerebral venous and intracranial pressure
	Decreased functional residual capacity (lung function)
	Decreased lung compliance
Prone	Venous congestion of face, tongue, and neck
	Decreased lung compliance
	Venocaval compression
Lateral decubitus	Decreased compliance of downside lung

of the propensity for the tongue to slide out of the mouth and kink the endotracheal tube. Nasotracheal intubation and placement of an oral bite/tongue may prevent these complications. Obese patients may be difficult to ventilate in the prone position and may benefit from a sitting position. In addition to the physiological sequelae of the sitting position, a whole spectrum of neurovascular compression and stretch injuries can occur.

Maintenance of Anesthesia

Given the possibility of iatrogenic cerebral hypoperfusion during surgery,[32] judicious dosing of anesthetic drugs is mandatory. Appropriate management of intraoperative blood pressure is hampered by the assumptions on a range of blood pressures that maintain adequate CBF and cerebral autoregulation in pediatric patients.[33] This hypothetical range of blood pressure is overly simplified and not necessarily supported by the original reports.[34] This requires vigilant monitoring of the blood pressure and adjusting the anesthetic dosing, fluid administration, and vasopressor support if needed. The exclusive use of specific anesthetic drugs and technique has no impact on outcome.[35] Chronic anticonvulsant therapy usually increases the dosage of neuromuscular blocking agents and opioids because of induced enzymatic metabolism.[36] Assessment of motor function during seizure and spinal cord surgery may preclude the use of neuromuscular blocking agents and should be discussed with the surgical and monitoring teams. Infants and children are especially susceptible to hypothermia during any surgical procedure because of their large surface-area-to-weight ratio. Active heating of the patient by increasing ambient temperature and use of radiant light warmers during induction of anesthesia, catheter insertion, and preparation and positioning of the patient are prophylactic measures against hypothermia. Forced hot air blankets and mattress and intravenous fluid warmers can also prevent intraoperative temperature loss and postoperative shivering.

Management of Fluids and Blood Loss

Hemodynamic stability during intracranial surgery requires careful maintenance of the patient's fluids and electrolytes to preserve neurological function. Since the lower limit of cerebral autoregulation in pediatric patients is unknown, they are at risk for cerebral hypoperfusion especially when they are deeply anesthetized during periods of massive blood loss.[33,37,38] Meticulous fluid and blood administration is essential in order to minimize hemodynamic instability. Stroke volume is relatively fixed in the neonate and infant, so the patient should be kept euvolemic. Normal saline is generally chosen because it is mildly hyperosmolar and should minimize cerebral edema, but rapid infusion of more than 60 mL/kg of normal saline may cause hyperchloremic acidosis.[39] The routine administration of glucose-containing solutions is generally avoided during neurosurgical procedures, except in patients who are at risk for hypoglycemia. Patients with diabetes mellitus or total parenteral alimentation and premature and small newborn infants may require glucose-containing intravenous fluids.

Maintaining euvolemia is crucial during craniotomies in infants and children by preserving the circulating blood volume with intravenous fluids and blood products. Premature neonates have a circulating blood volume of approximately 100 mL/kg total body weight; full-term newborns have a volume of 90 mL/kg; infants have a blood volume of 80 mL/kg. Maximal allowable blood loss (MABL) can be estimated using a simple formula: MABL = estimated circulating blood volume * (starting hematocrit − minimum acceptable hematocrit) / starting hematocrit.

Transfusion of 10 mL/kg of packed red blood cells increases hemoglobin concentration by 2 g/dl. Pediatric patients are susceptible to dilutional thrombocytopenia in the setting of massive blood loss and multiple red blood cell transfusions.[40] Administration of 5–10 mL/kg of platelets increases the platelet count by 50,000 to $100,000/mm^3$. The routine use of the antifibrinolytic tranexamic acid in surgical procedures with excessive blood loss has been shown to decrease blood loss in pediatric patients.[41]

Hemodynamic collapse due to massive blood loss or VAE looms as a catastrophic complication for any major craniotomy. Large-bore intravenous access and arterial blood pressure monitoring are therefore essential for these procedures. Massive blood loss should be aggressively treated with crystalloid and blood replacement and vasopressor therapy (e.g., dopamine, epinephrine, norepinephrine). Venous air embolism can occur during the surgery. Maintaining normovolemia minimizes this risk. Early detection of a VAE with continuous precordial Doppler ultrasound may allow treatment to be instituted before large amounts of air are entrained. Should a VAE produce hemodynamic instability, the operating table must be placed in the Trendelenburg position in order to improve cerebral perfusion and prevent further entrainment of intravascular air. Special risks exist in neonates and young infants since right-to-left cardiac mixing lesions can result in paradoxical emboli. In the case of severe cardiovascular collapse, some pediatric centers have rapid response extracorporeal membrane oxygenation (ECMO) teams that can provide cardiopulmonary support when the crisis is refractory to standard cardiopulmonary resuscitation algorithms.[42]

Postoperative Disposition of the Pediatric Neurosurgical Patient

Prompt examination of neurological function necessitates rapid emergence from general anesthesia. However, this may be complicated by hypertension, residual neuromuscular blockade, renarcotization, and airway edema. Hypertension during emergence from anesthesia can be controlled with vasodilator drugs such as labetalol. Neuromuscular blockade should be fully antagonized, and all anesthetic agents should be discontinued and, in the case of opioids, antagonized. Once the patient exhibits spontaneous ventilation and appropriate responses to verbal commands, the trachea can be extubated.

Premature extubation of the trachea can lead to airway obstruction due to laryngospasm or tracheal and upper airway edema. Both are major causes of postoperative morbidity and mortality.[21] Procedures in which several blood volumes have been lost and replaced with crystalloid and blood are associated with increased morbidity and mortality,[43] frequently result in airway and facial edema and may lead to postextubation airway obstruction. In addition, operations that disrupt cranial nerve nuclei or brainstem may lead to impairment of airway reflexes and respiratory drive. If anesthetic causes of delayed awakening are not apparent, neurological conditions should be strongly considered and evaluated with a CT scan of the head. Transportation to the CT suite requires maintenance of general anesthesia and continuous hemodynamic monitoring. In these circumstances, it is often safer for the patient's trachea to remain intubated. Therefore, patients who are at risk of these complications require closer observation in an intensive care unit (see Chapter 21).

Summary

The approach to the pediatric neurosurgical patient is based on developmental stage and surgical lesion. The evolving maturational changes of the various organ systems have a significant impact on the drugs and techniques used for the safe conduct of anesthesia.

References

1. Chumas P, Kenny T, Stiller C. Subspecialisation in neurosurgery—does size matter? *Acta Neurochir (Wien).* 2011;**153**:1231–6.

2. Hansen TG, Pedersen JK, Henneberg SW, Morton NS, Christensen K. Neurosurgical conditions and procedures in infancy are associated with mortality and academic performances in adolescence: a nationwide cohort study. *Paediatr Anaesth.* 2015;**25**:186–92.

3. Campbell E, Beez T, Todd L. Prospective review of 30-day morbidity and mortality in a paediatric neurosurgical unit. *Childs Nerv Syst.* 2017;**33**:483–9.

4. Kuo BJ, Vissoci JR, Egger JR, Smith ER, Grant GA, Haglund MM, Rice HE. Perioperative outcomes for pediatric neurosurgical procedures: analysis of the National Surgical Quality Improvement Program-Pediatrics. *J Neurosurg Pediatr.* 2017;**19**: 361–71.

5. Stolwijk LJ, Lemmers PM, Harmsen M, Groenendaal F, de Vries LS, van der Zee DC, et al. Neurodevelopmental outcomes after neonatal surgery for major noncardiac anomalies. *Pediatrics.* 2016;**137**:e20151728.

6. Sarnat HB, Flores-Sarnat L, Pinter JD. Neuroembryology. In: Winn HR, ed. *Youmans Neurological Surgery*, 6th ed. Philadelphia: Elsevier; 2011:78–97.

7. McClain CD, Soriano SG. The central nervous system: pediatric neuroanesthesia. In: Holzman RS, Mancuso TJ, Polaner DM, eds. *A Practical Approach to Pediatric Anesthesia*, 2nd ed. Philadelphia: Wolters Kluwer;2016: 226–64.

8. Pryds O. Control of cerebral circulation in the high-risk neonate. *Ann Neurol.* 1991;**30**:321–9.

9. Wintermark M, Lepori D, Cotting J, Roulet E, van Melle G, Meuli R, et al. Brain perfusion in children: evolution with age assessed by quantitative perfusion computed tomography. *Pediatrics.* 2004;**113**:1642–52.

10. Lee JK. Cerebral perfusion pressure: how low can we go? *Paediatr Anaesth.* 2014;**24**:647–8.

11. Tsuji M, Saul JP, du Plessis A, Eichenwald E, Sobh J, Crocker R, Volpe JJ. Cerebral intravascular oxygenation correlates with mean arterial pressure in critically ill premature infants. *Pediatrics.* 2000;**106**: 625–32.

12. Rhee CJ, Fraser CD III, Kibler K, Easley RB, Andropoulos DB, Czosnyka M, et al. Ontogeny of cerebrovascular critical closing pressure. *Pediatr Res.* 2015;**78**:71–5.

13. Kennedy C, Sokoloff L. An adaptation of the nitrous oxide method to the study of the cerebral circulation in children: normal values for cerebral blood flow and cerebral metabolic rate in childhood. *J Clin Invest.* 1957;**36**:1130–7.

14. Chugani HT, Phelps ME, Mazziotta JC. Positron emission tomography study of human brain functional development. *Ann Neurol.* 1987;**22**:487–97.

15. Pryds O, Andersen GE, Friis-Hansen B. Cerebral blood flow reactivity in spontaneously breathing, preterm infants shortly after birth. *Acta Paediatr Scand.* 1990;**79**:391–6.

16. Rahilly PM. Effects of 2% carbon dioxide, 0.5% carbon dioxide, and 100% oxygen on cranial blood flow of the human neonate. *Pediatrics.* 1980;**66**:685–9.

17. Saugstad OD, Aune D. Optimal oxygenation of extremely low birth weight infants: a meta-analysis and systematic review of the oxygen saturation target studies. *Neonatology.* 2014;**105**:55–63.

18. Shapiro K, Marmarou A, Shulman K. Characterization of clinical CSF dynamics and neural axis compliance using the pressure-volume index: I. The normal pressure-volume index. *Ann Neurol.* 1980;**7**:508–14.

19. Besunder JB, Reed MD, Blumer JL. Principles of drug biodisposition in the neonate. A critical evaluation of the pharmacokinetic-pharmacodynamic interface (Part I). *Clin Pharmacokinet.* 1988;**14**:189–216.

20. Cohen MM, Cameron CB, Duncan PG. Pediatric anesthesia morbidity and mortality in the perioperative period. *Anesth Analg.* 1990;**70**:160–7.

21. Habre W, Disma N, Virag K, Becke K, Hansen TG, Johr M, et al. Incidence of severe critical events in paediatric anaesthesia (APRICOT): a prospective multicentre observational study in 261 hospitals in Europe. *Lancet Respir Med.* 2017;**5**:412–25.

22. Ferrari LR, Rooney FM, Rockoff MA. Preoperative fasting practices in pediatrics. *Anesthesiology.* 1999;**90**: 978–80.

23. McCann ME, Kain ZN. The management of preoperative anxiety in children: an update. *Anesth Analg.* 2001;**93**:98–105.

24. Vanderhaegen J, Naulaers G, Van Huffel S, Vanhole C, Allegaert K. Cerebral and systemic hemodynamic effects of intravenous bolus administration of propofol in neonates. *Neonatology.* 2010;**98**:57–63.

25. Stricker PA, Lin EE, Fiadjoe JE, Sussman EM, Pruitt EY, Zhao H, Jobes DR. Evaluation of central venous pressure monitoring in children undergoing craniofacial reconstruction surgery. *Anesth Analg.* 2013;**116**:411–19.

26. Cucchiara RF, Bowers B. Air embolism in children undergoing suboccipital craniotomy. *Anesthesiology.* 1982;**57**:338–9.

27. Westergaard B, Classen V, Walther-Larsen S. Peripherally inserted central catheters in infants and children—indications, techniques, complications and clinical recommendations. *Acta Anaesthesiol Scand.* 2013;**57**:278–87.

28. Lee M, Rezai AR, Chou J. Depressed skull fractures in children secondary to skull clamp fixation devices. *Pediatr Neurosurg.* 1994;**21**:174–7; discussion 178.

29. Vitali AM, Steinbok P. Depressed skull fracture and epidural hematoma from head fixation with pins for craniotomy in children. *Childs Nerv Syst.* 2008;**24**: 917–23; discussion 925.

30. McClain CD, Soriano SG, Goumnerova LC, Black PM, Rockoff MA. Detection of unanticipated intracranial hemorrhage during intraoperative magnetic resonance image-guided neurosurgery. Report of two cases. *J Neurosurg.* 2007;**106**:398–400.

31. Gupta N. A modification of the Mayfield horseshoe headrest allowing pin fixation and cranial immobilization in infants and young children. *Neurosurgery.* 2006;58; discussion ONS-E181.

32. McCann ME, Schouten AN, Dobija N, Munoz C, Stephenson L, Poussaint TY, et al. Infantile postoperative encephalopathy: perioperative factors as a cause for concern. *Pediatrics.* 2014;**133**:e751–7.

33. McCann ME, Schouten AN. Beyond survival: influences of blood pressure, cerebral perfusion and anesthesia on neurodevelopment. *Paediatr Anaesth.* 2014;**24**:68–73.

34. Drummond JC. The lower limit of autoregulation: time to revise our thinking? *Anesthesiology.* 1997;**86**: 1431–3.

35. Todd MM, Warner DS, Sokoll MD, Maktabi MA, Hindman BJ, Scamman FL, Kirschner J. A prospective, comparative trial of three anesthetics for elective supratentorial craniotomy. Propofol/fentanyl, isoflurane/nitrous oxide, and fentanyl/nitrous oxide. *Anesthesiology.* 1993;**78**:1005–20.

36. Soriano SG, Martyn JAJ. Antiepileptic-induced resistance to neuromuscular blockers: mechanisms and clinical significance. *Clin Pharmacokinet.* 2004;**43**:71–81.

37. Williams M, Lee JK. Intraoperative blood pressure and cerebral perfusion: strategies to clarify hemodynamic goals. *Paediatr Anaesth.* 2014;**24**:657–67.

38. Vavilala MS, Lee LA, Lam AM. The lower limit of cerebral autoregulation in children during sevoflurane anesthesia. *J Neurosurg Anesthesiol.* 2003;**15**:307–12.

39. Scheingraber S, Rehm M, Sehmisch C, Finsterer U. Rapid saline infusion produces hyperchloremic acidosis in patients undergoing gynecologic surgery. *Anesthesiology.* 1999;**90**:1265–70.

40. Cote CJ, Liu LM, Szyfelbein SK, Goudsouzian NG, Daniels AL. Changes in serial platelet counts following massive blood transfusion in pediatric patients. *Anesthesiology.* 1985;**62**:197–201.

41. Faraoni D, Goobie SM. The efficacy of antifibrinolytic drugs in children undergoing noncardiac surgery: a systematic review of the literature. *Anesth Analg.* 2014;**118**:628–36.

42. Turek JW, Andersen ND, Lawson DS, Bonadonna D, Turley RS, Peters MA, et al. Outcomes before and after implementation of a pediatric rapid-response extracorporeal membrane oxygenation program. *Ann Thorac Surg.* 2013;**95**:2140–6; discussion 2146–7.

43. Goobie SM, DiNardo JA, Faraoni D. Relationship between transfusion volume and outcomes in children undergoing noncardiac surgery. *Transfusion.* 2016;**56**: 2487–94.

Developmental Cerebrovascular Physiology

Jennifer K. Lee and Ken M. Brady

Introduction

The foundation for evaluating a child's risk of brain injury includes frequent neurologic evaluations. If unable to conduct neurologic evaluations, the anesthesiologist must instead modulate physiologic parameters to ensure that the brain receives a constant supply of oxygen and glucose. The cerebrovascular system dilates and constricts to regulate cerebral blood flow (CBF) at the global level in pressure autoregulation. At the regional level of the neurovascular unit—the interface between neurons, vessels, and astrocytes—neurovascular coupling induces rapid and fine regional adjustments in CBF to meet local metabolic demands. Anesthesia and aberrancies in hemodynamic, blood gas, or glucose management can disrupt pressure autoregulation and neurovascular coupling. Therefore, the anesthesiologist must understand CBF regulation and the effects of anesthesia and intracranial lesions on cerebrovascular physiology.

Blood Pressure Autoregulation

Cerebrovascular autoregulation is the physiologic mechanism that maintains relatively constant CBF across changes in cerebral perfusion pressure (CPP). The CPP is calculated as the difference between the mean arterial blood pressure (MAP) and intracranial pressure (ICP). If the central venous pressure exceeds the ICP, the CPP is the difference between MAP and the central venous pressure. Cerebrovascular reactivity refers to the vasoconstriction and vasodilation of resistance vessels within the brain that constrain or increase CBF. This global autoregulatory vasoreactivity is functional in term newborns. Premature infants may have underdeveloped cerebral vasculature with limitations in vascular responsiveness.

Autoregulation functions within a specific range of CPP along the "autoregulatory plateau." When CPP is below the lower limit of autoregulation (LLA), CBF falls in a manner that is passive to the decreasing blood pressure. This places the patient at risk of cerebral ischemia. CPP levels above the upper limit of autoregulation exceed the vasoconstrictive capacity of the vasculature, which places the brain at risk of hyperemic injury. Volatile anesthetics uncouple CPP and CBF and alter pressure autoregulation responses, thereby resulting in more pressure-passive CBF than that observed during intravenous anesthesia.[1] However, no large clinical studies have compared inhaled and intravenous anesthetic techniques in children with neurologic lesions. Therefore, either an inhaled or intravenous anesthetic technique is generally considered acceptable for neurosurgical procedures that do not include a neuromonitoring method that warrants specific anesthetic regimens, such as intravenous techniques for electrophysiology monitoring.

The autoregulation curve is traditionally illustrated with (1) a horizontal CBF plateau at blood pressure levels within the range that produces pressure-reactive CBF, (2) a discrete cutoff at the LLA with a decline in CBF at pressures below the LLA, and (3) a cutoff at the upper limit of autoregulation with increasing CBF above that point. This representation is based on pooling CBF responses to fluctuations in CPP from multiple studies. In reality, the autoregulatory plateau for an individual does not have a slope of precisely zero, and the limits of autoregulation are smooth inflections on a curve (Figures 2.1 and 2.2). When blood pressure crosses below the LLA, cerebral arteries and arterioles may continue to dilate, but to a degree that is insufficient to maintain steady CBF. Likewise, when blood pressure exceeds the upper limit of autoregulation, additional cerebrovascular constriction might occur but be inadequate to maintain constant CBF. With extreme increases in arterial pressure, passive dilation of arteries can transmit pulsatile pressure to the cerebral microcirculation.

The blood pressure limits of autoregulation during general anesthesia are unknown in infants and children. Available data suggest that the LLA among healthy, American Society of Anesthesiologists (ASA) level I children of different ages without brain injury may be at a MAP of approximately 50–65 mmHg.[2] Young children (median age 2 years) on hypothermic cardiopulmonary bypass may have LLAs at a MAP of approximately 40 mmHg.[3] The effects of acute and chronic intracranial lesions on the blood pressure limits of autoregulation are not well studied in children. Anesthesia decreases the cerebral metabolic rate, an effect that might confer some level of protection during lower blood pressures. Nonetheless, the anesthesiologist should make every effort to maintain the patient's blood pressure close to the preoperative baseline.

Intracranial Hypertension and Pressure Autoregulation

The blood pressure limits of autoregulation are dynamic and may shift with intracranial lesions. For example, elevations in ICP with or without acute trauma shift the LLA to a higher CPP.[4,5] The treatment guidelines for pediatric traumatic brain injury provide level III recommendations that clinicians should maintain a patient's ICP at less than 20 mmHg and CPP greater than 40–50 mmHg. The target CPP may need to be increased for older children and adolescents.[6] Invasive arterial blood pressure monitoring is required to continually measure the CPP. When invasive ICP monitoring is unavailable but the anesthesiologist suspects that the patient has intracranial hypertension, he or she can estimate the ICP, for example 20–25 mmHg, and subtract this value from the MAP to obtain a rough assessment of the CPP until an ICP monitor can be placed.

The anesthesiologist must sometimes raise the arterial blood pressure to bring the CPP within a range that supports autoregulation. There is much debate about which vasopressor should be used to support CPP. Evidence in animal models suggests that sex may influence the autoregulatory response to vasopressors. In a piglet model of traumatic brain injury, dopamine supports autoregulation in both males and females after trauma,[7] whereas norepinephrine and phenylephrine may affect autoregulatory function differently in males and females.[8,9] Because evidence is currently limited to preclinical models, we cannot make clinical recommendations for which vasopressor is optimal. Raising the arterial blood pressure to support CPP must be balanced against the risks of increasing myocardial oxygen demand with cardiopulmonary compromise and decreasing splanchnic perfusion. Intravenous fluid boluses, blood products,

and colloids are also appropriate methods to raise the CPP. Using volume resuscitation to support the blood pressure is preferable to vasopressors in patients who have vascular malformations and are at risk of CBF dysregulation or vasospasm.

When supporting the CPP in patients with intracranial hypertension, the anesthesiologist should consider treatments to lower the ICP. The intracranial space conceptually consists of three volume compartments: the brain parenchyma, cerebrospinal or extracellular fluid, and cerebral blood volume. The rate at which ICP rises depends on how quickly the intracranial mass lesion develops. Slowly growing intracranial tumors or hydrocephalus will produce a slower rise in ICP than an acute hematoma from brain trauma. The growing cranium and widening sutures of infants and young children will allow an increase in head circumference with slowly growing intracranial lesions. It is important to note, however, that an open fontanelle and sutures do not protect an infant from intracranial hypertension or cerebral herniation. Infants and young children may have very little intracranial reserve when they become symptomatic from brain tumors or hydrocephalus. The risk of cerebral herniation after traumatic brain injury is greater in infants than in older children.[10]

When autoregulation is functional, there is an inverse relationship between MAP and ICP. When the arterial blood pressure increases, the cerebral vasculature constricts to constrain CBF. The consequent decrease in cerebral blood volume lowers the ICP (Figure 2.3A). Therefore, raising the blood pressure may lower the ICP when autoregulation is functional. However, when autoregulation becomes impaired, changes in blood pressure are directly transmitted as fluctuations in cerebral blood volume and ICP. In this situation, increases in arterial blood pressure will raise the ICP as well (Figure 2.3B).

Additional methods to lower the ICP include hyperventilation, hypertonic saline, deepening the intravenous anesthetic, or administering barbiturates. The latter two interventions will decrease the cerebral metabolic rate and CBF. Increasing the concentration of a volatile agent, however, could increase CBF by uncoupling CBF from CPP and cerebral metabolic rate. Moderate hypothermia decreases metabolic demand and may also lower CBF and therefore the ICP. Decompressive craniectomy must be considered in severe cases of refractory intracranial hypertension.

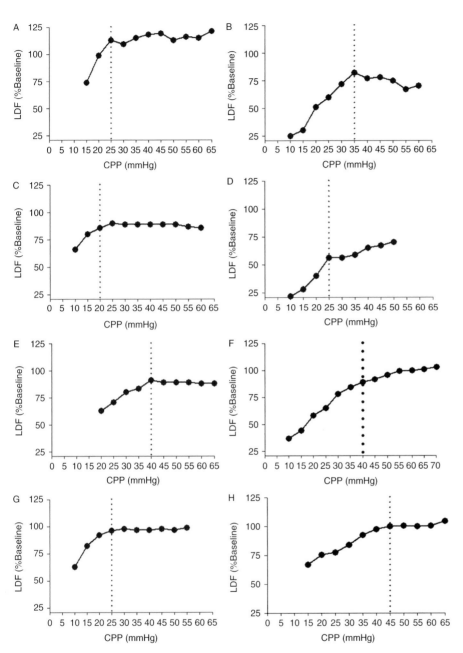

Figure 2.1. Examples of individual cerebral blood flow (CBF) autoregulation curves measured with laser Doppler flowmetry (LDF) in eight piglets as hypotension was slowly induced. The calculated cerebral perfusion pressure (CPP) lower limit of autoregulation (LLA) is demarcated with a dotted line. Variation among individual animals is observed in the CBF curve during hypotension. The left column illustrates piglets with relatively horizontal autoregulatory plateaus (panels A, C, E, and G). The right column illustrates piglets that did not have horizontal LDF curves when CPP exceeded the LLA (panels B, D, F, and H). Piglets in panels C, F, G, and H display smooth inflections in CBF that are often observed when blood pressure crosses below the LLA. Panels are reprinted with permission from *J Appl Physiol*, volume 115, Larson AC, Jamrogowicz JL, Kulikowicz E, Wang B, Yang ZJ, Shaffner DH, Koehler RC, Lee JK, Cerebrovascular autoregulation after rewarming from hypothermia in a neonatal swine model of asphyxic brain injury, pages 1433–42, copyright 2013, with permission from The American Physiological Society.

Hyperventilation should be reserved only for intracranial hypertensive crises and impending brain herniation. Hypocapnia induces vasoconstriction, which decreases the cerebral blood volume and lowers the ICP. However, sustained vasoconstriction from prolonged hyperventilation can cause cerebral ischemia.

When simultaneously treating intracranial hypertension and raising the arterial blood pressure to maintain CPP, controlling the ICP is paramount. Intracranial compliance decreases as ICP rises. Any increase in the intracranial volume, such as from bleeding or vasodilation from pain, hypercapnia, or seizures, could significantly increase the ICP and risk cerebral herniation. Because high ICP shifts the blood pressure LLA to a higher pressure,[4] lowering the ICP would also better support autoregulatory function at the same level of CPP.

Neurovascular Coupling

Neurovascular coupling with metabolic autoregulation occurs at the level of the neurovascular unit, which is typically characterized as the neuron, vessel, and astrocyte. Neurovascular coupling causes rapid and fine changes in CBF to meet local neural metabolic demands for oxygen and glucose. These fine changes in regional CBF are mediated by local release of nitric oxide, adenosine, prostaglandins, arachidonic acid, and other vasoactive compounds.[11] The effects of different anesthetics on neurovascular coupling are difficult to examine in clinical studies. Available data indicate that neurovascular coupling remains functional during propofol administration with a decrease in cerebral metabolic rate that decreases in linear correlation with decreases in CBF.[12] Volatile agents are classically considered to induce cerebral vasodilation that is uncoupled from the low cerebral metabolic rate during anesthesia.

Carbon Dioxide, Oxygen, and Glucose

The cerebral vasculature is exquisitely sensitive to the partial pressure of arterial CO_2 ($PaCO_2$). Acute changes in $PaCO_2$ rapidly trigger cerebral vasodilation or vasoconstriction by altering CO_2 diffusion in the cerebrospinal fluid. A 1-mmHg decrease in $PaCO_2$ from normocapnia reduces CBF by 1–3%, and a 1-mmHg increase in $PaCO_2$ raises CBF by 3–6%.[11] The cerebral vasoconstrictive response to hyperventilation generally lasts less than 3–6 hours and therefore cannot be used to control intracranial hypertension for long periods of time. However, brief periods of hyperventilation can be used to facilitate a neurosurgical procedure. For example, hyperventilation to induce cerebral vasoconstriction and reduce the cerebral blood volume may assist surgeons during craniotomies and duraplasties.

It must be remembered that prolonged hyperventilation can cause cerebral ischemia; therefore, the anesthesiologist must return the patient to normocarbic levels as soon as possible. The guidelines for treatment of pediatric traumatic brain injury state that hyperventilation to $PaCO_2$ <30 mmHg should be avoided, and that hyperventilation should be reserved for treatment of an intracranial hypertensive crisis and impending cerebral herniation.[6] Persistent hypercapnia causes cerebral hyperemia that may not return to baseline after normocarbia is restored.

The autoregulatory plateau is also influenced by hypocapnia. Although the LLA does not change during hypocapnia, the slope of $\Delta CBF/\Delta CPP$ may decrease. This likely reflects the vasoconstrictive effect of hypocapnia on overall CBF regulation. Moreover, the cerebral vascular response to changes in $PaCO_2$ may be diminished at birth and increase with gestational age.[13]

CBF remains constant overall at partial pressures of arterial O_2 (PaO_2) between approximately 60 and 300 mmHg. Decreases in oxygen delivery at a PaO_2 below ~50 mmHg, which corresponds to a hemoglobin oxygen saturation of 85%, are met by rapid cerebral vasodilation. This hypoxic vasodilation is

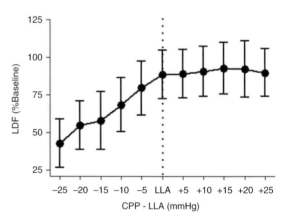

Figure 2.2. Data from the eight piglets in Figure 2.1 were combined to generate a single cerebral blood flow (CBF) autoregulation curve. Each piglet's lower limit of autoregulation (LLA; dotted line) is centered at zero on the x-axis to permit comparison of each LLA relative to the cerebral perfusion pressure (CPP). When CBF data from multiple individuals are pooled together, the autoregulatory plateau appears horizontal, and a cut point in CBF is observed at the LLA. Data are displayed as means with standard deviations.
LDF, laser Doppler flowmetry. Reprinted with permission from *Paediatr Anaesth*, volume 24, Williams M, Lee JK, Intraoperative blood pressure and cerebral perfusion: strategies to clarify hemodynamic goals, pages 657–67, copyright 2014, with permission from John Wiley & Sons, Ltd.

global. CBF may increase by up to 400%,[13] with a corresponding and potentially catastrophic increase in ICP. The CBF–PaO_2 curve shifts to the right with anemia,[13] resulting in cerebral vasodilation at higher PaO_2 levels. Therefore, hypoxia must be avoided in any child with intracranial hypertension or other risk of neurologic compromise.

The brain has limited glycogen reserves and therefore requires a constant supply of glucose. Plasma and brain glucose levels have a direct linear relationship, even at very low plasma glucose levels.[14] Hypoglycemia may preferentially induce cerebral vasodilation in specific brain regions rather than globally. Although exact glucose thresholds for cerebral vasodilation have not been defined, cerebral vasodilation may occur at serum glucose levels below 30 mg/dL in neonates without alterations in consciousness.[15]

Conclusions

The anesthesiologist must remain vigilant to avoid physiologic perturbations that could compromise pressure autoregulation and neurovascular coupling. Maintaining the patient's CPP within a range that supports autoregulation can be achieved by treating the ICP and using vasopressors and intravenous volume resuscitation. Normocapnia should be maintained, and hyperventilation should be reserved only for intracranial hypertensive crises. Hypoxia and hypoglycemia must be strictly avoided. Available data suggest that intravenous anesthetic techniques preserve pressure autoregulation and neurovascular coupling better than volatile agents, but clinical evidence is insufficient to recommend one type of anesthetic over the other.

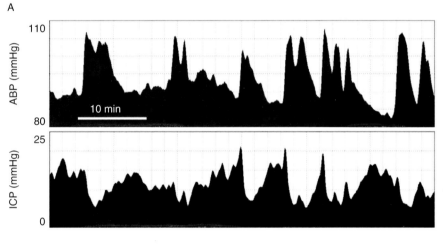

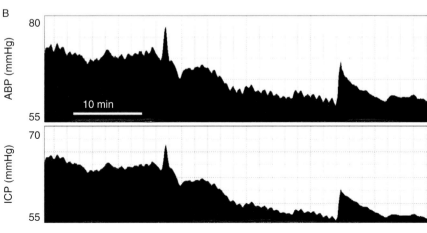

Figure 2.3. Example of cerebrovascular pressure reactivity in two children with traumatic brain injury. **(A)** When autoregulation is functional, arterial blood pressure (ABP) and intracranial pressure (ICP) are inversely related. Increases in the ABP will result in cerebral vasoconstriction and a decrease in ICP. **(B)** When autoregulation becomes impaired, fluctuations in ABP are directly transmitted to the cerebral vasculature, resulting in pressure-passive changes in cerebral blood volume and ICP. Increases in ABP will cause the ICP to rise. Reprinted with permission from *Pediatrics*, volume 124, Brady KM, Shaffner DH, Lee JK, Easley RB, Smielewski P, Czosnyka M, Jallo GI, Guerguerian AM, Continuous monitoring of cerebrovascular pressure reactivity after traumatic brain injury in children, pages e1205–12, copyright 2009, with permission from the American Academy of Pediatrics.

References

1. Bruins B, Kilbaugh TJ, Margulies SS, Friess SH. The anesthetic effects on vasopressor modulation of cerebral blood flow in an immature swine model. *Anesth Analg.* 2013;**116**(4):838–44.

2. Vavilala MS, Lee LA, Lam AM. The lower limit of cerebral autoregulation in children during sevoflurane anesthesia. *J Neurosurg Anesthesiol.* 2003;**15**(4):307–12.

3. Brady KM, Mytar JO, Lee JK, Cameron DE, Vricella LA, Thompson WR, et al. Monitoring cerebral blood flow pressure autoregulation in pediatric patients during cardiac surgery. *Stroke.* 2010;**41**(9):1957–62.

4. Brady KM, Lee JK, Kibler KK, Easley RB, Koehler RC, Czosnyka M, et al. The lower limit of cerebral blood flow autoregulation is increased with elevated intracranial pressure. *Anesth Analg.* 2009;**108**(4):1278–83.

5. Nusbaum D, Clark J, Brady K, Kibler K, Sutton J, Easley RB. Alteration in the lower limit of autoregulation with elevations in cephalic venous pressure. *Neurol Res.* 2014;**36**(12):1063–71.

6. Kochanek PM, Carney N, Adelson PD, Ashwal S, Bell MJ, Bratton S, et al. Guidelines for the acute medical management of severe traumatic brain injury in infants, children, and adolescents—second edition. *Pediatr Crit Care Med.* 2012;**13**(suppl 1):S1–82.

7. Armstead WM, Riley J, Vavilala MS. Dopamine prevents impairment of autoregulation after traumatic brain injury in the newborn pig through inhibition of up-regulation of endothelin-1 and extracellular signal-regulated kinase mitogen-activated protein kinase. *Pediatr Crit Care Med.* 2013;**14**(2):e103–11.

8. Armstead WM, Riley J, Vavilala MS. Preferential protection of cerebral autoregulation and reduction of hippocampal necrosis with norepinephrine after traumatic brain injury in female piglets. *Pediatr Crit Care Med.* 2016;**17**(3):e130–7.

9. Armstead WM, Kiessling JW, Riley J, Kofke WA, Vavilala MS. Phenylephrine infusion prevents impairment of ATP- and calcium-sensitive potassium channel-mediated cerebrovasodilation after brain injury in female, but aggravates impairment in male, piglets through modulation of ERK MAPK upregulation. *J Neurotrauma.* 2011;**28**(1):105–11.

10. Guerra SD, Carvalho LF, Affonseca CA, Ferreira AR, Freire HB. Factors associated with intracranial hypertension in children and teenagers who suffered severe head injuries. *J Pediatr (Rio J).* 2010;**86**(1):73–9.

11. Phillips AA, Chan FH, Zheng MM, Krassioukov AV, Ainslie PN. Neurovascular coupling in humans: physiology, methodological advances and clinical implications. *J Cereb Blood Flow Metab.* 2016;**36**(4):647–64.

12. Oshima T, Karasawa F, Satoh T. Effects of propofol on cerebral blood flow and the metabolic rate of oxygen in humans. *Acta Anaesthesiol Scand.* 2002;**46**(7):831–5.

13. Tasker RC. Intracranial pressure and cerebrovascular autoregulation in pediatric critical illness. *Semin Pediatr Neurol.* 2014;**21**(4):255–62.

14. van de Ven KC, van der Graaf M, Tack CJ, Heerschap A, de Galan BE. Steady-state brain glucose concentrations during hypoglycemia in healthy humans and patients with type 1 diabetes. *Diabetes.* 2012;**61**(8):1974–7.

15. Pryds O, Greisen G, Friis-Hansen B. Compensatory increase of CBF in preterm infants during hypoglycaemia. *Acta Paediatr Scand.* 1988;**77**(5):632–7.

Chapter 3

Neuroprotective Strategies in the Pediatric Patient

Rebecca Dube and Jason T. Maynes

Introduction

The pediatric brain utilizes a delicate homeostatic balance to ensure proper regional blood flow for nutrient delivery and waste removal. When homeostatic mechanisms are dysfunctional, normal neuronal activity and development are compromised, predisposing the maturing brain to morbidity. In the perioperative environment, pediatric cerebral injury may include focal (regional stroke) or global (hypoxic-ischemic encephalopathy; HIE) damage, resulting from surgical factors and alterations to control mechanisms induced by disease/patient or iatrogenic considerations. Over the course of the past 60 years, with the development of preclinical models of brain injury, our understanding of the mechanisms underlying this phenomenon has increased remarkably, as has our understanding of therapeutic interventions conferring a neuroprotective benefit. Neuroprotection refers to the preservation, recovery, or regeneration of neuronal tissue, and diverse perioperative interventions have been investigated for their neuroprotective benefit.

Mechanisms of Brain Injury in the Perioperative Setting

In the pediatric population, the primary initiators of neuronal injury in the perioperative setting are ischemia/hypoxia and inflammation, creating local excitotoxicity and the generation of reactive oxygen species (ROS) that potentially extend damage outside the initial at-risk area.[1,2] Global exposure to hypoxia, a particular concern for infants with less developed cerebral autoregulation, can lead to the development of HIE, epilepsy, cerebral palsy, and mild to severe developmental delay.[3]

During ischemia/hypoxia, the cell has a relative deficiency of oxygen, reducing high-efficiency aerobic metabolism (mitochondrial) in favor of lower efficiency anaerobic metabolism, and disrupting the cell's ability to maintain normal homeostatic balance. Neurons have

a particularly high energetic demand to maintain membrane potential, and the failure of important ionic pumps in the cell membrane that normally consume significant ATP can occur during hypoxia (i.e., Na/K ATPase), leading to cell depolarization and excess release of glutamate,[4] the primary excitatory neurotransmitter. Increased glutamate can trigger an excitotoxic cascade, via activation of N-methyl-D-aspartate (NMDA) and alpha-amino-3-hydroxyl-5-methyl-4-isoxazole-propionate (AMPA) receptor,[5] characterized by calcium influx into the cell, further mitochondrial dysfunction, increased intracellular nitric oxide, and the production of reactive oxygen and nitrogen species.[2,4,5] Irreversible cell damage from excitotoxicity, progressing over a period of minutes to days, can trigger apoptotic pathways, resulting in cell death both in and around the original area that experienced the oxygen/nutrient deficit.[5]

The developing brain is particularly sensitive to excitotoxic damage.[4] In preterm infants, between 23 and 32 weeks of gestational age, the release of excitotoxic neurotransmitters can lead to oligodendrocyte progenitor and neuronal cell death[1,2,4] and white matter injury.[1,2] This susceptibility to excitotoxicity is relevant for anesthesia in premature infants, as the gamma-aminobutyric acid type A (GABA-A) channel is excitotoxic through parts of development, and inhalational anesthetics may then exacerbate neuronal damage. Peroxisomes are used to help clear ROS in the cell, and are needed for the maturation of oligodendrocyte progenitor cells.[2] Interestingly, inflammation in the developing brain can reduce peroxisomal proliferation and prevent oligodendrocyte maturation, as a potential mechanism for white matter damage and adverse changes to developing nerve myelination.[2] Through the described mechanisms, ischemia/hypoxia, excitatory neurotransmitters, and inflammation form a damaging triad, each being caused by and exacerbating the other to induce neuronal dysfunction and death. Strategies to protect the pediatric brain during the perioperative period then focus on the prevention of hypoxia, and the mitigation of excitotoxicity, oxidative damage, and inflammation.

Physiologic Neuroprotective Interventions

Under anesthesia, mechanisms of cerebral autoregulation may be impaired, and oxygen/nutrient supply and demand must be matched to prevent ischemic or hypoxic injury. To this end, physiologic interventions, such as hyperventilation, osmodiuresis, glucose management, and hypothermia, are frequently used interventions in neuroanesthesia management.

As intracranial pressure (ICP) accumulates, cerebral perfusion may fall due to the fixed volume of the calvarium (with the Monro-Kellie doctrine, cerebral blood volume and perfusion are compromised at the expense of the enlarging brain).[6] Increasing ICP also compromises the ability of the local vasculature to regulate blood flow. As such, maintenance of normal ICP is a cornerstone of neuroanesthetic management to ensure both regional (in particular watershed) and global cerebral nutrient supply-demand matching. Reducing ICP may be accomplished by a number of mechanisms, including osmodiuresis, patient positioning (reverse Trendelenburg), and hyperventilation/hypocapnea.

Hyperventilation with hypocapnea induces a transient reduction in cerebral blood volume and blood flow in an attempt to emergently reduce ICP and (somewhat paradoxically) improves neuronal nutrient supply-demand by partially restoring autoregulation. Deliberate hyperventilation to an arterial carbon dioxide pressure of 25 to 30 mm Hg is a standard of care in the management of increased ICP.[7] Chapter 2 provides a comprehensive discussion of the effect of hypocapnea on cerebral blood flow.

Osmodiuretics are employed in neuroanesthesia to reduce ICP, provide brain relaxation, improve surgical conditions, and prevent neurologic deterioration. The effectiveness of osmodiuretics is linked to their "reflection coefficient," which defines the relative ability of the agent to cross the blood-brain barrier (where a coefficient of 0 indicates free flow across the blood-brain barrier, and a coefficient of 1 indicates complete impermeability). Mannitol and hypertonic saline are two common osmotic diuretics used in neuroanesthesia. The reflection coefficient of mannitol is 0.9 and that of hypertonic saline is 1.0, indicating that hypertonic saline may be a superior osmodiuretic to mannitol, producing less rebound cerebral edema with agent removal.[8] Recently, it has been demonstrated that hypertonic saline preserves cerebral microcirculation in an animal model,[9] and is more effective than mannitol in reducing ICP during neurosurgical procedures.[8] All osmodiuretic agents may be less effective in damaged areas of the brain since the reflection coefficient in that area may be altered, adversely allowing for the agent to cross the vasculature.

Patient positioning can also impact ICP. The use of 10 degree reverse Trendelenburg position has been shown to reduce ICP and, in pediatric patients undergoing craniotomy, the supine position has been demonstrated to reduce ICP compared to the prone position.[10]

To prevent neuronal damage not necessarily associated with an increased ICP (like neonatal hypoxic brain injury), there is strong evidence for the neuroprotective benefit of hypothermia.[11] Multiple randomized trials have demonstrated the effectiveness of therapeutic hypothermia initiated within 6 hours of neurological injury in reducing neurodevelopmental disability at 18 months of age in the setting of moderate to severe HIE,[11] a benefit that appears to be preserved into middle childhood.[12] The mechanisms underlying this neuroprotection are thought to include a reduction of cerebral metabolic rate (better balancing of nutrient supply-demand) and a reduction of excitotoxic free radicals.[12] The beneficial effect of hypothermia for pediatrics contrasts with adult data, where hypothermia does not consistently show a beneficial effect for neuroprotection during anesthesia or outside the operating room.[13] This difference may be from the increased neuronal plasticity in the young, or may be related to the underlying physiology where (micro) vascular disease would be much more prominent in the adult population and flow would be quicker to cease and take longer to return.

Hyperthermia, however, has been associated with brain injury.[6] Hyperthermia may increase metabolic demand, depleting energy stores and increasing cerebral blood flow, which may exacerbate reperfusion injury.[6] Elevated temperature has been associated with excitotoxic glutamate release independent of neuronal cell death, the generation of free radicals, and the elevation of neuronal inflammatory markers. Preclinical studies have demonstrated that hyperthermia exacerbates ischemic brain injury, and human data in pediatrics and adults support this association.[6] The avoidance of hyperthermia is therefore imperative in neurosurgical anesthesia.

Hypoglycemia and hyperglycemia are both associated with poor neurologic outcomes in ischemic cerebral injury.[14] Elevated glucose levels in acute ischemic stroke are predictive of increased infarction size, more significant reperfusion injury, the production of proinflammatory mediators and ROS, and increased mortality.[14] Glucose is the most important energy substrate for the brain, and the majority of glucose uptake, under basal conditions, is used for maintenance of normal ionic balance. Seizures and hypoglycemic coma can ensue as blood glucose drops to 2.8 to 3.0 mmol/L, and neuronal death occurs in animal models when the electroencephalography (EEG) becomes isoelectric. Hypoglycemia increases excitatory neurotransmitters in the extracellular space, and generates ROS. As an example of the importance of glucose homeostasis in neuronal survival and function, it was observed that after ischemic stroke in adults, both high and low glucose level on admission correlated with poorer neurocognitive outcomes at 24 hours, with the optimal glucose at 5 mmol/L.[15] A prospective study in pediatric cardiac surgery, however, found an association between intraoperative hypoglycemia but not hyperglycemia with electroencephalographic seizures and slower electroencephalogram recovery, although long-term neurocognitive outcomes were unaffected in both groups.[16] Regardless, maintenance of reasonable normoglycemia during neuroanesthesia is advocated.

Ischemic conditioning refers to the application of a subtoxic ischemic challenge to a tissue, serving to limit cellular damage and death from a more lethal ischemic event through alterations to cellular physiology.[17] Ischemic conditioning may be performed prior to, during, or after an insult, referred to as ischemic pre-, per-, and postconditioning, respectively. While all three work via similar (but not exact) mechanisms, there are differences in the protection benefit they provide for a certain type of insult or stress. Remote ischemic preconditioning has demonstrated effectiveness in animal models,[17] conferring benefit through overlapping biomolecular pathways, including antioxidative and antiapoptotic effects, subcellular organelle-based ischemic tolerance (especially mitochondrial), downregulation of inflammatory mediators, and glutamate and NMDA receptor-mediated neuroprotection. Preconditioning

initiated after the induction of anesthesia but prior to surgical insult can be effective in reducing postoperative cognitive impairment.[18] An intervention with good feasibility, remote ischemic per-conditioning has been shown to reduce infarction when used as an adjunctive treatment in adult ischemic stroke.[19] Although more research is needed for routine practical implementation, remote ischemic conditioning shows promise as a neuroprotective strategy.

Pharmacologic Neuroprotective Interventions

Anesthetic Neuroprotection

The ability of anesthetic agents to protect the brain against neuronal injury was first identified in the 1960s, when it was demonstrated that general anesthesia reduced electroencephalogram seizure activity in the setting of carotid artery occlusion.[20] At the time, it was hypothesized that a decrease in cerebral metabolic rate with the use of anesthesia played a significant role in the observed neuroprotection. Since then, a considerable body of research has further characterized neuroprotection from volatile and intravenous anesthetic agents, and the mechanisms underlying their effect. Recently, however, concerns over anesthetic neurotoxicity have also emerged, focusing ongoing research toward the identification of the determinants of neuroprotection and neurotoxicity and how the causative pathways overlap (see Chapter 19).

Several biomolecular mechanisms have been implicated in anesthetic conditioning against ischemic cerebral injury.[21] Anesthetic agents stimulate inhibitory GABA receptors, preventing membrane depolarization and energy expenditure during ischemia, thereby reducing excitotoxicity.[21] Isoflurane reduces the release of glutamate during cerebral ischemia, and the drug has been linked to a reduced response to both NMDA and AMPA in neurons. Activation of mitochondrial potassium ATP (mito$_{KATP}$) channels has also been shown to be enhanced by volatile anesthetics, leading to mitochondrial membrane hyperpolarization and inhibition of metabolic expenditure.[21] Exposure to volatile and intravenous anesthetics has been associated with an upregulation of antiapoptotic factors and a reduction of apoptotic cell death, via mitochondrial and calcium-dependent mechanisms. Other implicated pathways for anesthesia neuroprotection include an upregulation of antioxidant enzymes, a reduction of cerebral oxidative stress, diminished central nervous system catecholamines, and an increase in cerebral blood flow.[21–23]

Neuroprotection by Volatile Anesthetic Agents

The neuronal protection conferred by volatile anesthetic agents to hypoxia/ischemia has been well established in preclinical studies. In animal models of cerebral ischemia and excitotoxicity, both short- and long-term neuroprotection have been demonstrated with global and focal insults. Although robust evidence for improved short-term neurocognitive outcomes with the use of inhalational anesthetics exists, consensus on the long-term neuroprotective effects of volatile agents has yet to be reached.[21] Inhalational agents can confer neuroprotection when administered prior to, during, or shortly after a neurotoxic insult (similar to ischemic conditioning, referred to as pre-, per-, and postconditioning). Current evidence does not support the use of significantly delayed (>1 hour) anesthetic postconditioning. Whether volatile anesthetics provide neurocognitive protection in the clinical setting is the subject of ongoing research.[21] In the pediatric population, where concerns of volatile anesthetic agent neurotoxicity in the developing brain exist (see Chapter 19), the elucidation of factors mediating both neurotoxicity and neuroprotection of anesthetic agents is of prime importance.

The neuroprotective properties of isoflurane have been well documented in the literature.[24–26] Isoflurane has been demonstrated to provide dose-dependent neuroprotection in in vitro and in vivo models of cerebral ischemia when used prior to, during, or after the ischemic insult.[23,25] Exposure to a GABA-A receptor antagonist markedly attenuates the neuroprotection conferred by isoflurane, suggesting a role for the receptor in isoflurane's beneficial effect (not off-target). Long-term neurocognitive benefit from isoflurane conditioning, however, remains uncertain. Several groups have demonstrated the lack of long-term neurocognitive or histologic benefit from isoflurane as early as 3 weeks post-ischemic injury.[21,24]

As with isoflurane, sevoflurane preconditioning prior to focal or global ischemia demonstrates a neuroprotective effect in a dose-dependent manner.[23] Immediate postconditioning with sevoflurane, resulting in reductions in infarct size and apoptotic cell death and improvement in neurocognitive function, has been demonstrated.[27] Long-term neurocognitive benefit, persisting up to 4 weeks after ischemic injury, was seen with sevoflurane alone, or in combination with xenon.[27] Neuroprotection with the volatile anesthetic desflurane has received less attention, but available evidence demonstrates similar neuroprotection to other inhalational agents. When administered prior to an ischemic insult in animal models, desflurane demonstrated greater neuroprotective benefit than halothane, but comparable to isoflurane.[26,28]

Nitrous oxide is an inhalational anesthetic agent with anti-NMDA properties.[29] In vivo models have described both the neuroprotective and neurotoxic effects of nitrous oxide, similar to the stroke literature, where NMDA antagonists have been trialed for decades for recovery after an ischemic insult, with mixed results. Nitrous oxide demonstrated dose-dependent neuroprotection from the excitotoxic effects of subcutaneous racemic NMDA injection in rats, and exposure of neonatal rats to 70% nitrous oxide for 6 hours did not result in apoptotic neurodegeneration.[29,30] However, the dose-dependent neurotoxic properties of nitric oxide have also been demonstrated. In one in vitro model, this effect was attenuated by GABAergic drugs such as scopolamine or thiopental, suggesting a GABA-mediated mechanism.[29] Overall, however, the body of literature supporting a role for nitrous oxide in cerebral neuroprotection is less robust compared to that for other inhaled anesthetics.

Xenon is a noble gas with general anesthetic properties. As an anesthetic, it exerts its effect primarily via NMDA receptor antagonism, although AMPA and kainite receptors have also been implicated in xenon's mechanism of action.[31] The neuroprotective properties of xenon have been demonstrated in in vitro and in vivo models.[23,31,32] Xenon reduced neuronal death in the cortex and striatum via an NMDA-dependent mechanism in an in vivo model of ischemic brain injury.[32] When administered 1 hour post-global ischemic injury in a rodent model, xenon attenuated damage to neurons.[33] In models of HIE secondary to perinatal asphyxia, xenon has been used in combination with hypothermia to provide neuroprotection in in vitro and in vivo animal models.[34] A feasibility study investigating the safety of 50% xenon in conjunction with mild hypothermia in infants with neonatal encephalopathy using a closed-circuit delivery system found no adverse respiratory or cardiac effects with xenon treatment.[35] Evidence suggests that xenon is an anesthetic agent that may provide significant neuroprotection, warranting further investigations to improve its practical utility.

Neuroprotection by Intravenous Anesthetic Agents

The use of intravenous anesthetic agents for neuroprotection began gaining interest in the literature in the early 1970s, when barbiturates were demonstrated to provide neuroprotection after transient or permanent focal cerebral ischemia in animal models.[5] To date, the neuroprotective properties of a range of intravenous agents have been investigated.

Thiopental demonstrates neuroprotection in animal models of focal cerebral ischemia, but evidence for neuroprotection after global cerebral ischemia in animals remains controversial.[5] While multiple preclinical studies support thiopental's neuroprotective effect, robust evidence for a neuroprotective benefit in humans has not been demonstrated.[5,23] In the setting of cardiac surgery, a randomized trial of 300 adults who were administered thiopental titrated to burst suppression, or placebo, during cardiopulmonary bypass failed to detect a reduction in postoperative neurocognitive outcomes.[36] Thiopental was also ineffective in improving mortality or long-term neurocognitive outcomes in the setting of HIE in neonates. Overall, the neuroprotective benefit seen with thiopental in preclinical studies has not been demonstrated in humans.

Propofol, a phenolic derivative and widely used intravenous anesthetic agent, activates GABA type A receptors directly, reduces extracellular glutamate, and modulates intracellular calcium.[23] In vitro models have documented a neuroprotective effect of propofol in reducing neuronal injury. In animal models of focal ischemic injury, propofol has also been shown to reduce infarction size, comparable to isoflurane.[37] Sustained neuroprotection, persisting at 28 days post-ischemic injury has been reported, associated with reduced apoptosis in an animal model of cerebral ischemia.[38] However, this preclinical neuroprotective benefit has not translated to the clinical setting, where no data demonstrate an improvement in neurocognitive outcomes with propofol use in the setting of cerebral ischemia.[39] A randomized trial investigating propofol titrated to burst suppression in cardiac surgery showed no improvement in neuropsychiatric or neurocognitive outcomes, compared to control.[40] Similar to thiopental, propofol has demonstrated short- and long-term neuroprotection in preclinical studies, but this benefit has not translated to clinical practice.

The dissociative intravenous anesthetic agent ketamine has seen a resurgence of use, in particular for its potentially mood-enhancing properties. Ketamine is an enantiomeric molecule, and differential neuroprotection has been demonstrated according to the stereoisomer administered, whereby the more potent enantiomer, S(+), demonstrates enhanced neuroprotection compared to the R(-) stereoisomer.[41] In vitro and in vivo studies point to a neuroprotective mediated by a reduction of excitotoxicity, modulation of apoptotic factors, improvement in cerebral blood flow during ischemia, and a reduction in the inflammatory response to ischemia.[22,42,43] In adults, a small study of patients undergoing cardiac surgery demonstrated a reduction in postoperative cognitive decline with a bolus dose of ketamine at induction of anesthesia, although a subsequent study did not replicate these findings.[43]

Ketamine's potential neuroprotective properties have been tempered by concerns regarding the anesthetic agent's neurotoxicity, particularly in the developing brain. Experimental data point to dose- and exposure time-dependent neurodegeneration in developing animals.[23] In the developing rat brain, ketamine may induce aberrant cell cycle reentry, leading to apoptotic cell death.[44] Conflicting evidence regarding its neuroprotective properties combined with a concern for neurotoxicity in the developing brain have mitigated clinical research on ketamine-mediated neuroprotection.

Lidocaine, a local anesthetic and antiarrhythmic drug, has been demonstrated to provide neuroprotection in preclinical trials. Antiarrhythmic doses of lidocaine administered 45 minutes after a focal ischemic event in rats conferred a neurocognitive benefit, and prevented neuronal loss in the ischemic penumbra.[45] Lidocaine's neuroprotective properties may involve its ability to attenuate sodium influx, ATP depletion, and intracellular calcium increase in neuronal cells, reducing apoptotic cell death.[45] Although significant heterogeneity limits the interpretation of the data, some evidence supports the perioperative use of lidocaine, continued for 48 hours postoperatively, in preventing postoperative cognitive decline in nondiabetic patients undergoing cardiac surgery.[22]

Dexmedetomidine is an alpha-2 receptor agonist with a broad range of clinical applications in pediatrics, including anxiolysis, sedation, and management of postoperative delirium. Preclinical studies indicate a neuroprotective benefit for dexmedetomidine, administered prior to, or after, global and focal ischemic insults.[46,47] The neuroprotective properties of dexmedetomidine may be mediated by a reduction in oxidative stress, inflammation, and apoptotic neuronal cell death.[47] In particular, dexmedetomidine was found to attenuate isoflurane-induced neurodegeneration and long-term memory impairment in the developing brain in an animal model.[47] Dexmedetomidine itself does not produce long-term cognitive impairment in developing animal brains in clinically relevant doses. Although the results of preliminary studies investigating dexmedetomidine's neuroprotective properties in humans are promising,[48] the evidence supporting the clinical use of dexmedetomidine for neuroprotection is still in its infancy.

In general, preclinical studies consistently demonstrate the neuroprotective properties of both intravenous and inhalational anesthetics. A number of biomolecular mechanisms have been implicated in the cerebral protection conferred by these agents, including a reduction in ischemia-induced excitotoxicity, a decrease in inflammation and the inhibition of apoptotic cell death. For all agents, consistent and conclusive evidence in the clinical setting is lacking at the present time and no anesthetic agent may be definitively recommended for the purpose of neuroprotection. Complicating the analysis and translation to clinical utility is that the mechanisms anesthetic agents may use to provide neuroprotection are likely the same mechanisms by which they induce neuronal toxicity (for example mito$_{KATP}$ activation and mitochondrial depolarization), the physiological result depending on drug dose, timing, and the nature of the initial insult.

Summary

Brain injury in the perioperative period can occur because of patient pathology, surgical intervention, or anesthetic complications. Although more plastic, the developing brain is at a higher risk of injury from immature defense and repair mechanisms, including less responsive cerebral autoregulation. Damage is primarily mediated through excitotoxicity and the generation of ROS, and both preventative and responsive therapies should be targeted to reduce the generation of these damaging agents. Although the protective effects of both physiologic maneuvers (normalizing ICP, glycemic control, temperature management, patient positioning) and anesthetic pharmaceuticals (inhalational and intravenous agents) are well based in preclinical models, only the former has so far translated into solid clinical evidence for utility. The complexity of cerebral nutrient supply-demand regulation and the lack of ability to properly model this relationship for preclinical study have limited therapy development. Newer agents, like dexmedetomidine and xenon, show promise for implementation, but more work is needed for routine use.

References

1. Casaccia-Bonnefil P. Cell death in the oligodendrocyte lineage: a molecular perspective of life/death decisions in development and disease. *Glia*. 2000;**29**(2):124–35.

2. Chang E. Preterm birth and the role of neuroprotection. *BMJ*. 2015;**350**:g6661.

3. Shea KL, Palanisamy A. What can you do to protect the newborn brain? *Curr Opin Anaesthesiol*. 2015;**28**(3): 261–6.

4. Johnston MV. Excitotoxicity in perinatal brain injury. *Brain Pathol*. 2005;**15**(3):234–40.

5. Clarkson AN. Anesthetic-mediated protection/ preconditioning during cerebral ischemia. *Life Sci*. 2007;**80**(13):1157–75.

6. Kukreti V, Mohseni-Bod H, Drake J. Management of raised intracranial pressure in children with traumatic brain injury. *J Pediatr Neurosci*. 2014;**9**(3):207–15.

7. Laffey JG, Kavanagh BP. Hypocapnia. *N Engl J Med*. 2002;**347**(1):43–53.

8. Shao L, Hong F, Zou Y, Hao X, Hou H, Tian M. Hypertonic saline for brain relaxation and intracranial pressure in patients undergoing neurosurgical procedures: a meta-analysis of randomized controlled trials. *PLOS ONE*. 2015;**10**(1):e0117314.

9. Dostal P, Schreiberova J, Dostalova V, Tyll T, Paral J, Abdo I, et al. Effects of hypertonic saline and mannitol on cortical cerebral microcirculation in a rabbit craniotomy model. *BMC Anesthesiol*. 2015;**15**(1):88.

10. Stilling M, Karatasi E, Rasmussen M, Tankisi A, Juul N, Cold GE. Subdural intracranial pressure, cerebral perfusion pressure, and degree of cerebral swelling in supra- and infratentorial space-occupying lesions in children. *Acta Neurochir Suppl*. 2005;**95**:133–6.

11. Jacobs SE, Berg M, Hunt R, Tarnow-Mordi WO, Inder TE, Davis PG. Cooling for newborns with hypoxic ischaemic encephalopathy. *Cochrane Database Syst Rev*. 2013;(1):CD003311.

12. Azzopardi D, Strohm B, Marlow N, Brocklehurst P, Deierl A, Eddama O, et al. Effects of hypothermia for perinatal asphyxia on childhood outcomes. *N Engl J Med.* 2014;**371**(2):140–9.

13. Hindman BJ, Bayman EO, Pfisterer WK, Torner JC, Todd MM, IHAST Investigators. No association between intraoperative hypothermia or supplemental protective drug and neurologic outcomes in patients undergoing temporary clipping during cerebral aneurysm surgery: findings from the Intraoperative Hypothermia for Aneurysm Surgery Trial. *Anesthesiology.* 2010;**112**(1):86–101.

14. Sonneville R, Vanhorebeek I, Hertog den HM, Chrétien F, Annane D, Sharshar T, et al. Critical illness-induced dysglycemia and the brain. *Intensive Care Med.* 2015;**41**(2):192–202.

15. Ntaios G, Egli M, Faouzi M, Michel P. J-shaped association between serum glucose and functional outcome in acute ischemic stroke. *Stroke.* 2010;**41**(10):2366–70.

16. de Ferranti S, Gauvreau K, Hickey PR, Jonas RA, Wypij D, Plessis du A, et al. Intraoperative hyperglycemia during infant cardiac surgery is not associated with adverse neurodevelopmental outcomes at 1, 4, and 8 years. *Anesthesiology.* 2004;**100**(6):1345–52.

17. Fairbanks SL, Brambrink AM. Preconditioning and postconditioning for neuroprotection: the most recent evidence. *Best Pract Res Clin Anaesthesiol.* 2010;**24**(4):521–34.

18. Hudetz JA, Patterson KM, Iqbal Z, Gandhi SD, Pagel PS. Remote ischemic preconditioning prevents deterioration of short-term postoperative cognitive function after cardiac surgery using cardiopulmonary bypass: results of a pilot investigation. *J Cardiothorac Vasc Anesth.* 2015;**29**(2):382–8.

19. Zwerus R, Absalom A. Update on anesthetic neuroprotection. *Curr Opin Anaesthesiol.* 2015;**28**(4):424–30.

20. Wells BA, Keats AS, Cooley DA. Increased tolerance to cerebral ischemia produced by general anesthesia during temporary carotid occlusion. *Surgery.* 1963;**54**:216–23.

21. Matchett GA, Allard MW, Martin RD, Zhang JH. Neuroprotective effect of volatile anesthetic agents: molecular mechanisms. *Neurol Res.* 2009;**31**(2):128–34.

22. Bilotta F, Stazi E, Zlotnik A, Gruenbaum SE, Rosa G. Neuroprotective effects of intravenous anesthetics: a new critical perspective. *Curr Pharm Des.* 2014;**20**(34):5469–75.

23. Schifilliti D, Grasso G, Conti A, Fodale V. Anaesthetic-related neuroprotection: intravenous or inhalational agents? *CNS Drugs.* 2010;**24**(11):893–907.

24. Elsersy H, Sheng H, Lynch JR, Moldovan M, Pearlstein RD, Warner DS. Effects of isoflurane versus fentanyl-nitrous oxide anesthesia on long-term outcome from severe forebrain ischemia in the rat. *Anesthesiology.* 2004;**100**(5):1160–6.

25. Elsersy H, Mixco J, Sheng H, Pearlstein RD, Warner DS. Selective gamma-aminobutyric acid type A receptor antagonism reverses isoflurane ischemic neuroprotection. *Anesthesiology.* 2006;**105**(1):81–90.

26. Engelhard K, Werner C, Reeker W, Lu H, Möllenberg O, Mielke L, et al. Desflurane and isoflurane improve neurological outcome after incomplete cerebral ischaemia in rats. *Br J Anaesth.* 1999;**83**(3):415–21.

27. Lai Z, Zhang L, Su J, Cai D, Xu Q. Sevoflurane postconditioning improves long-term learning and memory of neonatal hypoxia-ischemia brain damage rats via the PI3 K/Akt-mPTP pathway. *Brain Res.* 2016;**1630**:25–37.

28. Haelewyn B, Yvon A, Hanouz JL, MacKenzie ET, Ducouret P, Gérard JL, et al. Desflurane affords greater protection than halothane against focal cerebral ischaemia in the rat. *Br J Anaesth.* 2003;**91**(3):390–6.

29. Jevtovic-Todorovic V, Todorović SM, Mennerick S, Powell S, Dikranian K, Benshoff N, et al. Nitrous oxide (laughing gas) is an NMDA antagonist, neuroprotectant and neurotoxin. *Nat Med.* 1998;**4**(4):460–3.

30. Haelewyn B, David HN, Rouillon C, Chazalviel L, Lecocq M, Risso J-J, et al. Neuroprotection by nitrous oxide: facts and evidence. *Crit Care Med.* 2008;**36**(9):2651–9.

31. Wilhelm S, Ma D, Maze M, Franks NP. Effects of xenon on in vitro and in vivo models of neuronal injury. *Anesthesiology.* 2002;**96**(6):1485–91.

32. David HN, Leveille F, Chazalviel L, MacKenzie ET, Buisson A, Lemaire M, et al. Reduction of ischemic brain damage by nitrous oxide and xenon. *J Cereb Blood Flow Metab.* 2003;**23**(10):1168–73.

33. Metaxa V, Lagoudaki R, Meditskou S, Thomareis O, Oikonomou L, Sakadamis A. Delayed post-ischaemic administration of xenon reduces brain damage in a rat model of global ischaemia. *Brain Inj.* 2014;**28**(3):364–9.

34. Ma D, Hossain M, Chow A, Arshad M, Battson RM, Sanders RD, et al. Xenon and hypothermia combine to provide neuroprotection from neonatal asphyxia. *Ann Neurol.* 2005;**58**(2):182–93.

35. Dingley J, Tooley J, Liu X, Scull-Brown E, Elstad M, Chakkarapani E, et al. Xenon ventilation during therapeutic hypothermia in neonatal encephalopathy: a feasibility study. *Pediatrics*. 2014;**133**(5):809–18.

36. Zaidan JR, Klochany A, Martin WM, Ziegler JS, Harless DM, Andrews RB. Effect of thiopental on neurologic outcome following coronary artery bypass grafting. *Anesthesiology*. 1991;**74**(3):406–11.

37. Gelb AW, Bayona NA, Wilson JX, Cechetto DF. Propofol anesthesia compared to awake reduces infarct size in rats. *Anesthesiology*. 2002;**96**(5):1183–90.

38. Engelhard K, Werner C, Eberspächer E, Pape M, Stegemann U, Kellermann K, et al. Influence of propofol on neuronal damage and apoptotic factors after incomplete cerebral ischemia and reperfusion in rats: a long-term observation. *Anesthesiology*. 2004;**101**(4):912–17.

39. Adembri C, Venturi L, Pellegrini-Giampietro DE. Neuroprotective effects of propofol in acute cerebral injury. *CNS Drug Rev*. 2007;**13**(3):333–51.

40. Roach GW, Newman MF, Murkin JM, Martzke J, Ruskin A, Li J, et al. Ineffectiveness of burst suppression therapy in mitigating perioperative cerebrovascular dysfunction. Multicenter Study of Perioperative Ischemia (McSPI) Research Group. *Anesthesiology*. 1999;**90**(5):1255–64.

41. Proescholdt M, Heimann A, Kempski O. Neuroprotection of S(+) ketamine isomer in global forebrain ischemia. *Brain Res*. 2001;**904**(2):245–51.

42. Hudetz JA, Pagel PS. Neuroprotection by ketamine: a review of the experimental and clinical evidence. *J Cardiothorac Vasc Anesth*. 2010;**24**(1):131–42.

43. Hudetz JA, Patterson KM, Iqbal Z, Gandhi SD, Byrne AJ, Hudetz AG, et al. Ketamine attenuates delirium after cardiac surgery with cardiopulmonary bypass. *J Cardiothorac Vasc Anesth*. 2009;**23**(5):651–7.

44. Soriano SG, Liu Q, Li J, Liu J-R, Han XH, Kanter JL, et al. Ketamine activates cell cycle signaling and apoptosis in the neonatal rat brain. *Anesthesiology*. 2010;**112**(5):1155–63.

45. Lei B, Popp S, Capuano-Waters C, Cottrell JE, Kass IS. Effects of delayed administration of low-dose lidocaine on transient focal cerebral ischemia in rats. *Anesthesiology*. 2002;**97**(6):1534–40.

46. Ren X, Ma H, Zuo Z. Dexmedetomidine postconditioning reduces brain injury after brain hypoxia-ischemia in neonatal rats. *J Neuroimmune Pharmacol*. 2016;**11**(2):238–47.

47. Sanders RD, Xu J, Shu Y, Januszewski A, Halder S, Fidalgo A, et al. Dexmedetomidine attenuates isoflurane-induced neurocognitive impairment in neonatal rats. *Anesthesiology*. 2009;**110**(5):1077–85.

48. Ge Y-L, Li X, Gao JU, Zhang X, Fang X, Zhou L, et al. Beneficial effects of intravenous dexmedetomidine on cognitive function and cerebral injury following a carotid endarterectomy. *Exp Ther Med*. 2016;**11**(3): 1128–34.

Neuropharmacology

Charu Mahajan, Indu Kapoor, and Hemanshu Prabhakar

Introduction

The most apparent difference between children and adults is size, but along with anatomical differences, significant variations exist also in pharmacokinetics and pharmacodynamics of the drugs. Rapid growth and development in early years may lead to alteration in uptake, distribution, metabolism, and elimination of drugs. These pharmacokinetic and -dynamic differences in pediatric population depend on age, developmental stage, and genetic factors (see Chapter 1).

Body composition determines the volume of distribution of hydrophilic and lipophilic drugs. Neonates and infants have greater total body and extracellular water, resulting in increased distribution volume for water-soluble drugs. Body fat content starts increasing at birth, peaks at 9 months, and then again starts decreasing. Decreased plasma protein binding may result in increased free drug, resulting in enhanced effect. Glomerular filtration rate and renal tubular secretion reaches the adult level by 8–12 and 6–12 months, respectively. Several anesthetic drugs depend on the liver for clearance. During the first 3 months, activity of hepatic cytochrome enzymes is markedly low and gradually increases to adult levels by 1 year. The hepatic blood flow is also low in neonates.

The minimum alveolar concentration (MAC) of halogenated agents rises during the first month and peaks at 1 year, after which it starts declining. Sevoflurane is an exception as MAC is highest in neonates.

For the ethical constraints, most of the evidence for usage of drugs in children has been extrapolated from results obtained from studies carried out in adults. The anesthetic management of children undergoing neurosurgery requires knowledge of drug actions on different systems (especially on central nervous system) and of its metabolism. In this chapter we primarily discuss the common drugs used in neuroanesthesia practice. The neurotoxicity of these anesthetic drugs is discussed elsewhere in the book (see Chapter 19).

Inhaled Anesthetic Agents

Inhaled anesthetics are the most common agents used for induction and maintenance of anesthesia in children. Presence of anatomical and physiological differences affects wash-in of inhalational agents, therefore it varies with age. Infants have a higher wash-in as compared to older children and adults. Agents that are less blood soluble are affected the least.

Nitrous oxide is highly insoluble in blood, which enables its rapid wash-in and wash-out. It has an anesthetic sparing and analgesic action when combined with other agents. Table 4.1 summarizes the properties and systemic effects of nitrous oxide. An ongoing controversy regarding its use especially in neurosurgical patients arises from the fact that it increases cerebral blood flow (CBF), cerebral metabolic rate ($CMRO_2$), and intracranial pressure (ICP) and impairs cerebral autoregulation. Carbon dioxide (CO_2) reactivity is preserved during nitrous oxide anesthesia. The vasodilatory effect can be countered by hyperventilation and administration of intravenous anesthetic agents like propofol and thiopentone. However, in clinical use, much of these effects are variable and depend on the volatile agent being concomitantly used and level of arterial CO_2. Rise in ICP makes it a less approved agent for use in conditions with reduced intracranial compliance, though it has not been confirmed by various studies. Use of nitrous oxide has also not shown to increase the incidence of venous air embolism in sitting position, but it must be discontinued as soon as it is detected.[1] Nitrous oxide has the ability to diffuse into air containing cavities and expand them. Omission of nitrous oxide does not warrant that pneumocephalus will not develop.[2] Some amount of intracranial air may persist for several days even after surgery is completed.[3] For this reason,

Table 4.1 Properties and Systemic Effects of Inhalational Agents

Anesthetic Agent	MAC (2 yrs)	Blood-Gas Partition Coefficient	% Metabolized	MAP	CBF	ICP	CMRO$_2$	CPP	SSEP	MEP
Nitrous oxide	Unknown	0.47	—	0	↑	↑	↑↓	↓	0↓	↓
Halothane	0.97	2.4	20	↓	↑↑	↑↑	↓	↑↑	↓	↓
Isoflurane	1.6	1.4	0.2	↓	↑	↑	↓	↑	↓	↓
Sevoflurane	2.6	0.66	5	↓	↑	0–↑	↓	↑	↓	↓
Desflurane	8.7	0.42	0.02	↓	↑	↑	↓	↑	↓	↓
Xenon	Unknown	0.115	0	0	↑↓	↑	↓	↑	Unknown	Unknown

MAC = minimum alveolar concentration; MAP = mean arterial pressure; CBF = cerebral blood flow; ICP = intracranial pressure; CMRO$_2$ = cerebral metabolic rate of oxygen; CPP = cerebral perfusion pressure; SSEP = somatosensory evoked potential; MEP = motor evoked potential; ↓ = decreases; ↑ = increases; 0 = no effect.

it should be avoided for 4–6 weeks in cases of redo craniotomy, lest it expand the air cavity before dura is opened. There is no literature available on use of nitrous oxide in children having cerebral ischemia. Results extrapolated from animal studies and adult human population show no deleterious effect of its use on neurologic function.[4,5] During intraoperative recording of evoked potentials, it is best to omit nitrous oxide as it can reduce the signal amplitude. Prolonged exposure to nitrous oxide inhibits vitamin B_{12}-dependent enzymes affecting myelin formation, DNA synthesis, homocysteine, and folate metabolism. A short intraoperative exposure is unlikely to result in toxicity. However, it should be avoided in children having methionine synthetase deficiency. On the basis of the current literature, there is still no strong evidence to discontinue nitrous oxide in pediatric neurosurgical cases.

Halogenated Anesthetic Agents

The mechanisms of action of these agents include antagonism of N-methyl-D-aspartic acid (NMDA) receptor, activation of gamma-aminobutyric acid (GABA) and glycine receptors, inhibition of ionic channels, and alteration of cellular proteins. All volatile inhalational agents decrease systemic blood pressure and increase heart rate in a dose-dependent manner (except halothane, which causes an increase in heart rate). All of these depress ventilatory drive and decrease tidal volume. All produce bronchodilatation, but evidence is not strong enough for desflurane.[6] They may all trigger malignant hyperthermia in susceptible children. Preconditioning with isoflurane, sevoflurane, and desflurane provides neurologic protection. However, all of them have also been implicated in neurotoxicity though to a varying extent.

Isoflurane is the most common volatile anesthetic for the maintenance of general anesthesia. However, it is not used for induction of anesthesia as it has a pungent odor that may irritate the airway and may even cause laryngospasm. All halogenated volatile anesthetic agents increase CBF and decrease $CMRO_2$. At 1 MAC, CO_2 reactivity and cerebral autoregulation is preserved. It does not affect CSF production but facilitates CSF reabsorption. At a low concentration, it increases the EEG frequency and decreases the voltage. At higher concentrations, it decreases frequency and increases amplitude. It can even produce burst suppression and isoelectric pattern on electroencephalography

(EEG). Isoflurane is the most potent suppressant of cortical somatosensory evoked potentials (SSEPs) and should be used in concentration <0.5 MAC for successful recording. Motor evoked potentials (MEPs) are diminished even at 0.2–0.5 MAC isoflurane. Many experimental and clinical models of cerebral ischemia suggest that isoflurane exerts a neuroprotective effect.[7,8]

Sevoflurane has been the gold standard agent for inhaled inductions because of its pleasant and non-irritating scent and low blood solubility, enabling its rapid uptake and wash-off. The recovery profile is better with sevoflurane as compared to isoflurane.[9] Rapid wash-off of sevoflurane at time of awakening may cause emergence delirium, which is comparable to that of desflurane.[10] It causes dose-dependent cerebral vasodilation resulting in raised CBF. It decreases $CMRO_2$ and preserves cerebrovascular reactivity to CO_2. It maintains cerebral autoregulation up to 1.5 MAC. Epileptiform EEG pattern has been seen at high concentration of sevoflurane.[11] The age-related brain developmental process like synaptogenesis and myelination affects the electroencephalogram (EEG) dynamics in response to sevoflurane especially in children less than 1 year.[12] The degradation of sevoflurane to produce inorganic fluoride and compound A rarely results in problems in clinical practice. Sevoflurane decreases the amplitude and increases latency of SSEPs, albeit at a higher concentration of 1–1.5 MAC. Sevoflurane has an action similar to isoflurane on MEPs. Under specific conditions it produces antiapoptotic effects, increased mitochondrial phosphorylation, activation of K (TREK-1) channel, and inhibition of caspase-3, thus imparting neuroprotection.[13–15] Sevoflurane can be associated with a higher incidence of emergence delirium when compared to other halogenated anesthetics.[16]

Desflurane has the most rapid wash-in and wash-off among the available inhalational anesthetic agents owing to its lowest blood:gas partition coefficient. It is not used for induction of anesthesia as it may incite laryngospasm and breath holding because of its pungent odor. It boils at room temperature (23.5°C), so requires a special heated vaporizer for its delivery. Similar to other volatile agents, it causes cerebral vasodilatation, impairs autoregulation at 1.0 MAC, increases ICP, and preserves CO_2 reactivity. Isoflurane, sevoflurane, and desflurane 0.5–1.0 MAC in nitrous oxide when administered to children all increase ICP and decrease minimum alveolar concentration (MAP) and cerebral perfusion pressure (CPP) in a dose-dependent manner.[17] The degree of increase in ICP with various agents is in the following order: desflurane >isoflurane > sevoflurane.[18] It suppresses EEG activity and can induce burst suppression at 1.24 MAC.[19] At 1.5 MAC desflurane, SSEP and MEP are suppressed. The amount of carbon monoxide production in the presence of desiccated soda lime or baralyme is greatest with desflurane and least with sevoflurane. Neuroprotection and cardioprotection with desflurane has been observed in several studies.[20,21] While few studies report more neuroapoptosis with desflurane than sevoflurane or isoflurane in neonatal animal studies, others are equivocal.[22,23]

Intravenous Anesthetic Agents

Most intravenous anesthetic agents exert their effect by binding to different subunits of gamma-aminobutyric acid type A (GABA$_A$) receptors and potentiating their inhibitory action. GABA$_A$ receptors form chloride channels, and when activated, they lead to postsynaptic hyperpolarization and inhibition of neuronal activity. The cerebrovascular effects of various agents are depicted in Table 4.2.

Sodium thiopenthal is an ultrashort-acting barbiturate used as an induction agent. It is highly lipid soluble and protein bound (80%). It is a direct myocardial depressant and decreases MAP, resulting in baroreceptor activation and an increase in heart rate. The degree of blunting of airway reflexes is less than propofol, predisposing to laryngospasm and bronchospasm. It has a favorable profile by decreasing CBF, cerebral blood volume, CMRO$_2$, and ICP. It does not impair cerebral autoregulation and CO$_2$ reactivity. It decreases the amplitude and latency of cortical SSEPs and inhibits

MEP. It has been found to have a neuroprotective effect in the treatment of focal cerebral ischemia. The induction dose of sodium thiopental in neonates (ED$_{50}$ = 3.4 mg/kg) is less than in infants (ED$_{50}$ = 6.3 mg/kg).[24] Small children have more vessel-rich tissue, which hastens uptake and achieves a rapid effect and prompt redistribution and elimination. Early awakening after a single intravenous bolus occurs by redistribution from brain to other tissues. It may also be administered as an infusion in children having refractory epilepsy. The dose is 3–5 mg/kg bolus, followed by an infusion of 3–5 mg/kg/hr. Hypotension is an important side effect and requires administration of vasopressors. Elimination from adipose tissue may be prolonged after administration of continuous infusion. Porphyria is an absolute contraindication to barbiturate administration.

Propofol is available as 1% aqueous emulsion containing soya bean oil, egg lecithin, and glycerol. The addition of disodium edetate helps in controlling bacterial growth. It is rapidly redistributed and metabolized by liver glucuronidation and other extrahepatic mechanisms. It decreases cardiac contractility, systemic vascular resistance (SVR), and preload, resulting in hypotension and reactionary increase in heart rate. It depresses the respiration and obtunds upper airway reflexes. It decreases CBF, CMRO$_2$, and ICP. Cerebral autoregulation and CO$_2$ reactivity are preserved. As a part of a total intravenous anesthesia technique, it is the preferred agent for somatosensory and MEP monitoring.[25] Propofol is helpful in controlling seizures and may be administered as an infusion. It has an additional advantage of having an antiemetic effect. ED$_{50}$ of propofol for older children is 2.4 mg/kg and for infants is 3 mg/kg. However, these doses can lead to

Table 4.2 Systemic Effects of Intravenous Agents

Anesthetic Agent	MAP	CBF	ICP	CMRO$_2$	CPP	SSEP	MEP
Sodium thiopentone	↓↓	↓↓↓	↓↓↓	↓↓↓	↑↑↑	↓A↑L	↓↓
Propofol	↓↓↓	↓↓↓	↓↓	↓↓↓	↑↑	↓A	↓
Etomidate	0–↓	↓↓	↓↓	↓↓↓	↑↑	↑A	↑
Ketamine	↑	↑↑	↑↑	↑	↓	↑A	0
Benzodiazepines	0–↓	↓↓	0	↓↓	↑	0	↓↓↓
Opioids	0–↓	↓	0–↓	↓	↓↑	↓A↑L	0

MAP = mean arterial pressure; CBF = cerebral blood flow; ICP = intracranial pressure; CMRO$_2$ = cerebral metabolic rate of oxygen; CPP = cerebral perfusion pressure; SSEP = somatosensory evoked potential; MEP = motor evoked potential; ↓ = decreases; ↑ = increases; 0 = no effect; A = amplitude; L = latency.

hypotension for as long as 30 minutes in unstimulated neonates and infants. Propofol infusion more than 10mg/kg/hr lasting for more than 48 hours if administered in critically ill patients may result in propofol infusion syndrome,characterized by metabolic acidosis, rhabdomyolysis, and renal and heart failure. For this reason, and associated hypotension, propofol is not used for intensive care unit (ICU) sedation in pediatric head injury patients. Pain on injection is a common side effect, and thus it is often mixed with lidocaine to reduce pain intensity.

Etomidate is a short-acting nonbarbiturate agent used primarily for induction of anesthesia. When used for this purpose it causes negligible hemodynamic perturbations but is commonly associated with myoclonic movements. It is also associated with pain at the injection site, which can be minimized by use of a formulation containing medium- and long-chain triglycerides. The cerebrovascular action comprises reduction of CBF, $CMRO_2$, and ICP. Absence of negative ionotropic effect maintains the blood pressure, which is advantageous in setting of intracranial hypertension.[26] It increases the amplitude of cortical SSEP and MEP during evoked potential monitoring. Etomidate has proconvulsant action and can produce epileptiform discharges. A major side effect is adrenal suppression, which may occur after continuous infusion or even a single induction dose. It blocks 11β-hydroxylase, thus inhibiting steroid synthesis. The dose used is 0.2–0.3 mg/kg. A pyrrole analog of etomidate known as carboetomidate does not affect steroid synthesis as well as maintains hemodynamic stability.[27]

Ketamine is an effective sedative and analgesic that produces dissociative anesthesia. It is a noncompetitive NMDA receptor antagonist. It preserves the upper airway reflexes and maintains respiration and blood pressure. The dose is 2 mg/kg, and requirement increases with decreasing age. Below the age of 3 months, its metabolism and clearance are reduced and half-life is prolonged. It can be administered through oral, intravenous, and intramuscular routes. It is a cerebral vasodilator and increases intraocular pressure (IOP), CBF, $CMRO_2$, and ICP. For these reasons it is generally not preferred in neurosurgical patients at risk of intracranial hypertension. Ketamine increases the amplitude of cortical SSEP and enables monitoring of myogenic MEP. It produces electroencephalographic seizure activity at low doses by blocking the inhibitory interneurons. At higher doses, it also blocks the excitatory neurons, thus acting as an anticonvulsant. It has been used as an effective antiepileptic in pediatric refractory status epilepticus patients without causing any complications.[28] However, significant controversy exists regarding its effect on ICP and neurotoxicity. Ketamine has even been shown to possess ICP-lowering action when administered to patients of head trauma being ventilated and sedated with propofol.[29] The effect of ketamine on ICP in severe head injury patients was assessed in 101 adult and 55 pediatric patients with severe head injury. ICP did not increase during ketamine administration when patients were sedated and ventilated.[30] On the basis of the available evidence, ketamine administration increases global CBF and rCBF in humans, but the level of evidence is 2b (grade C). Thus, it should not be routinely prohibited in all neurologically ill patients.[31] Ketamine may provide neuroprotection by virtue of NMDA receptor antagonism, antiapoptotic effect, and interference with the inflammatory reaction to injury. In several animal models, it has been shown to induce neuroapoptosis, but this has not been confirmed in humans who clinically receive much lower dose and exposure time. Hallucinations, euphoria, and dysphoria are common excitatory reactions seen after ketamine administration and may be lessened by coadministration of midazolam.

Benzodiazepines are GABA agonists that produce sedation and amnesia. Midazolam is a short-acting benzodiazepine that is often used as a premedicant, sedative, and inducing and antiepileptic agent. It causes anxiolysis, sedation, and anterograde amnesia, which makes it an ideal premedicant. It causes respiratory depression in a dose-dependent manner. It decreases SVR and blood pressure and increases heart rate. It decreases CBF and $CMRO_2$ but has a plateau effect beyond which it cannot further decrease $CMRO_2$ and produce isoelectric EEG. CO_2 reactivity is maintained and has no effect on ICP. It can be administered through various routes like oral, sublingual, intranasal, intravenous, intramuscular, and rectal. Midazolam has minimal effect on cortical SSEP but suppresses MEP even at small doses.[25] It is an effective anticonvulsant and can be used as an infusion for control of status epilepticus in children.[32] Dose for intravenous bolus and oral use is 0.05–0.1 mg/kg and 0.3–0.75 mg/kg. Low incidence of paradoxical reactions may be observed in children, which may require administration of other agents like propofol, ketamine, and benzodiazepine antagonist flumazenil (0.3–0.5 mg). However, fluma-zenil should be avoided in children having a history of seizures or elevated ICP because rapid reversal of midazolam effect may lead to a rebounding increase in CBF and ICP.

Opioids

Commonly used opioids in children are fentanyl and remifentanil. Fentanyl is 150 times more potent than morphine but is shorter acting and maintains more hemodynamic stability. It has little effect on blood pressure but at high doses can depress the baroreceptor control of heart rate in response to both increase or decrease in blood pressure. Remifentanil is an ultrashort-acting opioid that ensures rapid arousal even after long surgical time. It requires supplementation with another analgesic at the end of surgery to prevent breakthrough pain. At low doses, opioids do not affect cerebral hemodynamics. At high doses, opioids decrease CBF and $CMRO_2$. Cerebral autoregulation and CO_2 reactivity are maintained at all doses. Generally it is believed that overall opioids have no effect on ICP if MAP is maintained. Administration of fentanyl does not reduce ICP in pediatric patients having severe traumatic brain injury.[33] Opioids as a component of total intravenous anesthesia techniques are used during recording of evoked potentials. A slight reduction in amplitude and increase in latency of late cortical responses may be seen. High doses of remifentanil may produce a decrease in amplitude of SSEP. In clinical-used doses, opioids do not affect MEP. Fentanyl may be administered via oral, nasal, and intravenous routes, but because of predictability, intravenous is considered safer. The analgesic doses of fentanyl and remifentanil are 1–2 µg/kg and 0.05–2 µg/kg. Rapid administration may lead to chest rigidity or myoclonus. Other side effects of opioids that may be observed are nausea, vomiting, respiratory depression, pruritis, and constipation.

Dexmedetomidine is an α2 adrenoreceptor agonist that provides anxiolysis, sedation, and analgesia and induces normal sleep without any respiratory depression. It is used for procedural sedation, monitored anesthesia care, and ICU sedation and as an adjuvant during general anesthesia.[34] It has also been shown to be effective for prevention of emergence delirium after anesthesia. It is administered in loading dose of 0.5–1 µg/kg over 10 minutes followed by infusion of 0.3–0.5 µg/kg. Transient hypertension occurs after its bolus administration owing to its direct α2 stimulation. More common responses seen are bradycardia and hypotension. Animal studies have shown reduction in CBF that was not accompanied by reduction in $CMRO_2$.[35] Later it was shown by Drummond et al. that it decreases both CBF and $CMRO_2$ in healthy subjects.[36] Hypotension should be avoided as it can lead to a decrease in CBF. The effect on ICP is negligible if MAP is maintained. The neuroprotective effects of dexmedetomidine may be explained by decreased levels of catecholamines, increased production of neurotrophic factors, and decreasing cell necrosis and apoptosis.[37] It has no suppressive effect on evoked potentials. When used along with sevoflurane in children undergoing spinal surgery, it resulted in a more favorable recovery profile with less pain and excitatory reactions.[38] Food and Drug Administration (FDA) approval for its use pertains to sedation of intubated and ventilated patients in ICU settings for up to 24 hours and for in-hospital sedation. Withdrawal reactions may be seen in pediatric ICU patients who receive it for a prolonged duration.

Muscle Relaxants

The neuromuscular system is incompletely developed at birth. Infants less than 6 months have more slow twitch fibers, and infants less than 2 months have a lower train-of-four ratio and increased fade. This makes neonates and infants very sensitive to muscle relaxants. In general, muscle relaxants have no sedative, hypnotic, or analgesic action or any direct effect on cerebral hemodynamics. Succinylcholine is a rapid- and short-acting depolarizing muscle relaxant that produces ideal intubating conditions within 60 seconds. The initial dose is 2 mg/kg in infants and small children and 1 mg/kg in older children. It is associated with bradycardia, raised IOP, ICP, possible risk of inducing hyperkalemia in patients with neuromuscular disorders, and malignant hyperthermia in susceptible patients. Hyperkalemia after head injury may occur as early as 24–48 hours after injury.[39] For these reasons it is not generally used in children except for emergency situations and rapid sequence intubation. The cerebral stimulatory effect and increase in ICP are usually transient and can be minimized by a prior defasciculation dose. Moreover, in case of emergency a secure airway supersedes any transient risk of increase in ICP. Vecuronium and rocuronium are non-depolarizing muscle blockers (NDMBs) that act as long-acting agents in neonates and young infants. Rocuronium has a rapid onset and is a good alternative to succinylcholine for intubation. NDMBs have no direct effect on CBF and ICP but if associated with histamine release may lead to a decrease in MAP and cerebral vasodilation and increased ICP. The paretic side is usually resistant to non-depolarizing agents and should not be used for neuromuscular block monitoring. Maintenance dose is usually one-third to one-fourth of intubation dose. In patients receiving anticonvulsants, response to neuromuscular blocking agents (NMBA) varies depending on whether it is acute or chronic. Acute administration increases the duration of block while chronic use of all enzyme inducers shortens the duration of action.[40] This effect holds true for phenytoin, carbamazepine, and phenobarbital. Atracurium is metabolized by non-specific esterases and Hofmann degradation and is not affected by these interactions. The main side effects of non-depolarizing agents are related to cardiovascular changes in response to histamine release, bronchospasm, and anaphylaxis. The amount of histamine release is less in children than in adults.

Conclusion

Basic understanding of neuropharmacology and the effect of various anesthetic drugs and their interactions are essential for managing pediatric patients with neurological problems. Other than the direct cerebrovascular action, the majority of anesthetic drugs reduce blood pressure and, if not taken care of, may reduce cerebral perfusion pressure and precipitate cerebral ischemia.[41] This knowledge is extremely important for reducing perioperative morbidity and mortality.

References

1. Losasso TJ, Muzzi DA, Dietz NM, Cucchiara RF. Fifty percent nitrous oxide does not increase the risk of venous air embolism in neurosurgical patients operated upon in the sitting position. *Anesthesiology.* 1992;**77**:21–30.

2. Jain V, Prabhakar H, Rath GP, Sharma D. Tension pneumocephalus following deep brain stimulation surgery with bispectral index monitoring. *Eur J Anaesthesiol.* 2007;**24**:203–4.

3. Reasoner DK, Todd MM, Scamman FL, Warner DS. The incidence of pneumocephalus after supratentorial craniotomy. Observations on the disappearance of intracranial air.*Anesthesiology.* 1994;**80**:1008–12.

4. Yokoo N, Sheng H, Mixco J, Homi HM, Pearlstein RD, Warner DS. Intraischemic nitrous oxide alters neither neurologic nor histologic outcome: a comparison with dizocilpine. *Anesth Analg.* 2004;**99**:896–903.

5. Pasternak JJ, McGregor DG, Lanier WL, Schroeder DR, Rusy DA, Hindman B, et al. Effect of nitrous oxide use on long-term neurologic and neuropsychological outcome in patients who received temporary proximal artery occlusion during cerebral aneurysm clipping surgery. *Anesthesiology.* 2009;**110**: 563–73.

6. Goff MJ, Arain SR, Ficke DJ, Uhrich TD, Ebert TJ. Absence of bronchodilation during desflurane anesthesia: a comparison to sevoflurane and thiopental. *Anesthesiology.* 2000;**93**:404–8.

7. Zhao P, Ji G, Xue H, Yu W, Zhao X, Ding M, et al. Isoflurane postconditioning improved long-term neurological outcome possibly via inhibiting the mitochondrial permeability transition pore in neonatal rats after brain hypoxia-ischemia. *Neuroscience.* 2014;**280**:193–203.

8. Burchell SR, Dixon BJ, Tang J, Zhang JH. Isoflurane provides neuroprotection in neonatal hypoxic ischemic brain injury. *J Investig Med.* 2013;**61**: 1078–83.

9. Singh D, Rath GP, Dash HH, Bithal PK. Sevoflurane provides better recovery as compared with isoflurane in children undergoing spinal surgery. *J Neurosurg Anesthesiol.* 2009;**21**:202–6.

10. Gupta P, Rath GP, Prabhakar H, Bithal PK. Comparison between sevoflurane and desflurane on emergence and recovery characteristics of children undergoing surgery for spinal dysraphism. *Indian J Anaesth.* 2015;**59**:482–7.

11. Kreuzer I, Osthaus WA, Schultz A, Schultz B. Influence of the sevoflurane concentration on the occurrence of epileptiform EEG pattern. *PLOS ONE.* 2014;**9**:e89191.

12. Akeju O, Pavone KJ, Thum JA, Firth PG, Westover MB, Puglia M, et al. Age-dependency of sevoflurane-induced electroencephalogram dynamics in children. *Br J Anaesth.* 2015;**115**(suppl 1):i66–76.

13. Ye Z, Xia P, Cheng ZG, Guo Q. Neuroprotection induced by sevoflurane-delayed post-conditioning is attributable to increased phosphorylation of mitochondrial GSK-3β through the PI3K/Akt survival pathway. *J Neurol Sci.* 2015;**348**(1–2):216–25.

14. Tong L, Cai M, Huang Y, Zhang H, Su B, Li Z, Dong H. Activation of K(2)P channel-TREK1 mediates the neuroprotection induced by sevoflurane preconditioning. *Br J Anaesth.* 2014;**113**(1):157–67.

15. Wang H, Shi H, Yu Q, Chen J, Zhang F, Gao Y. Sevoflurane preconditioning confers neuroprotection via anti-apoptosis effects. *Acta Neurochir Suppl.* 2016;**121**:55–61.

16. Costi D, Cyna AM, Ahmed S, Stephens K, Strickland P, Ellwood J, et al. Effects of sevoflurane versus other general anaesthesia on emergence agitation in children. *Cochrane Database Syst Rev.* 2014;**12**(9).

17. Sponheim S, Skraastad Ø, Helseth E, Due-Tønnesen B, Aamodt G, Breivik H. Effects of 0.5 and 1.0 MAC isoflurane, sevoflurane and desflurane on intracranial and cerebral perfusion pressures in children. *Acta Anaesthesiol Scand.* 2003;47(8):932–8.

18. Holmstrom A, Akeson J. Desflurane increases intracranial pressure more and sevoflurane less than isoflurane in pigs subjected to intracranial hypertension. *J Neurosurg Anesthesiol.* 2004;**16**: 136–43.

19. Rampil IJ, Lockhart SH, Eger EI, Yasuda N, Weiskopf RB, Cahalan MK. The electroencephalographic effects of desflurane in humans. *Anesthesiology.* 1991;74:434–9.

20. Wise-Faberowski L, Raizada MK, Sumners C. Desflurane and sevoflurane attenuate oxygen and glucose deprivation-induced neuronal cell death. *J Neurosurg Anesthesiol.* 2003;15:193–9.

21. Loepke AW, Priestley MA, Schultz SE, McCann J, Golden J, Kurth CD. Desflurane improves neurologic outcome after low-flow cardiopulmonary bypass in newborn pigs. *Anesthesiology.* 2002;97:1521–7.

22. Kodama M, Satoh Y, Otsubo Y, Araki Y, Yonamine R, Masui K, Kazama T. Neonatal desflurane exposure induces more robust neuroapoptosis than do isoflurane and sevoflurane and impairs working memory. *Anesthesiology.* 2011;**115**(5):979–91.

23. Istaphanous GK, Howard J, Nan X, Hughes EA, McCann JC, McAuliffe JJ, et al. Comparison of the neuroapoptotic properties of equipotent anesthetic concentrations of desflurane, isoflurane, or sevoflurane in neonatal mice. *Anesthesiology.* 2011;**114**:578–87.

24. Davis PJ, Bosenberg A, Davidson A. Pharmacology of pediatric anesthesia. In: Davis PJ, Cladis FP, Motoyama EK, eds. *Smith's Anesthesia for Infants and Children*, 8th ed. Philadelphia: Elsevier Mosby; 2011:179–261.

25. Bithal PK. Anaesthetic considerations for evoked potentials monitoring. *J Neuroanaesthesiol Crit Care.* 2014;**1**:2–12.

26. Bramwell KJ, Haizlip J, Pribble C, VanDerHeyden TC, Witte M. The effect of etomidate on intracranial pressure and systemic blood pressure in pediatric patients with severe traumatic brain injury. *Pediatr Emerg Care.* 2006;**22**:90–3.

27. Cotten JF, Forman SA, Laha JK, Cuny GD, Husain SS, Miller KW, et al. Carboetomidate: a pyrrole analog of etomidate designed not to suppress adrenocortical function. *Anesthesiology.* 2010;**112**:637–44.

28. Ilvento L, Rosati A, Marini C, L'Erario M, Mirabile L, Guerrini R. Ketamine in refractory convulsive status epilepticus in children avoids endotracheal intubation. *Epilepsy Behav.* 2015;**49**:343–6.

29. Albanèse J, Arnaud S, Rey M, Thomachot L, Alliez B, Martin C. Ketamine decreases intracranial pressure and electroencephalographic activity in traumatic brain injury patients during propofol sedation. *Anesthesiology.* 1997;**87**:1328–34.

30. Zeiler FA, Teitelbaum J, West M, Gillman LM. The ketamine effect on ICP in traumatic brain injury. *Neurocrit Care.* 2014;**21**:163–73.

31. Zeiler FA, Sader N, Gillman LM, Teitelbaum J, West M, Kazina CJ. The cerebrovascular response to ketamine: a systematic review of the animal and human literature. *J Neurosurg Anesthesiol.* 2016;**28**: 123–40.

32. Abend NS, Loddenkemper T. Management of pediatric status epilepticus. *Curr Treat Options Neurol.* 2014;**16**:301.

33. Welch TP, Wallendorf MJ, Kharasch ED, Leonard JR, Doctor A, Pineda JA. Fentanyl and midazolam are ineffective in reducing episodic intracranial hypertension in severe pediatric traumatic brain injury. *Crit Care Med.* 2016;**44**:809–18.

34. Mahmoud M, Mason KP. Dexmedetomidine: review, update, and future considerations of paediatric perioperative and periprocedural applications and limitations. *Br J Anaesth.* 2015;**115**(2):171–82.

35. Zornow MH, Fleischer JE, Scheller MS, Nakakimura K, Drummond JC. Dexmedetomidine, an alpha 2-adrenergic agonist, decreases cerebral blood flow in the isoflurane-anesthetized dog. *Anesth Analg.* 1990;**70**:624–30.

36. Drummond JC, Dao AV, Roth DM, Cheng CR, Atwater BI, Minokadeh A, et al. Effect of dexmedetomidine on cerebral blood flow velocity, cerebral metabolic rate, and carbon dioxide response in normal humans. *Anesthesiology.* 2008;**108**:225–32.

37. Schoeler M, Loetscher PD, Rossaint R, Fahlenkamp AV, Eberhardt G, Rex S, et al. Dexmedetomidine is neuroprotective in an in vitro model for traumatic brain injury. *BMC Neurol.* 2012;**12**:20.

38. Gupta N, Rath GP, Prabhakar H, Dash HH. Effect of intraoperative dexmedetomidine on postoperative recovery profile of children undergoing surgery for spinal dysraphism. *J Neurosurg Anesthesiol*. 2013;**25**: 271–8.

39. Cooperman LH, Strobel GE Jr., Kennell EM. Massive hyperkalemia after administration of succinylcholine. *Anesthesiology*. 1970;**32**:161–4.

40. Soriano SG, Martyn JA. Antiepileptic-induced resistance to neuromuscular blockers: mechanisms and clinical significance. *Clin Pharmacokinet*. 2004;**43**(2):71–8.

41. McCann ME, Schouten AN, Dobija N, Munoz C, Stephenson L, Poussaint TY, et al. Infantile postoperative encephalopathy: perioperative factors as a cause for concern. *Pediatrics*. 2014;**133**:e751–7.

Blood Sparing Techniques

Susan M. Goobie and David Faraoni

Introduction

Despite advances made in surgical techniques, infants and children undergoing neurosurgical procedures remain at increased risk for perioperative bleeding and frequently require blood product transfusions. Among the surgeries performed, hemispherectomies, craniotomies, and cranioplasties are associated with the highest blood product transfusion rates.[1,2] Multimodal and multidisciplinary bleeding management approaches have been developed over the past decade and aim to maintain hemodynamic stability, preserve oxygen carrying capacity, and define optimal transfusion strategies based on both surgical and patients' characteristics. Prevention, detection, and goal-oriented treatment of hyperfibrinolysis and coagulopathy play a central role and are imperative in improving outcome. In this chapter, we review the background and the step-by-step approach for the prevention and management of significant blood loss in infants and children undergoing neurosurgical procedures.

Scope of Neurosurgical Bleeding

Among the surgical procedures regularly performed in children, hemispherectomies, tumor resection, traumatic subdural/epidural hematoma decompression, resection of cerebral aneurysms, and arteriovenous malformations present the highest risk for significant blood loss, with high exposure rates to allogeneic blood products. Highly vascular neoplasms, such as meningiomas or glomus tumors, can be associated with substantial blood loss. Tumor involvement and extension into cranial sinuses and veins increase the likelihood of massive blood loss. In children undergoing craniotomy for brain tumor resection, age <4 years, surgery duration >270 minutes, and preoperative hemoglobin <12.2 g/dL have been defined as important predictors for massive bleeding and blood products transfusion.[3] Despite improvements in surgical techniques such as functional vs. anatomical hemispherectomy, blood loss

for hemispherectomies can exceed more than one blood volume.[4,5] Cranial vault remodeling for craniosynostosis repair is associated with substantial bleeding, with blood losses varying between 0.5 to 4 blood volumes.[6] In this specific population, age <18 months, body weight <10 kg, American Society of Anesthesiologists (ASA) physical status classification ≥ 3, craniofacial syndromes, pansynostosis, operating time > 5 hours, redo operations, and the presence of high intracranial pressure have been shown to significantly increase the bleeding risk.[7]

Etiology of Hemostatic Derangement during Surgery in the Bleeding Child

Hemostatic changes observed during pediatric neurosurgery may be caused by a variety of factors. In children less than 1 year old, the potential immaturity of the hemostatic/coagulation system can increase perioperative bleeding. Indeed, some pivotal clotting factors are either not effectively produced or not fully active, minimizing the abilities of natural clotting and, therefore, increasing perioperative bleeding.[8] For example, levels of coagulation factors II, VII, XIII are reduced to about 50% of normal adult values at birth.[9] Neonatal platelet levels are similar to normal adult values at birth, but platelet function is decreased. In addition, other factors, like preexisting coagulation disorders (e.g., acquired or congenital), intraoperative activation of fibrinolysis, tissue factor activation through large surfaces of tissue injury, activation of coagulation and consumption of coagulation factors (e.g., fibrinogen), and the presence of surgical bleeding may lead to a significant amount of blood loss that further activates coagulopathy through the increased loss of coagulation factors and the development of a dilutional coagulopathy.

Neurosurgical patients may have a hypercoaguable state perioperatively.[10] However, during major neurosurgery, the coagulation and fibrinolytic systems are activated and the delicate balance between clot formation and clot lysis can be disrupted, increasing clot instability and bleeding tendency. Tissue injury and destruction of the blood-brain barrier can lead to vascular liberation of tissue activators (tissue plasminogen activator, tissue thromboplastin, urokinase, and kallikrein) that elicit the conversion of plasminogen into plasmin, an important trigger of the fibrinolytic activation.[11] When activated, the fibrinolysis decreases clot stability and increases bleeding tendency, by increasing consumption of fibrinogen and coagulation factors. In addition, plasmin induces many other responses that contribute to coagulopathy and bleeding, including activation of thrombin generation, platelets, and the inflammatory response. Together, this cascade can place the child into a vicious cycle of deteriorating hemostasis[12] (Figure 5.1).

When the child starts bleeding, the administration of crystalloids and/or colloids may lead to a dilutional coagulopathy, defined as the loss and consumption of coagulation factors and the dilution-dependent reduction of these factors in circulating blood. Its severity depends on the degree of blood loss and the concomitant amount and type of fluids administered.[13] Acquired fibrinogen deficiency may be the leading determinant in the development of perioperative dilutional coagulopathy; fibrinogen being the first coagulation factor that reaches a critically low value during massive blood loss,[14] while platelet count will reach a plateau when 50% of the circulating blood is lost due to the mobilization of the platelets pooled in the body.[15] It is also important to keep in mind that extremely severe degrees of hemodilution (e.g., up to 95%) are required before the effect of other clotting factors will be affected, and thrombin generation will be abolished.[16]

Last but not least, the hemostatic potential might be further deteriorated by hypothermia, acidosis, and hypocalcemia.

Scope and Associated Morbidity and Mortality of Transfusion

In a bleeding child, the transfusion of blood products may be life-saving and crucial in maintaining hemodynamic stability, preserving oxygen delivery to vital tissues and organs, and treating coagulopathy. Given that the most common identifiable cause of anesthesia-related cardiac arrest in children is hypovolemia due to blood loss, timely and appropriate management of blood loss in the bleeding child is imperative.[17] However, inappropriate transfusion of blood products may also be associated with nonnegligible complications. Despite improvements in hemovigilance and the significant reduction in the risk of transfusion-related infections, the reported incidence of noninfectious transfusion-associated complications has increased in children.[18] The Serious Hazards of Transfusion (SHOT) report states an incidence of 13 adverse events per 100,000 units of red blood cells transfused in adults, while the incidence is 18:100,000 in patients <18 years old and 37:100,000 in children <1 year.[19] Furthermore, there is strong evidence that transfusion-related side effects are associated with increased morbidity and mortality in children, with two cases of death reported every 100,000 blood products transfused.[20,21] Transfusion-related acute lung injury (TRALI), transfusion-related acute circulatory overload (TACO), and hemolytic transfusion reactions

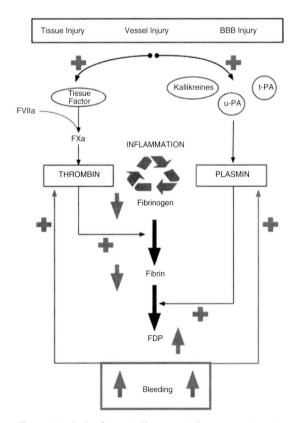

Figure 5.1. Cycle of potential hemostatic derangement in major pediatric surgery. BBB = blood-brain barrier; t-PA = tissue plasminogen activator; u-PA = urinary plasminogen activator (urokinase); FDP = fibrin degradation products.

are the main culprits, with mortality rates as high as 15–30%. Other risks include transfusion-transmitted infection and transfusion-related immunomodulation (TRIM), in addition to the risk of transfusion errors, which remains a major issue. Massive blood transfusion in pediatric trauma, surgery, and critical care has been identified as an independent predictor of multiple organ failure, systemic inflammatory response syndrome, increased infection, and increased mortality.[22,23] Furthermore, transfusion volume strongly correlates with an increased morbidity and mortality.[24] As a consequence, to avoid excessive and inappropriate transfusion, all efforts should be made to define preventative measures and ensure early recognition and appropriate, timely treatment of major blood loss. Before each transfusion, a careful assessment of the balance between the risk of non-transfusion, the risk associated with blood product administration, and the effectiveness of the transfusion should be recommended.

Patient Blood Management

Patient blood management (PBM) is the timely application of evidence-based medical concepts designed to optimize hemoglobin concentration, maintain hemostasis, and minimize blood loss through the development of multimodal and multidisciplinary (transfusion medicine specialists, surgeons, anesthesiologists, hematologists, and critical care specialists) management strategies.[25] Multimodal preventive strategies are emphasized to identify, evaluate, and manage anemia, to reduce iatrogenic blood losses, and to optimize hemostasis, utilizing pharmacological modalities and electronic ordering decision guidelines for appropriate blood product administration.[26]

PBM is recognized by the World Health Organization as a means to "promote the availability of transfusion alternatives."[27] To achieve these goals, European and North American health care institutions and accreditation and regulatory agencies have focused on blood management to improve clinical outcomes and patient safety. The United States Joint Commission developed PBM performance measures.[28] Following the guidelines published by the European Society of Anaesthesiology,[29] the American Society of Anesthesiologists Task Force on Perioperative Blood Management recently published updated guidelines that incorporate PBM initiatives.[30] The American Association of Blood Banks and the Society for the

Advancement of Blood Management also have well-established guidelines for PBM.[31] PBM programs reduce the need for allogeneic blood transfusions, reduce health care costs, and decrease morbidity and mortality.[32,33]

Blood Conservations Techniques

Preoperative

Even though the effectiveness of routine anemia screening and the implementation of specific preventive measures for children without anemia-related signs or symptoms has not been demonstrated,[34] high-risk neurosurgical children would benefit from the preoperative detection and treatment of anemia. This would allow for a preoperative optimization of the hemoglobin level, through the administration of oral or intravenous iron, sometimes in combination with recombinant human erythropoietin. Anemia is defined as a hemoglobin concentration less that the 5th percentile for the patient's age.[35] At least 25% of preschool-age children in industrialized countries are anemic,[36] with a global prevalence in children being 42.6%. The incidence of anemia in hospitalized children has not been reported, but up to 37% of neonates in US hospitals are anemic.[37,38] Severe anemia has a prevalence of 0.9 to 1.5% and is associated with substantially worse mortality and cognitive and functional outcomes. The common etiologies of preoperative anemia in children are nutritional, iron deficiency anemia, and iatrogenic blood loss (due to frequent in-hospital blood draws). Preoperative anemia is associated with increased mortality,[39] and has been shown to be an independent risk factor for postoperative mortality in neonates[40] (Figure 5.2) and children.[41]

Early detection and treatment of preoperative anemia include enteral or intravenous iron therapy. The dose of iron should be calculated based on the iron daily intake, and varies between 3 to 6 mg/kg/day divided in 3 doses. The maximal dose should not exceed 150 to 300 mg per day. Erythropoiesis stimulating agents (ESAs), such as recombinant human erythropoietin, increase the hemoglobin preoperatively, and may be a useful adjuvant in certain situations such as children at higher risk of bleeding and blood product transfusion requirement (e.g., weight < 10 kg, or a syndromic patient with comorbidities). ESA clinical protocols of epoetin alfa 600 IU kg/week subcutaneously for 3–4 weeks in divided doses, with iron, vitamin B12, vitamin E, and folic acid oral supplementation, have been described.[42] However, the

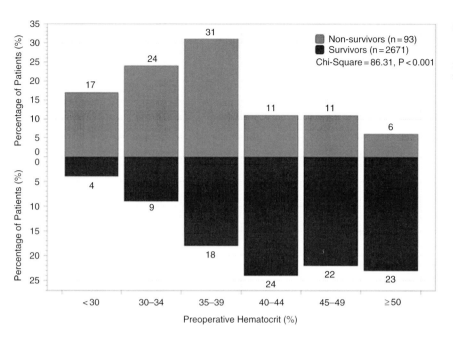

Figure 5.2. Distribution of preoperative hematocrit for neonates undergoing noncardiac surgery in US hospitals for survivors and nonsurvivors.

risk-benefit ratio (including risks of blood transfusion vs. risks of ESA) needs to be taken into account, since no large randomized studies have assessed the safety and efficacy of ESAs in the pediatric neurosurgical population. ESAs may cause rare complications such as red blood cell aplasia, infections, seizures, possible malignancy, hypertension, and venous thrombosis, which have led to its restricted use and a Food and Drug Administration (FDA)-mandated black box warning. Transfusion of blood may be a therapeutic modality to consider, but may also be associated with some important risks. Therefore, alternative strategies should be first and foremost utilized. The frequency and volume of blood draws and invasive procedures should be limited. Reducing blood draws directly correlates with reduced transfusion.

Careful preoperative preparation and optimization such as preoperative tumor vessel or arteriovenous malformation embolization or neoadjuvant chemotherapy, when appropriate, are important preemptive strategies.[43] Choosing an endoscopic approach, when feasible, is less invasive than an open operation. Surgical approach planning can be supplemented with preoperative imaging and 3D models of vessels and structures to plan appropriate, less invasive surgical options. A surgical navigation system can also be used to interface with magnetic resonance imaging (MRI) and computed tomography (CT) scans for preoperative planning.

Preoperative autologous blood donation may be offered in an older child. Most programs have a minimum weight of 20 kg, with a usual donation volume between 6 and 10 mL/kg. Disadvantages with this process include issues with rendering the patient anemic preoperatively, incomplete donations, wastage, clerical error, and blood storage issues. This technique is associated with substantial risks and costs, and therefore its routine use is not recommended, and should be limited to very specific conditions (e.g., alloantibodies).[44]

Intraoperative

During the intraoperative period, a number of options should be used, alone or in combination, to decrease the bleeding risk and the need for blood products transfusion.

Surgical techniques that can help control bleeding include the use of an intraoperative navigation system to localize and define vessels and lesions, minimally invasive surgery or endoscopic surgery, and the use of topical hemostatic agents. Surgical skills should be implemented to maintain meticulous hemostasis and control major vessels. Techniques to decrease bleeding in the surgical field include electric cautery, clips, careful dissection, and proper patient positioning to avoid venous congestion. Infiltration of a local vasoconstrictor and utilizing topical hemostatic agents, such as Gelfoam®, Floseal®, Fibrin Glue®, and

Surgicel®, are other adjuncts to minimize local bleeding; however randomized trials to prove efficacy in this area are lacking.[45]

Intraoperative blood salvage is another option that involves collecting autologous blood from the surgical site to be processed and given back to the patient during the surgery. Recently developed devices have a capacity as low as 30 mL, and are effective in reducing allogeneic blood transfusion in patients weighing as low as 10 kg.[46] The use of cell salvage is controversial in cancer surgery due to the potential risk of dissemination of tumor cells through the reinfusion of cell salvaged blood. However, recent studies have suggested that cell salvage can be used safely in cancer surgery[47] by utilizing white blood cell depletion filters and irradiating (50 Gy) cell salvage concentrate to minimize risks of tumor cell transfer. Contraindications include the use of agents that would result in red blood cell lysis (sterile water, alcohol, hydrogen peroxide), clotting agents (Surgicel and Gelfoam), contaminants (urine, bone, infection), and irrigating solutions (Betadine).[48]

Acute normovolemic hemodilution (ANH) and hypervolemic hemodilution (HH) are additional strategies. ANH involves removal of the patient's blood prior to surgery after induction of anesthesia and replacement with crystalloid or colloid to maintain normovolemia. It may be useful in older children and those who are difficult to cross match due to multiple antibodies. In younger patients this may not be feasible due to hemodynamic instability and anemia, and HH may be an option. HH involves initially hemodiluting the patient's blood to an acceptable Hct (usually about 25%) with approximately 15 mL/kg of colloid without blood removal and then subsequent fluid restriction during the case. HH is a technique that is useful when the starting Hct is >40% (as with ESA treatment preoperatively).

Anesthetized children are particularly prone to becoming hypothermic. Hypothermia, in combination with acidosis, inevitably leads to an impaired coagulation process and may worsen bleeding. Thus, forced-air warming should be rigorously used and temperature measured continuously.

Monitoring of Coagulopathy and Point of Care

Standard coagulation has been considered as the "gold standard" for the diagnosis of congenital and acquired coagulopathies, and to guide the administration of anticoagulation both in adults and children. Activated partial thromboplastin time (PTT), international normalized ratio (INR), and prothrombin time (PT) remain widely used to assess coagulation status pre-, intra-, and postoperatively. In addition, the standard Clauss method is also used to measure the plasmatic fibrinogen concentration. Unfortunately, those tests were not designed to monitor perioperative coagulopathy or to guide the administration of hemostatic agents in bleeding situations. As it takes 30–45 minutes to obtain the results from standard coagulation assays, limited information is provided by these tests in the context of acute bleeding.[49] In addition, standard laboratory tests are performed on platelet poor plasma (PPP) and do not allow for a global assessment of coagulation, giving no information about clot firmness and clot lysis.

Over the past decade thromboelastography (TEG®) and thromboelastometry (ROTEM®) have become more popular for the assessment of coagulation and to guide the administration of blood products in bleeding patients. With the thromboelastometry method, different assays are available and allow for assessment of the intrinsic pathway (INTEM), the extrinsic pathway (EXTEM), and the fibrinogen function (FIBTEM) (Figure 5.3). Thromboelastography also allows for the assessment of the intrinsic activation and the fibrinogen function. More recently, other tests have been developed to assess platelet function. Among the large number of parameters, viscoelastic assays measure clot initiation (e.g., clotting time), clot firmness (e.g., clot amplitude measured after 5, 10, 20, 30 minutes as well as the maximal amplitude), and clot stability (e.g., percentage of lysis after 30 or 60 minutes). This approach allows for a rapid assessment of the coagulopathy, and a recent study suggested that early values of clot amplitudes measured as soon as 5, 10, or 15 minutes after clotting time could be used to predict maximum clot firmness in all ROTEM® tests.[50]

Viscoelastic assays are now integrated in transfusion algorithms, and their use is recommended in all European and American guidelines. In children undergoing neurosurgery, both thromboelastography[51] and thromboelastometry[52] have been used successfully. A significant decrease in plasma and platelet transfusions after the implementation of a transfusion algorithm based on thromboelastometry and the use of factor concentrates (e.g., fibrinogen concentrate and concentrate of FXIII) have recently been reported.[53]

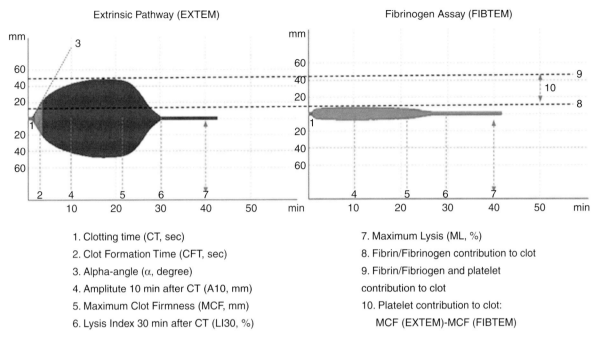

Figure 5.3. Thromboelastometry (ROTEM) tracings. EXTEM (screening test for extrinsic hemostatic system) and FIBTEM (fibrinogen assay) are shown.

1. Clotting time (CT, sec)
2. Clot Formation Time (CFT, sec)
3. Alpha-angle (α, degree)
4. Amplitute 10 min after CT (A10, mm)
5. Maximum Clot Firmness (MCF, mm)
6. Lysis Index 30 min after CT (LI30, %)

7. Maximum Lysis (ML, %)
8. Fibrin/Fibrinogen contribution to clot
9. Fibrin/Fibriogen and platelet
contribution to clot
10. Platelet contribution to clot:
MCF (EXTEM)-MCF (FIBTEM)

Antifibrinolytics

Antifibrinolytic drugs include the lysine analogs that competitively inhibit the activation of plasminogen to plasmin, tranexamic acid (TXA) and epsilon aminocaproic acid (EACA). TXA is the most common antifibrinolytic agent used since EACA is not available in many countries (such as Canada, New Zealand, and most of Europe). There is strong evidence that the implementation of a PBM strategy involving intraoperative prophylactic administration of TXA (and weaker evidence for EACA) is useful for decreasing blood loss and transfusion requirement in children undergoing major surgery[12] including craniofacial surgery.[54,55] TXA has been used successfully in high-risk pediatric neurosurgical tumor surgery.[56] Even though different dose schemes have been described, recent pharmacokinetic data[57] and pharmacodynamic data[58] support the use of lower doses. Based on recent data, a TXA dose of 10 mg/kg LD followed by a continuous infusion of 5 mg/kg/hr is recommended[57] (Figure 5.4). Regarding EACA, a loading dose of 100 mg/kg followed by a continuous infusion of 40 mg/kg/hr is recommended in infants undergoing craniofacial surgery.[59] A retrospective study supports the efficacy of EACA craniofacial surgery, but a well-designed prospective trial is yet to be done.[60]

TXA and EACA have side effects such as seizures; the incidence is low and likely dose related. Antifibrinolytics should be considered if massive blood loss is anticipated such as in hemispherectomy surgery. TXA has been used successfully in choroid plexus papilloma resection surgery, a highly vascular tumor of infancy, as part of a multimodal blood conservation strategy.[56] There may be a role for TXA in treating subarachnoid hemorrhage in the prevention of rebleeding and improvement in neurological outcome, and an ongoing trial may answer this question.[61,62] Investigating further the efficacy, safety, appropriate dosing scheme, and pharmacokinetic profile of antifibrinolytics in children having neurosurgical procedures with a high potential for bleeding will have a positive impact on patient care.

Fluid Management

The goal of intraoperative fluid management should be to maintain normovolemia while avoiding hypervolemia, to minimize swelling, edema, and hemodilution. Recent studies have suggested that an

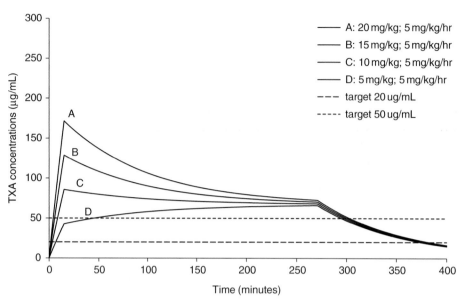

Figure 5.4. Tranexamic acid plasma concentration curve over time in pediatric craniofacial surgery. Dosage recommendations shown (A–D) for target tranexamic acid plasma levels 20 µg/mL and 50 µg/mL. Recommended dose of 10 mg/kg loading dose and 5 mg/kg/hr infusion for the duration of the surgery (5 hours on average).

intraoperative positive fluid balance may increase the need for transfusion and the incidence of postoperative fluid overload, both shown to significantly affect patients' outcomes.[63–65] Even though most of these studies were performed in children undergoing cardiac surgery, fluid overload should be avoided in children undergoing neurosurgery, and a careful monitoring of fluid administration should be recommended. Normal saline is commonly used as maintenance in intracranial neurosurgical procedures as it is mildly hyperosmolar (308 mOsm) and therefore may minimize brain edema.[66] However, if given in large volumes (> 60 mL/kg), it may lead to hyperchloremic metabolic acidosis.[67] Ringers lactate (273 mOsm) and PlasmaLyte (294 mOsm) are preferred especially when used in extracranial cases as they are associated with less severe acidosis. While some data suggested that colloid administration is associated with better hemodynamic effect with a less positive balance,[68] most of the studies were performed in children undergoing cardiac surgery and critically ill patients, and no randomized controlled trial has reported the superiority of colloids over crystalloids for perioperative fluid management in children undergoing neurosurgical procedures.[29] Certainly in the scenario of massive blood loss, colloids may have the advantage over crystalloids to better replace the volume lost and better restore normovolemia, preventing and treating hypotension together with other adjuncts such as vasopressors and blood product transfusion. Notably, in patients with a disrupted blood-brain barrier, caution regarding the liberal use of colloids should be mentioned, as the SAFE (Saline versus Albumin Fluid Evaluation) trial showed that in adult intensive care unit (ICU) patients, colloid administration was associated with a higher mortality in the head trauma subgroup.[69]

Transfusion of Red Blood Cells

While the international blood transfusion guidelines recommend against a single transfusion trigger, maintenance of a hemoglobin (Hb) level >8 g/dL is an accepted standard intraoperatively in an actively bleeding child,[29,30] while in stable critically ill or anesthetized children, a threshold of 7 g/dL is sufficient.[70] This trigger is supported by recent trials reporting no difference in morbidity and mortality when a restrictive transfusion strategy was compared with a more liberal one in critically ill children.[71,72] Caution should be mentioned regarding neonates as the optimum transfusion Hb trigger has not been determined by evidence-based prospective trials and a higher target may be necessary.[73]

Preoperative calculation of the circulating blood volume could help clinicians to estimate the importance of the blood loss, and help guide the administration of fluids and blood products. The blood volume of a preterm infant is 90–100 mL/kg, while the blood volume of a term neonate is 80–90 mL/kg. Above 3 months and until 1 year of age the blood volume will vary between 70 and 80 mL/kg, and will be considered as being 70 mL/kg in children older than 1 year. In addition to the estimation of the child's blood volume, the maximum allowable blood loss (MABL) is usually calculated using the circulating blood volume (CBV), the initial hematocrit or hemoglobin, and the minimum acceptable value:

MABL = CBV × (initial hematocrit – minimum acceptable hematocrit) / initial hematocrit.

This approach allows for the determination of the minimum hematocrit or hemoglobin tolerable for each patient and should be based on the child's comorbidities, ability to maintain adequate cardiac output and oxygen delivery, metabolic needs, and tolerance to anemia. In addition to the MABL, the CBV can also be used to estimate the volume of allogeneic red blood cell needed to reach a certain hematocrit or hemoglobin level.

RBC needed = (targeted hematocrit – current hematocrit) × CBV / hematocrit of the packed red blood cell.

Transfusion volume should be limited to the volume required to achieve a certain target and to correct intraoperative acute anemia. Overtransfusion should be avoided as adverse events are directly related to the volume administered, with higher incidences of complications reported following the administration of 40 mL/kg or more.[74] As a rule of thumb, the required transfusion volume in children could also be calculated as follows: bodyweight (kg) × desired increment in Hb (g/dL) × 5. The goal is to restore/maintain tissue oxygenation to vital organs and tissues and to consider the clinical status of the patient.

Transfusion of Platelets

In children undergoing neurosurgery, a preoperative platelet count varying from >50,000 to 100,000 cells/μL is suggested based on the bleeding risk, the type of procedure, and the patient's comorbidities. In case of active bleeding, platelet transfusion is recommended to maintain a minimal platelet count above 80,000 cells/μL. Platelet count can be expected to rise by approximately 50,000 cells/μL after transfusion of 5–10 mL/kg of an apheresis platelet concentrate. The transfusion of platelet concentrate carries the highest risk of side effects of all allogeneic blood products (bacterial contamination of platelet components is the second most common cause of transfusion-related deaths) and therefore should be performed cautiously.

Transfusion of Fresh Frozen Plasma

Accepted practice guidelines suggest replacing coagulation factor deficiency with fresh frozen plasma (FFP) when there is ongoing clinical microvascular bleeding and the PT >1.5 times normal, or INR > 2, or PTT >2 times normal or correction of excessive microvascular bleeding secondary to coagulation factor deficiency in patients transfused more than one blood volume (when laboratory values can't be obtained in a timely fashion) at a dose of 10–15 mL/kg.[30] However, this value may be too low, and therefore expert consensus recommends as much as 15–30 mL/kg FFP to replace coagulation factors in an actively bleeding child. Recent European guidelines highlight that while FFP transfusion is recommended to treat severe bleeding by several guidelines, high-quality evidence is lacking regarding the indication and dosing.[29] Certainly, severe risks have been reported including the noninfectious serious hazards of transfusion: TRALI, TACO, TRIM, and multiple organ failure.

The 2010 American Association of Blood Banks (AABB) Evidence-Based Practice Guidelines for plasma transfusion state, "We cannot recommend for or against transfusion of plasma for patients undergoing surgery in the absence of massive transfusion (quality of evidence = very low)." The AABB recommends that plasma be transfused to trauma patients requiring massive transfusion (quality of evidence = moderate). But the organization "cannot recommend for or against transfusion of plasma at a plasma: RBC ratio of 1:3 or more in trauma patients during massive transfusion (quality of evidence = low)." Furthermore these guidelines state, "It is unclear how this strategy pertains to managing massive blood loss in the pediatric surgical patient."[75]

However, prophylactic transfusion of plasma should not be recommended in a nonbleeding child and should certainly not be considered before an invasive procedure (e.g., lines removal) even in the presence of prolonged coagulation tests. Indeed, plasma remains frequently transfused in critically ill children or before a major surgery in the absence of bleeding. A recent audit of plasma transfusions in critically ill patients concluded that one-third of transfused patients were not bleeding and that plasma transfusion significantly improved the INR only in those patients with a severe derangement, indicated by an INR > 2.5.[76] Furthermore, coagulation tests are not sensitive to the increase in coagulation factors resulting from plasma transfusion. FFP is not recommended for volume expansion.

Cryoprecipitate or Fibrinogen Concentrate

Acquired fibrinogen deficiency is defined as fibrinogen below 150–200 mg/dL or maximum clot firmness (MCF) in the ROTEM® FIBTEM assay < 8 mm. Treatment, if clinically necessary, consists traditionally of transfusion of FFP and cryoprecipitate or administration of fibrinogen concentrate. Although frequently used, the recommended dosages for FFP of 10–15 mL/kg may not be adequate to achieve a clinically meaningful improvement in fibrinogen deficiency, and expert consensus recommends up to 30 mL/kg. The potential for volume overload and increasing noninfectious adverse effects such as TRALI and TACO may preclude increased dosing. Cryoprecipitate contains higher, but unpredictable, concentrations of fibrinogen as compared to FFP. This product was withdrawn from most European countries (while still used in North America) because of the risk of immunologic reactions and potential transmission of infectious agents. Cryoprecipitate (5 mL/kg) or fibrinogen concentrate (30–50 mg/kg) is recommended to increase plasma fibrinogen concentrations above trigger values of 150–200 g/dL or FIBTEM MCF > 7 mm in bleeding children.[29]

Factor Concentrates

Over the last couple of years, the use of concentrates of hemostatic factors has become popular in some European countries. Prothrombin complex concentrates (PCCs) contain the vitamin K-dependent clotting factors II, VII, IX, and X and are marketed as 3 or 4 factor-PCC formulations depending on the concentrations of factor VII. They are approved in Europe, Canada, and Australia for replacement of inherited and acquired coagulation factor deficiencies. PCCs are approved by the US Food and Drug Administration for replacement of factor IX (hemophilia B) and for the reversal of vitamin K antagonists in the setting of coagulopathy or bleeding. Even though there is a growing experience with off-label use of PCCs (25–50 Ui/kg) to treat bleeding in patients undergoing cardiac surgery or in traumatized patients,[77] no evidence supports the use of PCCs in children undergoing neurosurgery. Because of the powerful increase in thrombin generation associated with the administration of PCCs, they may be associated with an increased incidence of postoperative thromboembolic complications, and a careful monitoring and prevention of thrombotic complication should be recommended. Further studies are needed to better evaluate the safety and efficacy of PCCs before they can be recommended as part of perioperative coagulation treatment algorithms for refractory bleeding in children undergoing neurosurgical procedures.

Recombinant activated factor VII has also been used to treat massive bleeding in adults and children. However, the administration of this agent has been associated with a significant increase in the incidence of arterial and venous thrombosis[78] and should not be part of the bleeding management in children undergoing neurosurgery.

Massive Transfusion Protocol

The goal of a massive transfusion protocol (MTP) is to avoid coagulopathy as a consequence of platelet and clotting factor depletion secondary to transfusion restricted to packed red blood cells (PRBC). For the treatment of massive hemorrhage in adult trauma patients, early and aggressive transfusion of FFP in a 1:1 ratio with PRBC may improve survival. Such MTPs, using fixed ratios of blood products (RBC:FFP: platelets in a ratio of 1:1:1) may improve outcome in coagulopathic military and civilian adult trauma patients, but there is a paucity of data on the efficacy of MTP for pediatric trauma patients, whose mechanism of injury may differ from those in adults.[79,80] However, it is unclear how this strategy pertains to managing massive blood loss in the pediatric surgical patient.

Table 5.1 Pediatric Patient Blood Management Strategies[81]

Preoperative	Intraoperative	Postoperative
• Schedule optimal timing for procedure • Avoid unnecessary laboratory workup • Clear structured bleeding anamnesis • Early diagnosis and treatment of anemia • Stimulate erythropoiesis • Education of medical professionals in PBM goals • Implementation of PBM program	• Maximize tissue oxygen delivery • Minimize tissue oxygen consumption • Careful blood pressure management • Optimize fluid management; avoid hemodilution • Keep normothermia; avoid acidosis • Clear algorithm for bleeding management • Optimize surgical technique and consider blood sparing alternatives • Usage of topical hemostatic agents • Antifibrinolytics • Point-of-care assessment of hemostasis • Usage of cell salvage • Usage of purified coagulation factors whenever possible and when available • Restrictive transfusion practice • Transfusion of appropriate type and volume of blood products when necessary; avoid unnecessary and overtransfusion	• Optimize ventilation, cardiac output, and tissue oxygenation • Optimize fluid management; avoid hemodilution • Education of medical professional in PBM goals • Tolerate anemia if possible • Treat anemia with iron therapy • Stimulate erythropoiesis • Limit iatrogenic blood loss • Reduce amount and volume of laboratory blood draws • Clear algorithm for blood product transfusion • Avoid treatment of impaired standard laboratory tests without clinical relevance • Treat coagulopathy with vitamin K if indicated • Tolerate coagulopathy if possible • Consider antifibrinolytic treatment

Even if MTPs are feasible to perform in pediatrics, they are associated with increased blood product transfusion with no benefit in survival. The value of aggressive blood product transfusion using MTPs for the pediatric patient with massive hemorrhage requires further prospective validation.

Postoperative

Postoperatively, the avoidance of hemodilution, careful hemodynamic control, minimizing blood draws and other causes of iatrogenic blood loss, tolerating anemia and coagulopathy when not clinically significant, utilizing restrictive transfusion guidelines, and goal-directed blood product transfusion protocols should be considered.

Table 5.1 details these perioperative pediatric PBM strategies.

Conclusion

A comprehensive understanding of pathophysiology of hematologic derangements and a multimodal PBM strategy are crucial to safely managing anemia and coagulopathy associated with massive intraoperative blood loss during pediatric neurosurgery.

References

1. Keung CY, Smith KR, Savoia HF, Davidson AJ. An audit of transfusion of red blood cell units in pediatric anesthesia. *Paediatr Anaesth.* 2009;**19**(4): 320–8.

2. Vadera S, Griffith SD, Rosenbaum BP, Seicean A, Kshettry VR, Kelly ML, et al. National trends and in-hospital complication rates in more than 1600 hemispherectomies from 1988 to 2010: a nationwide inpatient sample study. *Neurosurgery.* 2015;**77**(2): 185–91; discussion 91.

3. Vassal O, Desgranges FP, Tosetti S, Burgal S, Dailler F, Javouhey E, et al. Risk factors for intraoperative allogeneic blood transfusion during craniotomy for brain tumor removal in children. *Paediatr Anaesth.* 2016;**26**(2):199–206.

4. Koh JL, Egan B, McGraw T. Pediatric epilepsy surgery: anesthetic considerations. *Anesthesiol Clin.* 2012;**30**(2):191–206.

5. Flack S, Ojemann J, Haberkern C. Cerebral hemispherectomy in infants and young children. *Paediatr Anaesth.* 2008;**18**(10):967–73.

6. White N, Marcus R, Dover S, Solanki G, Nishikawa H, Millar C, et al. Predictors of blood loss in fronto-orbital advancement and remodeling. *J Craniofac Surg.* 2009;**20**(2):378–81.

7. Goobie SM, Zurakowski D, Proctor MR, Meara JG, Meier PM, Young VJ, et al. Predictors of clinically significant postoperative events after open craniosynostosis surgery. *Anesthesiology*. 2015;**122**(5): 1021–32.

8. Guzzetta NA, Miller BE. Principles of hemostasis in children: models and maturation. *Paediatr Anaesth*. 2011;**21**(1):3–9.

9. Ignjatovic V, Ilhan A, Monagle P. Evidence for age-related differences in human fibrinogen. *Blood Coagul Fibrinolysis*. 2011;**22**(2):110–17.

10. Goobie SM, Soriano SG, Zurakowski D, McGowan FX, Rockoff MA. Hemostatic changes in pediatric neurosurgical patients as evaluated by thrombelastograph. *Anesth Analg*. 2001;**93**(4):887–92.

11. Gerlach R, Krause M, Seifert V, Goerlinger K. Hemostatic and hemorrhagic problems in neurosurgical patients. *Acta Neurochir (Wien)*. 2009;**151**(8):873–900.

12. Faraoni D, Goobie SM. The efficacy of antifibrinolytic drugs in children undergoing noncardiac surgery: a systematic review of the literature. *Anesth Analg*. 2014;**118**(3):628–36.

13. Haas T, Mauch J, Weiss M, Schmugge M. Management of dilutional coagulopathy during pediatric major surgery. *Transfus Med Hemother*. 2012;**39**(2):114–19.

14. Levy JH, Szlam F, Tanaka KA, Sniecienski RM. Fibrinogen and hemostasis: a primary hemostatic target for the management of acquired bleeding. *Anesth Analg*. 2012;**114**(2):261–74.

15. McLoughlin TM, Fontana JL, Alving B, Mongan PD, Bunger R. Profound normovolemic hemodilution: hemostatic effects in patients and in a porcine model. *Anesth Analg*. 1996;**83**(3):459–65.

16. Dunbar NM, Chandler WL. Thrombin generation in trauma patients. *Transfusion*. 2009;**49**(12):2652–60.

17. Bhananker SM, Ramamoorthy C, Geiduschek JM, Posner KL, Domino KB, Haberkern CM, et al. Anesthesia-related cardiac arrest in children: update from the Pediatric Perioperative Cardiac Arrest Registry. *Anesth Analg*. 2007;**105**(2):344–50.

18. Bolton-Maggs PH. Transfusion and hemovigilance in pediatrics. *Pediatr Clin North Am*. 2013;**60**(6): 1527–40.

19. Harrison E, Bolton P. Serious hazards of transfusion in children (SHOT). *Paediatr Anaesth*. 2011;**21**(1):10–13.

20. Lavoie J. Blood transfusion risks and alternative strategies in pediatric patients. *Paediatr Anaesth*. 2011;**21**(1):14–24.

21. Stainsby D, Jones H, Wells AW, Gibson B, Cohen H, SHOT Steering Group. Adverse outcomes of blood transfusion in children: analysis of UK reports to the serious hazards of transfusion scheme 1996–2005. *Br J Haematol*. 2008;**141**(1):73–9.

22. Demaret P, Tucci M, Karam O, Trottier H, Ducruet T, Lacroix J. Clinical outcomes associated with RBC transfusions in critically ill children: a 1-year prospective study. *Pediatr Crit Care Med*. 2015;**16**(6): 505–14.

23. Neff LP, Cannon JW, Morrison JJ, Edwards MJ, Spinella PC, Borgman MA. Clearly defining pediatric massive transfusion: cutting through the fog and friction with combat data. *J Trauma Acute Care Surg*. 2015;**78**(1):22–8; discussion 8–9.

24. Goobie SM, DiNardo JA, Faraoni D. Relationship between transfusion volume and outcomes in children undergoing non-cardiac surgery. *Transfusion*. 2016;**56**(10):2487–94.

25. Society for the Advancement of Blood Management. Patient blood management. Available at www.sabm .org.2012/.

26. Murphy MF, Goodnough LT. The scientific basis for patient blood management. *Transfus Clin Biol*. 2015;**22**(3):90–6.

27. World Health Organization. 63rd World Health Assembly. Availability, safety and quality of blood. Available at http://apps.who.int/gb/ebwha/pdf_files/ WHA63/A63_R12-en.pdf.

28. Joint Commission. Patient blood management performance measures. Available at www .jointcommission.org/patient_blood_management_ performance_measures_project/2012.

29. Kozek-Langenecker SA, Afshari A, Albaladejo P, Santullano CA, De Robertis E, Filipescu DC, et al. Management of severe perioperative bleeding: guidelines from the European Society of Anaesthesiology. *Eur J Anaesthesiol*. 2013;**30**(6):270–382.

30. American Society of Anesthesiologists Task Force on Perioperative Blood Management. Practice guidelines for perioperative blood management: an updated report by the American Society of Anesthesiologists Task Force on Perioperative Blood Management. *Anesthesiology*. 2015;**122**(2):241–75.

31. American Association of Blood Banks. Building a better patient blood management program. Identifying tools, solving problems and promoting patient safety. Available at www.aabb.org/pbm/Docu ments/AABB-PBM-Whitepaper.pdf.

32. Goodnough LT, Shander A. Patient blood management. *Anesthesiology*. 2012;**116**(6):1367–76.

33. Goobie SM, Haas T. Perioperative bleeding management in pediatric patients. *Curr Opin Anaesthesiol*. 2016;**29**(3):352–8.

34. Siu AL, US Preventive Services Task Force. Screening for iron deficiency anemia in young children: USPSTF

recommendation statement. *Pediatrics*. 2015;**136**(4): 746–52.

35. World Health Organization. Haemoglobin concentrations for the diagnosis of anaemia. 2011. Available at www.who.int/vmnis/indicators/haemoglobin/en/.

36. Stevens GA, Finucane MM, De-Regil LM, Paciorek CJ, Flaxman SR, Branca F, et al. Global, regional, and national trends in haemoglobin concentration and prevalence of total and severe anaemia in children and pregnant and non-pregnant women for 1995–2011: a systematic analysis of population-representative data. *Lancet Glob Health*. 2013;**1**(1):e16–25.

37. Janus J, Moerschel SK. Evaluation of anemia in children. *Am Fam Physician*. 2010;**81**(12):1462–71.

38. Bateman ST, Lacroix J, Boven K, Forbes P, Barton R, Thomas NJ, et al. Anemia, blood loss, and blood transfusions in North American children in the intensive care unit. *Am J Respir Crit Care Med*. 2008;**178**(1):26–33.

39. Fowler AJ, Ahmad T, Phull MK, Allard S, Gillies MA, Pearse RM. Meta-analysis of the association between preoperative anaemia and mortality after surgery. *Br J Surg*. 2015;**102**(11):1314–24.

40. Goobie SM, Zurakowski D, DiNardo JA. Preoperative anemia is an independent risk factor for postoperative mortality in neonates. *JAMA Pediatr*. 2016;**170**(9): 855–62.

41. Faraoni D, DiNardo DJ, Goobie SM. Relationship between preoperative anemia and in-hospital mortality in children undergoing non-cardiac surgery. *Anesth Analg*. 2016;**123**(6):1582–7.

42. Goodnough LT, Shander A. Update on erythropoiesis-stimulating agents. *Best Pract Res Clin Anaesthesiol*. 2013;**27**(1):121–9.

43. Schneider C, Kamaly-Asl I, Ramaswamy V, Lafay-Cousin L, Kulkarni AV, Rutka JT, et al. Neoadjuvant chemotherapy reduces blood loss during the resection of pediatric choroid plexus carcinomas. *J Neurosurg Pediatr*. 2015;**16**(2):126–33.

44. British Committee for Standards in Haematology TTF, Boulton FE, James V. Guidelines for policies on alternatives to allogeneic blood transfusion. 1. Predeposit autologous blood donation and transfusion. *Transfus Med*. 2007;**17**(5):354–65.

45. Goodnough LT, Shander A. Current status of pharmacologic therapies in patient blood management. *Anesth Analg*. 2013;**116**(1):15–34.

46. Fearon JA. Reducing allogenic blood transfusions during pediatric cranial vault surgical procedures: a prospective analysis of blood recycling. *Plast Reconstr Surg*. 2004;**113**(4):1126–30.

47. Kumar N, Chen Y, Zaw AS, Nayak D, Ahmed Q, Soong R, et al. Use of intraoperative cell-salvage for autologous blood transfusions in metastatic spine tumour surgery: a systematic review. *Lancet Oncol*. 2014;**15**(1):e33–41.

48. Waters JH. Indications and contraindications of cell salvage. *Transfusion*. 2004;**44**(12 suppl): 40S-44S.

49. Segal JB, Dzik WH. Transfusion Medicine/Hemostasis Clinical Trials Network. Paucity of studies to support that abnormal coagulation test results predict bleeding in the setting of invasive procedures: an evidence-based review.*Transfusion*. 2005;**45**(9):1413–25.

50. Perez-Ferrer A, Vicente-Sanchez J, Carceles-Baron MD, Van der Linden P, Faraoni D. Early thromboelastometry variables predict maximum clot firmness in children undergoing cardiac and non-cardiac surgery. *Br J Anaesth*. 2015;**115**(6):896–902.

51. Nguyen TT, Hill S, Austin TM, Whitney GM, Wellons JC III, Lam HV. Use of blood-sparing surgical techniques and transfusion algorithms: association with decreased blood administration in children undergoing primary open craniosynostosis repair. *J Neurosurg Pediatr*. 2015;**16**(5):556–563.

52. Luostarinen T, Silvasti-Lundell M, Medeiros T, Romani R, Hernesniemi J, Niemi T. Thromboelastometry during intraoperative transfusion of fresh frozen plasma in pediatric neurosurgery. *J Anesth*. 2012;**26**(5):770–4.

53. Haas T, Goobie S, Spielmann N, Weiss M, Schmugge M. Improvements in patient blood management for pediatric craniosynostosis surgery using a ROTEM®-assisted strategy—feasibility and costs. *Paediatr Anaesth*. 2014;**24**(7):774–80.

54. Goobie SM, Meier PM, Pereira LM, McGowan FX, Prescilla RP, Scharp LA, et al. Efficacy of tranexamic acid in pediatric craniosynostosis surgery: a double-blind, placebo-controlled trial. *Anesthesiology*. 2011;**114**(4):862–71.

55. Dadure C, Sauter M, Bringuier S, Bigorre M, Raux O, Rochette A, et al. Intraoperative tranexamic acid reduces blood transfusion in children undergoing craniosynostosis surgery: a randomized double-blind study. *Anesthesiology*. 2011;**114**(4):856–61.

56. Phi JH, Goobie SM, Hong KH, Dholakia A, Smith ER. Use of tranexamic acid in infants undergoing choroid plexus papilloma surgery: a report of two cases. *Paediatr Anaesth*. 2014;**24**(7):791–3.

57. Goobie SM, Meier PM, Sethna NF, Soriano SG, Zurakowski D, Samant S, et al. Population pharmacokinetics of tranexamic acid in paediatric patients undergoing craniosynostosis surgery. *Clin Pharmacokinet*. 2013;**52**(4):267–76.

58. Rozen L, Faraoni D, Sanchez Torres C, Willems A, Noubouossie DC, Barglazan D, et al. Effective tranexamic acid concentration for 95% inhibition of tissue-type plasminogen activator induced hyperfibrinolysis in children with congenital heart disease: a prospective, controlled, in-vitro study. *Eur J Anaesthesiol*. 2015;**32**(12):844–50.

59. Stricker PA, Zuppa AF, Fiadjoe JE, Maxwell LG, Sussman EM, Pruitt EY, et al. Population pharmacokinetics of epsilon-aminocaproic acid in infants undergoing craniofacial reconstruction surgery. *Br J Anaesth*. 2013;**110**(5):788–99.

60. Hsu G, Taylor JA, Fiadjoe JE, Vincent AM, Pruitt EY, Bartlett SP, et al. Aminocaproic acid administration is associated with reduced perioperative blood loss and transfusion in pediatric craniofacial surgery. *Acta Anaesthesiol Scand*. 2016;**60**(2):158–65.

61. Gaberel T, Magheru C, Emery E, Derlon JM. Antifibrinolytic therapy in the management of aneurismal subarachnoid hemorrhage revisited. A meta-analysis. *Acta Neurochir (Wien)*. 2012;**154**(1):1–9.

62. Germans MR, Post R, Coert BA, Rinkel GJ, Vandertop WP, Verbaan D. Ultra-early tranexamic acid after subarachnoid hemorrhage (ULTRA): study protocol for a randomized controlled trial. *Trials*. 2013;**14**:143.

63. Hazle MA, Gajarski RJ, Yu S, Donohue J, Blatt NB. Fluid overload in infants following congenital heart surgery. *Pediatr Crit Care Med*. 2013;**14**(1):44–9.

64. Hassinger AB, Wald EL, Goodman DM. Early postoperative fluid overload precedes acute kidney injury and is associated with higher morbidity in pediatric cardiac surgery patients. *Pediatr Crit Care Med*. 2014;**15**(2):131–8.

65. Seguin J, Albright B, Vertullo L, Lai P, Dancea A, Bernier PL, et al. Extent, risk factors, and outcome of fluid overload after pediatric heart surgery. *Crit Care Med*. 2014;**42**(12):2591–9.

66. Butterworth JF, Mythen MG. Should "normal" saline be our usual choice in normal surgical patients? *Anesth Analg*. 2013;**117**(2):290–1.

67. McCluskey SA, Karkouti K, Wijeysundera D, Minkovich L, Tait G, Beattie WS. Hyperchloremia after noncardiac surgery is independently associated with increased morbidity and mortality: a propensity-matched cohort study. *Anesth Analg*. 2013;**117**(2):412–21.

68. Van der Linden P, De Hert S, Mathieu N, Degroote F, Schmartz D, Zhang H, et al. Tolerance to acute isovolemic hemodilution. Effect of anesthetic depth. *Anesthesiology*. 2003;**99**(1):97–104.

69. Finfer S, Bellomo R, Boyce N, French J, Myburgh J, Norton R, et al. A comparison of albumin and saline for fluid resuscitation in the intensive care unit. *N Engl J Med*. 2004;**350**(22):2247–56.

70. Morley SL. Red blood cell transfusions in acute paediatrics. *Arch Dis Child Educ Pract Ed*. 2009;**94**(3):65–73.

71. Lacroix J, Hebert PC, Hutchison JS, Hume HA, Tucci M, Ducruet T, et al. Transfusion strategies for patients in pediatric intensive care units. *N Engl J Med*. 2007;**356**(16):1609–19.

72. Rouette J, Trottier H, Ducruet T, Beaunoyer M, Lacroix J, Tucci M, et al. Red blood cell transfusion threshold in postsurgical pediatric intensive care patients: a randomized clinical trial. *Ann Surg*. 2010;**251**(3):421–7.

73. Whyte RK. Neurodevelopmental outcome of extremely low-birth-weight infants randomly assigned to restrictive or liberal hemoglobin thresholds for blood transfusion. *Semin Perinatol*. 2012;**36**(4):290–3.

74. Goobie SM, DiNardo JA, Faraoni D. Relationship between transfusion volume and outcomes in children undergoing non-cardiac surgery. *Anesthesiology*. 2016;**56**(10):2487–94.

75. Roback JD, Caldwell S, Carson J, Davenport R, Drew MJ, Eder A, et al. Evidence-Based Practice Guidelines for plasma transfusion. *Transfusion*. 2010;**50**(6):1227–39.

76. Karam O, Demaret P, Shefler A, Leteurtre S, Spinella PC, Stanworth SJ, et al. Indications and effects of plasma transfusions in critically ill children. *Am J Respir Crit Care Med*. 2015;**191**(12):1395–402.

77. Ghadimi K, Levy JH, Welsby IJ. Prothrombin complex concentrates for bleeding in the perioperative setting. *Anesth Analg*. 2016;**122**(5):1287–300.

78. Levi M, Levy JH, Andersen HF, Truloff D. Safety of recombinant activated factor VII in randomized clinical trials. *N Engl J Med*. 2010;**363**(19):1791–800.

79. Chidester SJ, Williams N, Wang W, Groner JI. A pediatric massive transfusion protocol. *J Trauma Acute Care Surg*. 2012;**73**(5):1273–7.

80. Nosanov L, Inaba K, Okoye O, Resnick S, Upperman J, Shulman I, et al. The impact of blood product ratios in massively transfused pediatric trauma patients. *Am J Surg*. 2013;**206**(5):655–60.

81. Goobie SM, Haas T. Perioperative bleeding management in pediatric patients. *Curr Opin Anaesthesiol*. 2016;**29**(3):352–8.

Regional Anesthesia for Pediatric Neurosurgery

Ravi Shah and Santhanam Suresh

Introduction

Children who are undergoing neurosurgical procedures can benefit from regional anesthesia, which provides excellent analgesia with minimal adverse effects. Peripheral nerve blocks can blunt the surgical stress response, decrease anesthetic requirements, and minimize opioid-related side effects.

Most peripheral nerve blocks of the head and neck are simple to perform since anatomical landmarks are easily located. These blocks can facilitate a significant reduction in both analgesic requirements and the incidence of nausea, vomiting, pruritis, and respiratory depression.[1] The nerves undergoing blockade are terminal sensory branches, which can be effectively blocked with minimal volume of local anesthetic solution (Table 6.1). This decreases the likelihood of approaching toxic plasma levels, even in infants and neonates.[2]

Increased use of regional anesthesia has significantly improved the scope of pediatric pain management.[3]

Regional anesthetic techniques are often combined with general anesthesia to provide a synergistic multimodal approach to analgesia while maintaining hemodynamic stability. Suresh and Bellig reported a critically ill 700-g neonate who underwent Ommaya reservoir placement for hydrocephalus with adjunctive blockade of both the supraorbital and greater occipital nerves.[4] This approach provided good analgesia while minimizing opioid requirements. In the adult literature, blockade of the scalp innervation, which anesthetizes both the superficial and deep layers of the scalp, is considered an effective means to decrease hemodynamic responses to Mayfield head-holder application.[5] Nguyen and colleagues conducted a prospective, double-blinded, randomized controlled study to assess the role of scalp blocks in reducing postoperative pain after craniotomy.[6] They demonstrated that intraoperative scalp block decreases the severity of pain after craniotomy and that this effect is long lasting, possibly through a preemptive mechanism. Sebeo described the use of peripheral nerve blocks

Table 6.1 Head and Neck Blocks for Pediatric Neurosurgical Procedures

Nerve to Be Blocked	Neurosurgical Indications	Potential Complications
Trigeminal V1: Ophthalmic division	Frontal craniotomy Ventriculoperitoneal shunt Ommaya reservoir placement Scalp lesions	Hematoma formation Intravascular injection
Trigeminal V2: Maxillary division (infraorbital nerve)	Transsphenoidal hypophysectomy	Hematoma formation Persistent paresthesia of upper lip Damage to globe of the eye Intravascular injection
Trigeminal V3: Mandibular division (auriculotemporal nerve)	Craniotomy with temporal incisions	Hematoma formation Intravascular injection
Greater occipital nerve	Posterior fossa craniotomy Ventriculoperitoneal shunt Occipital craniotomy Occipital neuralgia	Intravascular injection Hematoma formation

of the scalp in children as a means to provide effective analgesia while maintaining stable hemodynamics.[7]

Sole regional anesthetic techniques have also been described in the pediatric neurosurgical literature. Uejima and Suresh reported three ex-premature infants who underwent successful placement of ventricular drainage devices using regional anesthesia alone.[8] The supraorbital nerve (trigeminal V1) and the zygomaticotemporal nerve (trigeminal V2) were designated as the sensory supply for the surgical operative site and blockade was performed with local anesthetic. All infants were swaddled in a blanket and were allowed to suck on a pacifier dipped in an oral glucose solution during the procedure. No patient required supplemental analgesics or sedative/hypnotic drugs. Sole regional anesthetic approaches may reduce the risk for postoperative apnea in neonates who may otherwise require postoperative ventilation after such procedures.[9] Batra and Rajeev have also described the successful use of peripheral nerve blocks as a sole anesthetic to perform burr hole drainage of a brain abscess in a medically complex child who was at an elevated risk for anesthetic complications.[10]

Safety of Head and Neck Blocks in Children

Peripheral nerve blocks of the head and neck are associated with a low incidence of adverse effects. In contrast to adult practice, most regional anesthetic techniques in children are performed under deep sedation or general anesthesia. Prospective and retrospective safety studies support this practice.[11] The Pediatric Regional Anesthesia Network (PRAN) is a multicenter collaborative effort that has facilitated the collection of detailed prospective data for research and quality improvement. Polaner and colleagues recently reported on the first three years of data registry, giving a favorable impression of the safety of current pediatric regional anesthesia practice with no reported complications or adverse events associated with head and neck blocks.[12]

Clinical Anatomy of the Head and Neck

The sensory supply of the head and neck is primarily derived from three major branches of the trigeminal nerve (cranial nerve V) along with the C2–C4 cervical roots, which supply the neck and the occipital portion of the scalp (Figure 6.1).

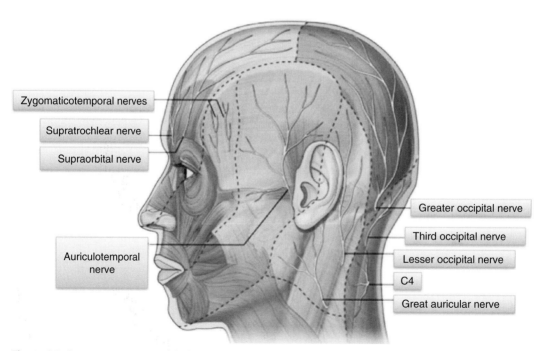

Figure 6.1. Cutaneous innervation of the head and neck.

Trigeminal Nerve

The sensory and motor roots of the trigeminal nerve arise from the ventral aspect of the base of the pons. Sensory branches are sent to the large semilunar ganglion, which gives rise to three main divisions: *V1 (ophthalmic), V2 (maxillary)*, and *V3 (mandibular)*. These three major divisions of the trigeminal nerve exit the cranium through three distinct foramina.

V1

The ophthalmic division of the trigeminal nerve provides sensory innervation to the scalp, forehead, upper eyelid, cornea of the eye, mucous membranes of the nasal cavity, the frontal sinuses, and parts of the meninges. The nerve enters the orbit through the superior orbital fissure, where it divides into three branches: (1) frontal (supraorbital n. and supratrochlear n.), (2) lacrimal, and (3) nasociliary.

V2

The mandibular nerve passes through the foramen rotundum and, after exiting the skull, courses anteriorly over the pterygopalatine fossa. The nerve enters the floor of the orbit and emerges through the infraorbital fissure as the infraorbital nerve. The infraorbital nerve carries sensory input from the lower eyelid, the upper lip, teeth, and gums, the nasal mucosa, the palate and roof of the mouth, the maxillary, ethmoid, and sphenoid sinuses, and parts of the meninges. Anatomical localization of the infraorbital nerve has gained recent attention in response to increasing indications for postoperative pain control. Bosenberg and Kimble examined 15 neonatal cadavers and applied their measurements to guiding successful blockade of the infraorbital nerve in four neonates undergoing cleft lip repair.[13] Suresh and colleagues evaluated computed tomography (CT) scans of 48 pediatric patients and demonstrated a linear correlation between age and the distance to the infraorbital foramen.[14] A mathematical formula (distance to infraorbital foramen from midline = 21 mm + 0.5 × age in years) can be utilized to locate the nerve in cases where palpation of the foramen is difficult.

V3

The mandibular nerve travels into the infratemporal fossa through the foramen ovale and divides into three major branches: (1) auriculotemporal nerve, (2) lingual nerve, and (3) inferior alveolar nerve. The auriculotemporal nerve provides sensory innervation to the external acoustic meatus and auricle of the ear,

the temporomandibular joint, and the scalp over the temple.

The terminal branches of the three trigeminal nerve divisions, the supraorbital, infraorbital, and mental nerves, exit the skull through the supraorbital, infraorbital, and mental foramina, respectively, and typically lie vertically in line with each other in the plane of the pupil.

Occipital Nerves

The posterior scalp is innervated by sensory fibers of the greater and lesser occipital nerves.

Greater Occipital Nerve

The greater occipital nerve originates from the posterior ramus of the second cervical spinal nerve (C2) and travels in a cranial direction, medial to the occipital artery, until it pierces the posterior cervical aponeurosis and provides branches medially to supply the posterior portion of the scalp (sensory) and the semispinalis capitis muscle (motor).

Lesser Occipital Nerve

The lesser occipital nerve is derived from the second (and occasionally also the third) anterior cervical ramus and traverses cephalad from the posterior edge of the sternocleidomastoid muscle. At this point, it pierces the deep fascia and travels up the scalp behind the auricle before it divides into several sensory branches.

The following section provides an overview of commonly performed regional anesthetic techniques for pediatric neurosurgical procedures. We describe the indications, landmarks and surface anatomy, technique, and potential complications of relevant head and neck blocks.

Trigeminal Nerve Blocks

Ophthalmic Nerve (V1: Supraorbital Nerve, Supratrochlear Nerve)

Indications

Indications include frontal craniotomy, ventriculoperitoneal shunt insertion/revision, Ommaya reservoir placement, scalp lesions.

Landmarks and Surface Anatomy

The ophthalmic nerve's largest branch is the frontal nerve, which divides into two terminal branches, the supraorbital and the supratrochlear nerves. These terminal branches can be blocked at the supraorbital foramen, which is located at the superior part of the orbital rim in the midline, in line with the pupil. The nerves are too superficial to visualize with ultrasound, however the foramina can be visualized with ultrasound by scanning sagitally in the medial to lateral direction. The absence of a hyperechoic bony structure indicates the position of the foramen.

Technique

After careful preparation with betadine or chlorhexidine (take caution to avoid the eyes), a 30-gauge needle is used to inject local anesthetic subcutaneously with the needle positioned toward the supraorbital notch. After careful aspiration, 0.1 mL/kg (max volume 2 mL) of 0.2% Ropivicaine with 1:200,000 epinephrine is injected (Figure 6.2). Gentle massage followed by pressure application to the injection site is provided to prevent hematoma formation. Epinephrine-containing solutions are useful to prevent excessive bleeding from the injection site. An additional block of the supratrochlear nerve is required if the field of anesthesia is to cross the midline of the forehead. This block is performed by directing the needle medially at the upper internal angle of the orbital rim.

Complications

Intravascular injection and hematoma formation are uncommon but potential complications. Persistent paresthesias are rare even if a paresthesia was elicited at the time of injection.

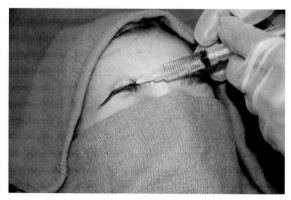

Figure 6.2. Supraorbital nerve block.

Infraorbital Nerve (V2)

Indications

Indications include transsphenoidal hypophysectomy.

Landmarks and Surface Anatomy

The infraorbital notch can be palpated along the base of the orbital rim in most children. This approach can, however, be challenging in neonates due to developing craniofacial configurations. In such situations, a small gauge needle may be used to gently probe and identify the foramen. Alternatively, the previously mentioned mathematical formula, distance from midline = 21 mm + 0.5 × age, can be utilized to estimate the location of the foramen.

Technique

The infraorbital nerve block can be performed by either an intraoral or extraoral approach. Local anesthetic solution is deposited at the level of the infraorbital foramen, where the maxillary division of the trigeminal nerve exits the skull. Advantages to the intraoral approach include (1) absence of an external needle stick and potential hematoma formation on the skin surface and (2) more adequate blockade of the maxillary division. The upper lip is everted and the mucosa is cleaned with sterile gauze. A 27-gauge needle is inserted and directed toward the infraorbital foramen. A finger is placed at the level of the infraorbital foramen to prevent the needle from advancing into the globe of the eye. After aspiration, 0.1 mL/kg of epinephrine-containing local anesthetic is injected. The extraoral approach is performed be palpating the floor of the orbital rim to identify the infraorbital foramen. A 30-gauge needle is advanced toward the foramen until bone is contacted. The needle is withdrawn 1–2 mm, aspiration is performed, and 0.5–1 mL of local anesthetic is injected.

The suprazygomatic maxillary nerve block is an advanced extraoral technique that requires deep needle insertion to perform accurate nerve blockade. The recommended insertion point is at the junction of the superior zygoma and posterior orbit. The needle is inserted perpendicularly to contact the greater wing of the sphenoid. After the bone is contacted, the needle is redirected slightly inferior and anterior in the plane of the philtrum and is advanced 3–4 cm further to enter the pterygopalatine fossa. Approximately 0.15 mL/kg of local anesthetic is injected after negative aspiration.

Nerve stimulation and ultrasound have both been reported as effective modalities to assist with block placement.[15] Sola and colleagues recently published a randomized, double-blinded study evaluating an ultrasound-guided approach to the suprazygomatic maxillary nerve block.[16] In their described technique, a linear array probe was placed in the infrazygomatic region to allow out of plane visualization of the needle tip and local anesthetic spread in the pterygopalatine fossa (Figure 6.3).

Complications

Potential complications of the infraorbital block include hematoma formation, persistent paresthesia of the upper lip, damage to the globe of the eye, and intravascular injection.

Mandibular Nerve (V3)

Indications

Indications include craniotomy with temporal incisions (auriculotemporal nerve).

Technique

The auriculotemporal nerve block is performed at the midpoint of a line drawn between the pinna and the angle of the eye. The nerve, which is located superficially, is easily blocked using subcutaneous injection through a 27-gauge needle. The needle is inserted in the medial direction immediately anterior to the superficial temporal artery (Figure 6.4).

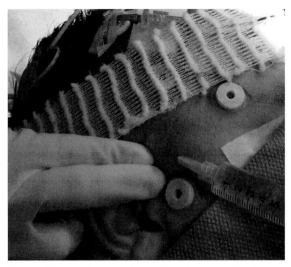

Figure 6.4. Auriculotemporal nerve block for ventriculoperitoneal shunt revision.

Complications

Hematoma formation and intravascular injection are both potential complications of the auriculotemporal nerve block.

Greater Occipital Nerve Block

Indications

Indications include posterior fossa craniotomy, VP shunt insertion or revision, occipital craniotomy, occipital neuralgia.

Landmarks and Surface Anatomy

The greater occipital nerve is typically located lateral (1–2 cm) and inferior (1–2 cm) to the external occipital protuberance. In adults, this is typically located one-third of the distance from the external occipital protuberance to the mastoid process. The nerve can also be identified by its medial location to the easily palpated occipital artery. The lesser occipital nerve is situated lateral to the greater occipital nerve along the inferior nuchal line.

Technique

Landmark-Based Approach — The occipital artery, located immediately lateral to the midline and inferior to the superior nuchal line, is identified by palpation. A 27-gauge needle is inserted subcutaneously at the midpoint of a line drawn between the mastoid process and the midline. The needle is fanned laterally and, after careful aspiration, local anesthetic (e.g., 1–2 mL

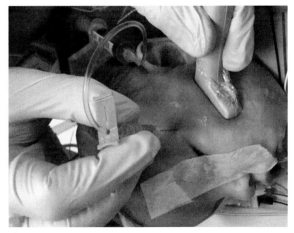

Figure 6.3. Ultrasound-guided suprazygomatic maxillary nerve block.

of 0.1–0.2% Ropivicaine with 1:200,000 epinephrine) is injected subcutaneously as the needle is withdrawn. Gentle massage of the area will promote adequate spread of local anesthetic.

Ultrasound-Guided Technique — Ultrasound-guided approaches to the occipital nerve block have also been described.[17,18] A linear probe is placed in the midline over the spinous process of the C1 vertebra and the probe is moved in the caudal direction toward the C2 vertebra, which is bifid in appearance. The probe is rotated laterally until the obliquus capitis muscle is identified. The greater occipital nerve, which is located superior to this muscle, can be blocked using an in-plane approach (Figure 6.5).

Complications

Potential complications include intravascular injection (decreased likelihood with ultrasound guidance) and local hematoma formation. Care must be taken to limit needle advancement in the anterior direction to avoid unintentional entrance into the foramen magnum. When performing the ultrasound-guided occipital nerve block at the C2 vertebra, it is important to utilize Doppler ultrasound to identify and avoid injection into the vertebral artery.

Regional anesthetic techniques have gained recent popularity since data have emerged to demonstrate their safety in children undergoing surgical procedures. Peripheral nerve blocks of the head and neck can serve as useful adjuncts to decrease anesthetic requirement, minimize opioid-related side effects, and blunt the surgical stress response. Recent publications illustrating new techniques for nerve localization combined with a thorough understanding of the

relevant anatomy may encourage more practitioners to perform these blocks in children.

References

1. Suresh S, Voronov P. Head and neck blocks in infants, children, and adolescents. *Paediatr Anaesth.* 2012;**22**(1):81–7.

2. Belvis D, Voronov P, Suresh S. Head and neck blocks in children. *Tech Reg Anesth Pain Manag.* 2007;**11**:208–14.

3. Shah RD, Suresh S. Applications of regional anaesthesia in paediatrics. *Br J Anaesth.* 2013;**111**(suppl 1):i114–24.

4. Suresh S, Bellig G. Regional anesthesia in a very low-birth-weight neonate for a neurosurgical procedure. *Reg Anesth Pain Med.* 2004;**29**(1):58–9.

5. Pinosky ML, Fishman RL, Reeves ST, et al. The effect of bupivacaine skull block on the hemodynamic response to craniotomy. *Anesth Analg.* 1996;**83**(6):1256–61.

6. Nguyen A, Girard F, Boudreault D, et al. Scalp nerve blocks decrease the severity of pain after craniotomy. *Anesth Analg.* 2001;**93**(5):1272–6.

7. Sebeo JOI. The use of "scalp block" in pediatric patients. *Open J Anesthesiol.* 2012; 270–3.

8. Uejima T, Suresh S. Ommaya and McComb reservoir placement in infants: can this be done with regional anesthesia? *Paediatr Anaesth.* 2008;**18**(9):909–11.

9. Liu LM, Cote CJ, Goudsouzian NG, et al. Life-threatening apnea in infants recovering from anesthesia. *Anesthesiology.* 1983;**59**(6):506–10.

10. Batra YK, Rajeev S. Regional anesthesia in a child with pulmonary arteriovenous malformation for a neurosurgical procedure. *Paediatr Anaesth.* 2007;**17**(9):910–12.

11. Giaufre E, Dalens B, Gombert A. Epidemiology and morbidity of regional anesthesia in children: a one-year prospective survey of the French-Language Society of Pediatric Anesthesiologists. *Anesth Analg.* 1996;**83**(5):904–12.

12. Polaner DM, Taenzer AH, Walker BJ, et al. Pediatric Regional Anesthesia Network (PRAN): a multi-institutional study of the use and incidence of complications of pediatric regional anesthesia. *Anesth Analg.* 2012;**115**(6):1353–64.

13. Bosenberg AT, Kimble FW. Infraorbital nerve block in neonates for cleft lip repair: anatomical study and clinical application. *Br J Anaesth.* 1995;**74**(5):506–8.

14. Suresh S, Voronov P, Curran J. Infraorbital nerve block in children: a computerized tomographic

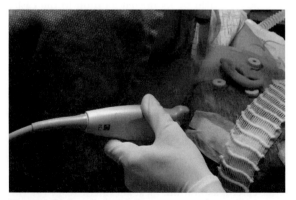

Figure 6.5. Ultrasound-guided greater occipital nerve block.

measurement of the location of the infraorbital foramen. *Reg Anesth Pain Med.* 2006;**31**(3):211–14.

15. Mesnil M, Dadure C, Captier G, et al. A new approach for peri-operative analgesia of cleft palate repair in infants: the bilateral suprazygomatic maxillary nerve block. *Paediatr Anaesth.* 2010;**20**(4):343–9.

16. Sola C, Raux O, Savath L, et al. Ultrasound guidance characteristics and efficiency of suprazygomatic maxillary nerve blocks in infants: a descriptive prospective study. *Paediatr Anaesth.* 2012;**22**(9):841–6.

17. Eichenberger U, Greher M, Kapral S, et al. Sonographic visualization and ultrasound-guided block of the third occipital nerve: prospective for a new method to diagnose C2-C3 zygapophysial joint pain. *Anesthesiology.* 2006;**104**(2):303–8.

18. Greher M, Moriggl B, Curatolo M, et al. Sonographic visualization and ultrasound-guided blockade of the greater occipital nerve: a comparison of two selective techniques confirmed by anatomical dissection. *Br J Anaesth.* 2010;**104**(5):637–42.

Anesthesia for Posterior Fossa Craniotomy

Audrice Francois and Sulpicio G. Soriano

Introduction

The posterior fossa is a common site for neurosurgical lesions in infants and children. It is one of three cranial fossae and contains the cerebellum, the pons, and the medulla oblongata. Given the limited confines of the posterior fossa, it is a critical location for pathology because space-occupying lesions (tumors, hemorrhages, and structural defects of the cerebellum) will impair cerebrospinal fluid (CSF) flow and compress brainstem structures, which can lead to obstructive hydrocephalus and cardiorespiratory derangements, respectively (Figure 7.1). These aberrations place patients undergoing posterior fossa craniotomies at increased risk of perioperative complications.[1,2]

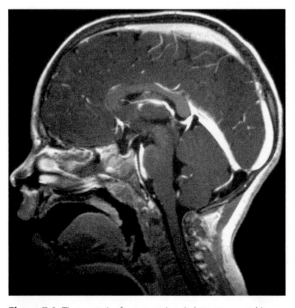

Figure 7.1. The posterior fossa contains vital structures and is a critical space for pathology because enlarging and invasive lesions can lead to obstructive hydrocephalus and cardiorespiratory derangements.

Neurosurgical Lesions in the Posterior Fossa

Tumors

The posterior fossa is the site of approximately 50% of all childhood brain tumors.[3] Patients frequently present with the triad of headache, vomiting, and lethargy. Cerebellar involvement manifests as truncal and limb ataxia. While bulbar or facial palsies herald brainstem infiltration. Symptoms in infants and preverbal toddlers include irritability, vomiting, and enlarged cranium. Posterior fossa tumors of childhood in decreasing order of incidence include medulloblastoma, cerebellar astrocytoma, ependymoma, brainstem glioma, and atypical teratoid or rhabdoid tumors. Surgery is most frequently the initial step in the treatment of these tumors for total or near total resection or to obtain a histological diagnosis.

Medulloblastomas frequently occur in the first decade and occur in the inferior medial zone (vermis) of the cerebellum. In the absence of infiltration of the subarachnoid space, gross total resection is the goal of surgery. However, it has a tendency to metastasize. Therefore, magnetic resonance imaging (MRI) of the entire spinal axis is crucial. Radiation therapy, chemotherapy, and surveillance MRI follow the initial surgical resection and frequently require sedation or general anesthesia for these procedures.

Cerebellar astrocytomas typically appear in the end of the first decade. The majority of these tumors arise in the cerebellum and can extend into the brainstem or cerebellar peduncles. These tumors are well circumscribed with both cystic and solid components. Total resection of the tumor is the standard operative course.

Ependymomas arise from the ependymal lining of the fourth ventricle and are situated either in the fourth ventricle or cerebellopontine angle. Half of these tumors present by 3 years of age and under. These tumors are invasive rather than infiltrative and can extend out of the confines of the posterior fossa and can predispose patients to massive blood loss and postoperative cranial nerve dysfunction.

Brainstem gliomas constitute 25% of posterior fossa tumors in children. These tumors produce cranial nerve palsies, cerebellar signs, and motor and sensory dysfunction due to their proximity to cranial nerve nuclei and corticospinal tracts. Given their poor prognosis and high potential for iatrogenic injury to vital brainstem structures, these tumors are typically treated with biopsies or focal resections followed by radiotherapy and chemotherapy.

Chiari Malformations

There are two types of hindbrain herniation or Chiari malformations due to structural defects of the cranium or cerebellum (Figure 7.2). Type I involves only the descent of the cerebellar tonsils and is often an isolated finding. Chiari malformation type II involves descent of the cerebellar vermis, medulla, and fourth ventricle, is strongly associated with hydrocephalus, and includes brainstem dysfunction (see Chapter 8). Structural anomalies of the craniocervical junction may form a CSF-filled cavity (syringomelia) in the spinal canal due to obstruction of CSF flow. Type I Chiari malformations can occur in healthy children without myelodysplasia. These defects also involve caudal displacement of the cerebellar tonsils below the foramen magnum (Figure 7.2). Symptoms such as headaches, neck

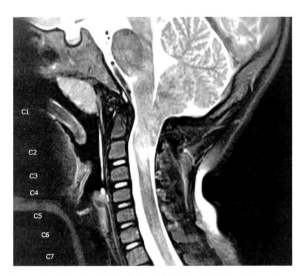

Figure 7.2. Midsagittal MRI of a child with a Chiari I malformation. Note the descent of the cerebellar tonsils through the foramen magnum.

pain, vertigo, paresthesia, hyperreflexia, paresis, or ataxia typically arise during adolescence. However, the diagnosis can be incidentally made during MRIs for the evaluation of scoliosis. The goal of surgery is to increase the size of the cisterna magna and normalize CSF flow. This involves decompression of the craniocervical junction by a suboccipital decompression, cervical laminectomies, and dural opening with a duraplasty.[4] Cauterization of the cerebellar tonsils and lysis of arachnoid adhesions may be considered in some cases.

The Arnold-Chiari malformation type II typically occurs in patients with myelodysplasia. This structural defect consists of caudal displacement of the cerebellar vermis, fourth ventricle, and lower brainstem below the plane of the foramen magnum. Medullary cervical cord compression can lead to vocal cord paralysis with stridor, apnea, dysphagia, pulmonary aspiration, opisthotonos, and cranial nerve deficits. Tracheostomy and gastrostomy are recommended in the most severe cases to secure the airway and to minimize chronic aspiration. Extreme head flexion should be avoided in these patients because it may cause brainstem compression. Early surgical decompression is recommended in order to minimize irreversible medullary dysfunction (cranial nerve palsies and disordered respiratory drive).

Perioperative Concerns

The major perioperative goals in the management of patients with pathological lesions in the posterior fossa are stabilizing intracranial pressure (ICP), preventing damage to the brainstem, and avoiding venous air embolism. In order to optimize the patient prior to surgery, complete preoperative evaluation and physical examination should be performed, as outlined in Chapter 1. Extensive MRI for surgical planning should be reviewed in depth and will require sedation or general anesthesia in uncooperative patients.

Patients with posterior fossa pathology have varying degrees of intracranial hypertension. Posterior fossa tumors obstruct CSF flow, which leads to obstructive hydrocephalus. Vasogenic edema from the tumor will also increase ICP. Treatment ranges from administration of dexamethasone for mild signs to placement of a ventricular catheter or shunt for severe symptoms. Patients should be positioned with the head at a 30-degree angle from horizontal to maximize cerebral venous drainage. Neonates and infants are particularly vulnerable to pharmacologic and physiologic insults. Hypoxia and hypotension are preventable conditions that can cause postoperative neurologic impairment. Therefore, optimizing cerebral perfusion and oxygenation during these intracranial surgical procedures is paramount. While the metabolic requirement of the brain ($CMRO_2$) decreases under anesthesia, the anesthetic agents utilized and positioning the patient may decrease cerebral perfusion pressure, especially since limits of cerebral autoregulation in infants and neonates are unclear (see Chapter 2). Furthermore, intracranial pathology itself can also potentially impair cerebral autoregulation.

Brainstem tumor infiltration and direct compression by adjacent structures can present as cranial nerve dysfunction, long-tract symptoms, and severe hydrocephalus (Figure 7.1), whereas tumors in the medulla oblongata (dorsal and ventral respiratory group) and pons (pneumotaxic and apneustic center) will disrupt generation and maintenance of respiration. Patients with severely impaired brainstem may have vocal cord paralysis, loss of the pharyngeal reflex, and disordered respiratory drive. These severely compromised patients may require tracheostomy and gastrostomy tubes and perioperative mechanical ventilation.

The presence of a congenital heart defect or patent foramen ovale can lead to catastrophic venous air embolism and should negate the use of the sitting position for surgery. Furthermore, prolonged nausea and vomiting and fluid restriction may lead to hypovolemia, which may compromise cerebral perfusion in the setting of intracranial hypertension. The patient's volume status should be optimized prior to surgery with intravenous fluid therapy.

Intraoperative Management

Induction and Maintenance of Anesthesia

Induction of anesthesia will depend on the infant or child's symptoms. If the patient's mental status is stable and he has no intravenous (IV) access, general anesthesia can be induced by mask with sevoflurane and oxygen. Alternatively, anesthesia can be induced with propofol in an existing IV. A non-depolarizing muscle relaxant, vecuronium, or rocuronium should be administered to facilitate intubation of the trachea. Patients who are lethargic or nauseated are at risk for aspiration pneumonitis and require a rapid-sequence

induction of anesthesia using cricoid pressure and succinylcholine or high-dose rocuronium. Etomidate and ketamine can be used to induce anesthesia in hemodynamically compromised patients.

Maintenance of General Anesthesia

Drugs for the maintenance of general anesthesia should be tailored to preserve hemodynamic stability and intraoperative neuromonitoring and facilitate rapid emergence. Since specific anesthetic drugs and technique have been shown to have no impact on outcome,[5] an opioid (fentanyl, sufentanil, or remifentanil) combined with low-dose isoflurane or sevoflurane or total intravenous anesthesia (TIVA) with propofol and remifentanil infusions are equally effective. However, intraoperative neuromonitoring favors TIVA techniques without the neuromuscular blockade.

Given the potential for massive blood loss and reduced access to the patient during surgery, large peripheral venous cannulae should be secured. Insertion of central venous cannulation may be necessary in patients with poor peripheral veins. The routine use of central venous catheters was not effective in determining volume status in pediatric patients.[6,7] Given the small caliber of infant central venous catheters, its utility as a conduit for aspiration of venous air embolism (VAE) is questionable.[8]

Airway Management

Patients in the prone position are at increased risk for intraoperative airway complications. These include kinking and dislodgement of the orotracheal tube and macroglosia from pressure injury and herniation through the mouth. Orotracheal tubes can kink at the base of the tongue when the head is flexed and result in airway obstruction. In the prone position, oral endotracheal tubes can cause direct pressure injury to the tongue. Therefore, nasotracheal tubes are best suited for these situations because they are secured to the nose and maxilla and are less likely to be kinked. A reinforced or armored oral endotracheal tube should be used when nasotracheal intubation is contraindicated, such as patients with pharyngeal flaps or choanal atresia. Oral airways are best avoided because they can cause edema of the tongue. A folded roll of gauze can be inserted between the lateral incisors to prevent the tongue from extruding and in cases where motor evoked potentials are used intraoperatively to prevent tongue lacerations.

Positioning

Patient positioning for surgery requires careful preoperative planning to allow adequate access to the patient for both the neurosurgeon and the anesthesiologist. Table 7.1 compares the physiologic sequelae of prone and sitting positions. Cranial stabilization is typically secured with skull clamps and age-appropriate cranial pins (Figure 7.3). Since neonates and small infants have thin skulls, head pinning systems are avoided because of increased risk of skull fractures and epidural hematomas.[9] Instead, there are a variety of non-pin-based headrests available such as pediatric horseshoe headrest and padded head clamps (Figure 7.4). Extreme head flexion should be avoided because it can result in brainstem compression, high cervical spinal cord ischemia, and kinking and obstruction of the endotracheal tube. Extremities should be well padded and secured in a neutral position.

Prone Position

The prone position is commonly used for posterior fossa and cervical spinal cord surgery. The torso should be supported to ensure free abdominal wall motion because increased intra-abdominal pressure may impair ventilation, cause vena cava compression, and increase epidural venous pressure and bleeding. This is achieved most easily by placing silicone rolls or rolled blankets laterally on each side of the child's chest running from the shoulders toward the pelvis. Placing the rolls in this position should also allow a precordial Doppler monitor to be easily placed on the anterior chest without undue pressure. Extremities should be well padded and secured in a neutral position.

Table 7.1 Physiologic Effects of Patient Positioning

Position	Physiologic Effect
Sitting	Enhanced cerebral venous drainage
	Decreased cerebral blood flow
	Increased venous pooling in the lower extremities
	Postural hypotension
Prone	Venous congestion of face, tongue, and oral mucosa
	Decreased lung compliance and venocaval compression from abdominal compression

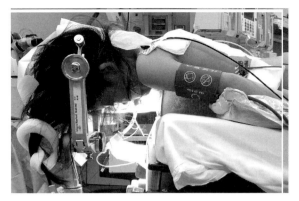

Figure 7.3. This 5-year-old child is in the prone position for posterior fossa surgery. Typically, a nasotracheal endotracheal is utilized to secure the airway. However, this child had a pharyngoplasty for the treatment of velopharyngeal insufficiency, in which a nasotracheal tube is contraindicated. An armored orotracheal tube was inserted in this surgery.

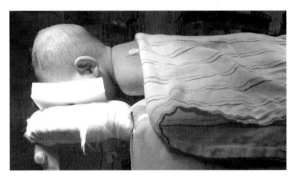

Figure 7.4. Neonates and infants have thin skulls that are susceptible to fractures and epidural/subdural hematomas from traditional skull clamp and pin systems. Typically, the head is placed prone on a cerebellar horseshoe headrest with foam padding.

Significant airway edema may develop in a child who is in the prone position for an extended period. Rarely, prophylactic postoperative intubation may be necessary if a great deal of facial swelling has developed during a prolonged surgery. Postoperative vision loss has been linked with prolonged spine surgery in the prone position and significant blood loss.[10] Avoidance of direct pressure on the globe of the eyes, staged procedures to decrease surgical time, and maintenance of stable hemodynamics with avoidance of excessive intraoperative fluid administration should be ensured in prone children.

Sitting Position

The sitting position is now used less commonly in pediatric neurosurgical procedures and is rarely used in children younger than 3 years of age. However, this position may be used for morbidly obese children who cannot tolerate the prone position due to excessive intrathoracic and abdominal pressures. The sitting position has several advantages including better surgical exposure with anatomic orientation and optimum access to midline posterior fossa and upper cervical spine lesions. It also provides improved blood and CSF drainage from the operative field. Complications associated with the sitting position are that it can produce significant hemodynamic instability, VAE, pneumocephalus, peripheral neuropathy, tetraplegia, and macroglossia. The use of a horizontal position, however, does not eliminate the risk of VAE and may have decreased CSF and blood drainage.

Monitoring

In addition to standard American Society of Anesthesiologists (ASA) monitoring, additional monitoring modalities are often employed in posterior fossa procedures. Arrhythmias and acute blood pressure changes may occur during surgical exploration, especially when the brainstem structures are manipulated. Given the risk of injury to cranial nerves V, VII, and X during posterior fossa surgery, the electrocardiogram, arterial waveform, and electromyogram (EMG) should be closely monitored (Table 7.2). Altered respiratory control may be masked by neuromuscular blocking drugs and mechanical ventilation.

Intraoperative neurophysiologic monitoring (IONM) is also used to monitor brainstem integrity (see Chapter 16). Somatosensory evoked potentials (SSEPs), motor evoked potentials (MEPs), and auditory brainstem responses (ABRs) assess the function of the brainstem or their vascular supply, to reduce the risk of iatrogenic damage to the nervous system and enable complete resections. These modalities typically require TIVA because they are sensitive to the depressant effects of volatile agents.

VAE is the entrainment of air or exogenous gas into the arterial or venous system. VAE is a potentially serious complication that is not eliminated by the prone or lateral position because head-up angles of 10 to 20 degrees are frequently used to improve cerebral venous drainage. Large head size relative to body size in infants and toddlers accentuates this problem. Entrained air can cause hemodynamic collapse, which may be difficult to discriminate from massive blood loss. Paradoxical air embolism can occur through

Table 7.2 Intraoperative Signs of Surgical Encroachment on Brainstem Structures

Brainstem Site	Signs
Trigeminal nerve CN V	Hypertension, bradycardia, and masseter muscle contraction
Facial nerve CN VII	Facial muscle contraction
Vagus nerve CN X	Hypotension, bradycardia
Medulla oblongata and pons	Loss of BAER and SSEP signals, hyper/hypotension, tachy/bradycardia

CN = cranial nerve nuclei; BAER = brainstem evoked potentials; SSEP = somatosensory evoked potentials.

a patent foramen ovale, which is present in many children. Standard monitoring will reveal decreases in end-tidal carbon dioxide and oxygen saturation.

Detection of VAE requires additional real-time monitoring modalities. The most sensitive device for monitoring VAE is transesophageal echocardiography (TEE), capable of detecting 0.02 mL/kg of air. However, it also detects microemboli that may be of no clinical significance and the probe may cause esophageal edema and injury. Precordial Doppler ultrasound is the most sensitive of the noninvasive monitors and can detect 0.05 mL/kg of air. It can be placed on the right or left sternal border, and its position confirmed by an injection or a bubble test. End-tidal carbon dioxide is readily available, is most convenient and practical, but is of moderate sensitivity and not very specific. End-tidal nitrogen is not available on all anesthesia monitors. Changes in oxygen saturation will be a late finding.

Postoperative Management

Since an immediate postoperative neurological examination is essential in assessment of the patient, the timing of extubation may be challenging following neurosurgical procedures in the posterior fossa. Infants, particularly those with Chiari II malformations or extensive tumor resections, may exhibit intermittent apnea, vocal cord paralysis, or other irregularities before resuming a stable respiratory pattern. Significant airway edema and postoperative obstruction can complicate prone procedures or those involving significant blood losses and large volume replacement. Lingual or supraglottic swelling may require direct laryngoscopy to assess the airway. Head-up positioning and gentle forced diuresis usually improve airway edema within 24 hours. Postoperative mechanical ventilation may be required after prolonged surgery and in situations where the respiratory centers have been injured. Nausea and vomiting are common after posterior fossa surgery and mandate extensive antiemetic drug treatment. Posterior fossa syndrome, which manifests as cerebellar mutism, absence of vocalization, has been observed in patients after posterior fossa surgery for midline tumors.[11] Patients may also exhibit dysarthria, hypotonia, dysphagia, and mood lability, as well as deficiencies in cognition. The onset may be immediate or delayed and may persist. It is thought to result from ischemia and edema due to retracted and manipulated dentate nuclei.

Conclusion

Posterior fossa operations require continuous vigilance of personnel dedicated to the care of these patients. Children under the age of 1 year are at the highest risk for morbidity and mortality and their vulnerability must be considered.[12] Complications are also higher in children with coexisting disorders. Often, these patients also have congenital cardiac anomalies, craniofacial disproportions, and respiratory disorders that add to their complexity. Preoperative evaluations, continuous perioperative physiologic surveillance, as well as comprehensive pain management regimens are paramount to their overall care.

References

1. Meridy HW, Creighton RE, Humphreys RP. Complications during neurosurgery in the prone position in children. *Can Anaesth Soc J.* 1974;**21**:445–53.

2. Aleksic V, Radulovic D, Milakovic B, Nagulic M, Vucovic D, Antunovic V, Djordjevic M. A retrospective analysis of anesthesiologic complications in pediatric neurosurgery. *Paediatr Anaesth.* 2009;**19**:879–86.

3. Pollack IF. Brain tumors in children. *N Engl J Med.* 1994;**331**:1500–7.

4. Durham SR, Fjeld-Olenec K. Comparison of posterior fossa decompression with and without duraplasty for the surgical treatment of Chiari malformation type I in pediatric patients: a meta-analysis. *J Neurosurg Pediatr.* 2008;**2**:42–9.

5. Todd MM, Warner DS, Sokoll MD, Maktabi MA, Hindman BJ, Scamman FL, Kirschner J. A prospective, comparative trial of three anesthetics for elective supratentorial craniotomy. Propofol/fentanyl, isoflurane/nitrous oxide, and fentanyl/nitrous oxide. *Anesthesiology.* 1993;**78**:1005–20.

6. Stricker PA, Lin EE, Fiadjoe JE, Sussman EM, Pruitt EY, Zhao H, Jobes DR. Evaluation of central venous pressure monitoring in children undergoing craniofacial reconstruction surgery. *Anesth Analg.* 2013;**116**:411–19.

7. Vavilala MS, Soriano SG, Krane EJ. Anesthesia for neurosurgery. In: Davis PJ, Cladis FP, eds. *Smith's Anesthesia for Infants and Children*, 9th ed. Philadelphia: Elsevier; 2017: 744–73.

8. Cucchiara RF, Bowers B. Air embolism in children undergoing suboccipital craniotomy. *Anesthesiology.* 1982;**57**:338–9.

9. Lee M, Rezai AR, Chou J. Depressed skull fractures in children secondary to skull clamp fixation devices. *Pediatr Neurosurg.* 1994;**21**:174–7.

10. Lee LA, Roth S, Posner KL, Cheney FW, Caplan RA, Newman NJ, Domino KB. The American Society of Anesthesiologists Postoperative Visual Loss Registry: analysis of 93 spine surgery cases with postoperative visual loss. *Anesthesiology.* 2006;**105**:652–9.

11. Avula S, Mallucci C, Kumar R, Pizer B. Posterior fossa syndrome following brain tumour resection: review of pathophysiology and a new hypothesis on its pathogenesis. *Childs Nerv Syst.* 2015;**31**: 1859–67.

12. Hansen TG, Pedersen JK, Henneberg SW, Morton NS, Christensen K. Neurosurgical conditions and procedures in infancy are associated with mortality and academic performances in adolescence: a nationwide cohort study. *Paediatr Anaesth.* 2015;**25**: 186–92.

Chapter 8

Congenital Neurosurgical Lesions

Cynthia Tung, Lazslo Vutskits, and Sulpicio G. Soriano

Introduction

The development of the central nervous system (CNS) occurs early in gestation and is orchestrated by a combination of transcriptional and mechanical factors.[1] A basic understanding of normal and abnormal development of the CNS is valuable for understanding the perioperative management of congenital lesions of the CNS.[2]

The primitive CNS originates from the neural plate, which folds and fuses dorsally. Primary neurulation occurs when the neural plate folds to form the neural tube. The walls of the neural tube give rise to the brain and spinal cord, while the canal develops into the ventricles and central canal of the brain and spinal cord, respectively. Fusion of the cranial neural folds and closure of the cranial neuropore, which give rise to the forebrain, midbrain, and hindbrain, arise from these structures. Closure starts near the cervical spine region and extends cephalad and caudad. Closure of the neural tube begins at gestational age 22–23 days, with complete closure around days 26–27. Failure of the anterior neuropore to close by day 24 results in anencephaly, while posterior defects lead to encephaloceles and myelomeningoceles. Therefore, most commonly defects occur along the thoracic or lumbosacral region but can occur along the cervical region. Secondary neurulation ensues when the neuroepithelium caudal to the posterior neuropore closes. Derangements in this progression can lead to spinal dysraphism (spinal bifida, myelomeningocele, and tethered cord). If left untreated, these congenital lesions can lead to chronic conditions such as hydrocephalus and caudal neurological deficits. The incidence of neural tube defects is approximately 2–5/1,000 live births. Outcome studies reveal increased perioperative morbidity, mortality, and cognitive deficits in neonates with congenital neurological lesions.[3–6]

Congenital Anomalies

Congenital CNS anomalies typically occur as midline defects. These neural tube defects may arise anywhere along the neural axis from the head (cranial dysraphism) to the spine (spinal dysraphism). They may be relatively minor and affect only superficial bony and membranous structures, or may include a large segment of malformed neural tissue. These lesions are associated with Arnold-Chiari malformations, hydrocephalus, and neurologic deficits. Cervical cord or brainstem compression are possible in patients with concomitant Arnold-Chiari malformations. After birth, the defects are usually covered with sterile, saline-soaked gauze in order to keep the lesion moist and clear. After birth, the patient is typically positioned prone to avoid direct pressure on the defect.

Cranial Dysraphism

Cranial dysraphisms or encephaloceles are characterized by a sac-like calvarial defect that arises anywhere from the nose to the occiput. The former can manifest as nasal polyps that protrude through the cribriform plate. Cranial meningoceles contain cerebrospinal fluid (CSF) and meninges, and the presence of neural elements classifies this cystic lesion as meningoencephalocele. Encephaloceles are classified by their location on the cranium, with sincipital lesions in the frontal calvarium and occipital encephaloceles sited posteriorly. Primary encephaloceles are often diagnosed in utero by fetal ultrasonography, with large encephaloceles delivered by elective cesarean section. Most small encephaloceles have minimal neurological deficits, whereas those with large lesions may present with cranial nerve abnormalities and subsequent developmental and growth delay, poor feeding, blindness, and seizures.

Preoperative diagnostic imaging is essential in delineating the content and margins of the lesion and require sedation or general anesthesia for computed tomography (CT) and magnetic resonance imaging (MRI) scans. Encephaloceles can be associated with hydrocephalus and other craniofacial and brain abnormalities such as anencephaly, microcephaly, ataxia, Meckel's, and amniotic band syndrome.

If the neonate is stable, encephaloceles will continue to enlarge and surgery can be delayed and performed in stages if the overlying skin is intact. Innovations in neonatal care and surgical techniques, including image guidance and multidisciplinary reconstruction techniques, have improved the outcome for these patients.

Sincipital encephaloceles usually contain fibrous tissue, which can be safely transected at the level of the skull and the defect closed primarily. Nasal or sphenoethmoidal encephaloceles are rare and characterized by a skull base defect around the sella turcica. Large lesions may obstruct the airway and compromise pituitary function. However, smaller lesions may be undetected during infancy. Other midline nasal masses including nasal polyps, dermoid sinus cyst, and tumors should be considered in the differential diagnosis of these lesions. Image guidance based on three-dimensional image reconstructions and radionuclide ventriculography are useful. The resection and closure can be difficult during transpalatal surgical approaches due to exposure and inadequate soft tissue for closure. Other surgical procedures include transcranial, subfrontal, and endoscopic transnasal approaches. The postoperative course may be complicated by CSF leaks, meningitis, visual impairments, and endocrine derangements.

Occipital encephaloceles may contain functional brain tissue that needs to be preserved. Most encephaloceles with substantial neural tissue herniating through large cranial defect may require an expansion cranioplasty and a plastic surgeon to create split thickness calvarial grafts. When primary closure is not possible, a staged secondary repair is an option. Large occipital encephaloceles may be associated with twisting of the brainstem, lobar herniation, and hydrocephalus.

Spinal Dysraphisms

Spinal dysraphisms are lesions where the dorsal midline structures fail to fuse during embryogenesis and are categorized into spina bifida aperta and spina bifida occulta. Spina bifida aperta is easily identifiable by the sac-like lesion containing meninges (meningocele) or neural tissue and meninges (myelomeningocele), while spina bifida occulta has no superficial cutaneous manifestations.

These spinal defects can occur anywhere along the vertebral column, although lumbar and low thoracic defects are most common. Rachischisis is the most severe form where the posterior neuropore fails to fuse. A protruding membranous sac containing meninges, CSF, nerve roots, and a dysplastic spinal cord often protrudes through the defect in meningocele or myelomeningocele.

Prenatal ultrasonography affords early diagnosis and elective cesarean delivery and closure of meningomyeloceles. These lesions may be repaired in utero at specialized fetal surgery centers (Chapter 10). In order to minimize the risk of infection, meningomyeloceles undergo primary closure of the defect within the first 24 hours of life. These lesions are often associated with a type II Chiari malformation where both the cerebellum and brainstem tissue protrude into the foramen magnum.

Since type II Chiari (Arnold-Chiari) malformations predispose these patients to hydrocephalus, insertion of a ventriculoperitoneal shunt may be combined with the initial surgery. Alternatively, a ventriculoperitoneal shunt may be inserted a few days later or deferred if there is no evidence of hydrocephalus at birth. Patients with thoracic lesions may have poor autonomic control below level of the defect.

Patients with myelodysplasia are chronically at high risk for latex sensitivity and anaphylaxis, due to repeated exposure to latex products encountered during frequent bladder catheterizations and multiple surgical procedures. These children should be managed in a latex-free environment from birth to minimize the chances of sensitization.[7] Latex allergy should be suspected if signs and symptoms of anaphylaxis develop during surgery. Suspected anaphylaxis should be treated with intravenous epinephrine in a dose of 1 to 10 μg/kg, as required.

Anesthetic Management

Preanesthetic Evaluation

Cranial and spinal dysraphisms are heterogeneous lesions and mandate an individualized approach based on the severity as well as its location. Therefore, a thorough review of the antenatal history, birth history, prematurity, other comorbidities, and other congenital anomalies should be completed prior to surgery (Chapter 1). Some patients with encephaloceles may have tenuous respiratory function due to direct airway obstruction or impairment of the pontomedullary respiratory control center. Depending on the size of the lesion and extent of the surgical procedure, significant blood loss should be anticipated during both the intra- and postoperative periods.

Intraoperative Management

Positioning the neonate for induction of anesthesia can be challenging. Anesthesia can be induced with a propofol, but hypotension and possible cerebral ischemia might ensue[8] due to the lack of surgical stimulation. In most cases, tracheal intubation can be performed with the neonate in the supine position and the patient's back or head supported with foam or gel head rings so there is no direct pressure on the lesion (Figure 8.1). Manipulation of these lesions should be limited because of the risk of rupturing the thin membranes. For very large defects, it may be necessary to place the infant in the left lateral decubitus position for induction of anesthesia and tracheal intubation.

Encephaloceles are associated with compromised airways by varying degrees. Effective mask ventilation may be impaired by protruding lesions of sincipital encephalocele and may hinder effective mask ventilation. In these patients, difficult airway precautions and techniques should be applied.[9] Gigantic encephaloceles may prohibit proper positioning of the patient for intubation of the trachea. Some fluid-filled encephaloceles can be decompressed by aspirating CSF with a sterile needle and syringe under ultrasound guidance. Alternatively, giant occipital encephaloceles can be suspended through a pediatric horseshoe headrest. Mask ventilation may be difficult in this position, so an assistant can support the head as the anesthesiologist applies a mask seal. Intubation may also be more difficult in the lateral position and may require the use of a flexible fiberoptic bronchoscope or video laryngoscope.

The surgical repair is performed in a prone position so the patient's face should be well supported by a padded foam on a horseshoe headrest to prevent direct pressure on the eyes and mouth (Figure 8.2). In this position, caution should be taken so that the endotracheal tube (ETT) is well secured to the patient. Since the airway will be inaccessible during repair of encephaloceles, a nasotracheal tube should be secured to minimize dislodgement. Prone positioning for the surgery also requires careful padding to prevent increased abdominal pressure.

Ensuring adequate oxygenation and perfusion of the developing brain is the cornerstone of neonatal anesthesia and critical care.[10,11] Typically, blood loss during the procedure is not significant enough to necessitate blood transfusions. However, the risk of bleeding and venous air embolization is greater in patients with larger cranial defects. Therefore, multiple intravenous and an arterial catheter should be inserted for these large lesions where large blood

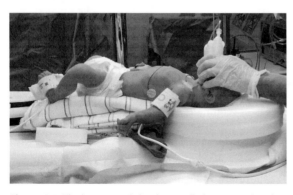

Figure 8.1. The large encephalocele is cradled in sponge head rings, while the rest of the body is elevated with soft towels. This positioning provides optimal conditions for managing the airway and tracheal intubation.

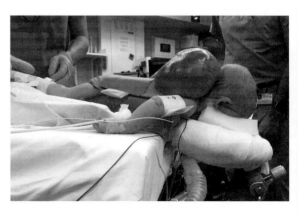

Figure 8.2. The patient is placed in the prone position with a soft sponge padding the head on the Mayfield headrest. The eyes, nose, and mouth are suspended thorough an opening in the sponge to avoid direct pressure. Note that the thorax and abdomen are hovering on lateral silicone rolls to prevent thoracoabdominal compression.

loss may be anticipated. Occasionally, rotational or myocutaneous flaps may be required for closure of large defects. Respiratory parameters and oxygenation should be carefully monitored during primary closure of large defects because tight skin closure may compromise tidal volume and reduce venous return. Significant hypotension is typically due to blood and CSF losses, but also can be a manifestation of hypothyroidism, adrenocortical deficiency, or diabetes insipidus. Patients who develop diabetes insipidus should be treated with a vasopressin infusion and urinary output replaced with crystalloid. Bladder catheter and arterial lines should be considered for any complex lesions. If risk for postoperative CSF leak is significant, a ventricular drain may be inserted.

Postoperative Management

Since a majority of these patients are neonates, postoperative observation should be in a neonatal intensive care setting. The decision for tracheal extubation is dictated by the degree of blood loss and fluid and blood administration and level of neurological status of the neonate. Patients with large sincipital encephaloceles should go to an intensive care unit postoperatively to be closely monitored for adrenal cortical deficiency, diabetes insipidus, and airway obstruction. Mild sedation may be required for some pediatric patients should tracheal intubation and mechanical ventilation be continued.

Persistent CSF leaks are not an uncommon complication in repaired encephaloceles and may be confused with normal sinus drainage. Some patients may need additional surgery or have a ventriculostomy drain placed. In some complex occipital encephalocele and large myelomeningocele repairs, it is preferable to recover the patient in the prone position in order to avoid pressure on the incision. The patient will often continue to lose blood into the surgical site, and hemoglobin should be measured during the postoperative period.

Spina Bifida Occulta

Spina bifida occulta or occult spinal dysaphism (OSD) encompasses a wide variety of spinal anomalies. Patients with OSD have skin covering over their underlying defect, which typically occurs over the lower lumbar region and presents as hair tufts, skin dimples, or fat pads. These lesions can functionally lead to tethered cord syndrome (TCS) and are due to

tension on and restricted movement of the spinal cord. Clinical presentation of TCS varies widely and may include motor weakness, sensory deficit, gait disturbances, scoliosis, pain, orthopedic deformities, and urologic dysfunction. Neonates and infants with midline cutaneous stigmata such as nevi or hairy tufts along the sacrum, sacral dimpling, lipomas, or anorectal malformations should be highly suspected for spinal cord tethering. Older children and adults may have a history of orthopedic surgeries, urologic surgeries, or trauma before a diagnosis of TCS is recognized.

Children who have had a meningomyelocele repaired after birth may also develop an ascending neurologic deficit from a tethered spinal cord. Most neurological deficits are caused by traction on the spinal cord and can progress to a permanent neurological deficit distal to the lesion if it is not surgically released.

Diagnosis of OSD and determining the extent of the lesion is highly dependent on MRI studies, which will reveal the heterogeneous abnormal anatomy that impinges on the spinal cord. The goal is to untether the spinal cord and release tension without causing further nerve damage. Surgical technique will vary depending on the cause of tethering. For example, a tethered cord after prior myelomeningocele repair may require release of the cord from scar tissue, whereas lipomas may require surgical debulking of the mass.

Anesthetic Considerations

Preanesthetic Evaluation

The most important issue is to determine, preoperatively, whether the OSD is causing traction on the spinal cord. A reliable history and physical exam can help make the diagnosis, otherwise a recent MRI may be required. It is also important to determine if the patient has any evidence of scoliosis, neurogenic bladder, incontinence, positional limitations, spasticity, back pain, or leg pain. Sometimes the excision of the OSD can worsen neurological function.

Intraoperative Management and Neuromonitoring

The modality of neuromonitoring will dictate the choice of anesthesia drugs utilized during the surgical untethering of the lesion (Chapter 10). A muscle relaxant can be used to facilitate intubation, followed by an anesthetic maintenance plan with no further muscle relaxation in order to facilitate neuromonitoring protocols. Since patients are placed in a prone position, pressure points should be appropriately padded. Soft rolls are generally used to elevate and support the lateral chest wall and hips in order to minimize abdominal and thoracic pressure, which will improve ventilation and decrease venous engorgement of the spine.

Tethered spinal cord syndrome occurs in myelomeningoceles, lipoma of the filum terminalis, spina bifida occulta, and adhesions from prior spinal surgery. Persistence of this anatomical anomaly can lead to cord or nerve root distortion and impaired perfusion resulting in progressive neurological deficits and chronic pain. Visualization and identification of functional nerve roots may be difficult and may result in an inadvertent injury during the surgical dissection. This can lead to fecal and urinary incontinence and exacerbation of lower extremity neurologic dysfunction. Electromyography (EMG) helps identity functional nerve roots. Placement of the EMG electrodes in the external anal and urethral (in females) sphincter allows continuous monitoring of the nerve roots supplying the pudenal nerves (S2–S4). Movement and evoked action potentials of the anterior tibialis and sural muscles can also be detected both visually and by EMG, respectively. Muscle contractions can be readily observed by using clear sterile plastic drapes. Muscle relaxation must be discontinued prior to stimulation in order to accurately detect motor activity. Volatile anesthetics and opioids do not appear to interfere with muscle action potentials, and the patient should be deeply anesthetized because direct nerve root stimulation often elicits a significant sympathetic response and pain management Muscle relaxants should be avoided or permitted to dissipate before intraoperative assessment. For simple OSD lesions that solely tether spinal roots, EMG is the standard monitoring technique. Complex OSD lesions that impinge on the spinal cord may benefit from somatosensory (SSEP), and motor evoked potentials (MEPs) may be useful to test the integrity of the neural pathways that are at risk of injury. Volatile anesthetics should be limited to 0.5 mean alveolar concentration (MAC). Opioids have a minimal effect on action potentials. Therefore, opioid infusions are popular techniques.

The use of lumbar neuroaxial catheters for uncomplicated management is controversial because of abnormal lumbosacral anatomy and unpredictable analgesic effect. Furthermore, abnormal epidural space predisposes these patients to inadvertent dural punctures.

Postoperative Management

Patients should lie flat to decrease the orthostatic pressure of CSF on the dural closure.

Chiari Malformations

There are several types of Chiari malformations. The Arnold-Chiari malformation (type II) usually coexists in children with myelodysplasia. This defect consists of a bony abnormality in the posterior fossa and upper cervical spine with caudal displacement of the cerebellar vermis, fourth ventricle, and lower brainstem below the plane of the foramen magnum. Medullary cervical cord compression can also occur. Vocal cord paralysis with stridor and respiratory distress, apnea, abnormal swallowing and pulmonary aspiration, opisthotonos, and cranial nerve deficits may be associated with the Arnold-Chiari malformation and usually manifest during infancy. Children with vocal cord paralysis or a diminished gag reflex may require tracheostomy and gastrostomy to secure the airway and to minimize chronic aspiration. Children of any age may have abnormal responses to hypoxia and hypercarbia because of cranial nerve and brainstem dysfunction.[12] Extreme head flexion may cause brainstem compression in otherwise asymptomatic children.

Surgical treatment usually involves a decompressive suboccipital craniectomy with cervical laminectomies. The anesthetic management of craniectomy for Arnold-Chiari malformations is discussed in Chapter 7.

Hydrocephalus

Hydrocephalus is the most common affliction of pediatric neurosurgical patients.[13] It has been defined as "an active distension of the ventricular system of the brain related to inadequate passage of CSF from its point of production within the ventricular system to its point of absorption into the systemic circulation."[14] This can be due primarily to buildup of CSF within the ventricular system by congenital lesions, tumors, or extrinsic factors. Communicating hydrocephalus occurs when the blockage of CSF flow is downstream of the ventricles, while noncommunicating hydrocephalus occurs when the flow of CSF is blocked along one of the passages connecting the ventricles. Pathological increases in CSF production or decreases in reabsorption are less common causes of hydrocephalus.

Hydrocephalus is ideally managed by ameliorating the underlying problem. If this is not possible, surgical implantation of a drain or shunt may be necessary. The most common place to drain CSF through an implanted shunt is the peritoneal cavity, but the right atrium or pleural cavity may also be used. Although implantation of a ventriculoperitoneal shunt is relatively straightforward, patients may be at increased risk for aspiration of gastric contents. Venous air embolism (VAE) may occur during placement of the distal end of a ventriculoatrial shunt if the operative site is above the heart. Acute obstruction of a ventricular shunt requires urgent treatment because an acute increase in intracranial pressure in the relatively small cranial vault of the infant and child can have devastating consequences.

Premature neonates are likely candidates for hydrocephalus secondary to intraventricular hemorrhages.[15,16] The severity of posthemorrhagic hydrocephalus is assessed by serial head ultrasounds. Accumulated CSF can be temporarily drained by placement of a ventricular reservoir or ventriculosubgaleal shunt. Diversion of CSF is the permanent treatment for hydrocephalus. However, placement of a ventriculoperitoneal shunt is limited by the size of the patient and increased risk of shunt failure.

Infants with hydrocephalus can be treated with the creation of a ventriculostomy on the floor of the third ventricle followed by cauterization of the choroid plexus to attenuate excessive production of CSF.[17,18] Precise insertion of ventricular shunt catheters can be facilitated with endoscopy as well. Recent advancements in endoscopic techniques are being utilized to perform endoscopic third ventriculostomy (ETV) with the option of cauterization of the choroid plexus.[17,18]

Anesthetic Management

The common symptoms of hydrocephalus include a rapid increase in head circumference, irritability, sleepiness, nausea and vomiting, and downward deviation of the eyes. Acute obstruction of a ventricular shunt requires urgent treatment because an acute increase in intracranial pressure in the relatively small cranial vault of the infant and child can have devastating consequences.

The anesthetic management of these patients depends on the acuity of the patient's symptoms. In a patient with an intact mental status or one in whom intravenous access cannot be established, an inhalation induction with sevoflurane and gentle cricoid pressure may be used. If the patient is obtunded, is at risk for herniation, or has a full stomach, intravenous access should be established in order to perform a rapid sequence induction followed by tracheal intubation. VAE may occur during placement of the distal end of a ventriculoatrial shunt if the operative site is above the heart.

Technological advances in minimally invasive surgery have entered the realm of pediatric neurosurgery. These techniques include endoscopy and stereotactic-guided insertion of intracranial devices. Given the relatively small size of the cranial vault in pediatric patients, life-threatening intracranial hypertension can occur insidiously.

Neuroendoscopic techniques have been utilized for treatment of hydrocephalus and tumor biopsies.[19] Infants with hydrocephalus can be treated with the creation of a ventriculostomy on the floor of the third ventricle followed by cauterization of the choroid plexus to attenuate excessive production of CSF.[17,18] Precise insertion of ventricular shunt catheters can be facilitated with endoscopy as well. Despite the relative safety of this procedure, hypertension, arrhythmias, and neurogenic pulmonary edema have been reported in conjunction with acute intracranial hypertension due to lack of egress of irrigation fluids and/or manipulation of the floor of the third ventricle.

Summary

The approach to the neonates and infants with congenital neurological lesion is based on a fundamental understanding of the surgical lesion and implications of maturational changes of the developing organ systems. Neonatal surgery is associated with increased perioperative morbidity, mortality, and cognitive deficits in this patient population.[3-6] Therefore a comprehensive course of preoperative evaluation, intraoperative care, and postoperative observation is indicated in this vulnerable patient group.

References

1. Stiles J, Jernigan TL. The basics of brain development. *Neuropsychol Rev.* 2010;**20**:327–48.

2. McClain CD, Soriano SG. The central nervous system: pediatric neuroanesthesia. In: Holzman RS, Mancuso TJ, Polaner DM, eds. *A Practical Approach to Pediatric Anesthesia*, 2nd ed. Philadelphia: Wolters Kluwer; 2016:226–64.

3. Campbell E, Beez T, Todd L. Prospective review of 30-day morbidity and mortality in a paediatric neurosurgical unit. *Childs Nerv Syst.* 2017;**33**:483–9.

4. Kuo BJ, Vissoci JR, Egger JR, Smith ER, Grant GA, Haglund MM, Rice HE. Perioperative outcomes for pediatric neurosurgical procedures: analysis of the National Surgical Quality Improvement Program—Pediatrics. *J Neurosurg Pediatr.* 2017;**19**:361–71.

5. Stolwijk LJ, Lemmers PM, Harmsen M, Groenendaal F, de Vries LS, van der Zee DC, et al. Neurodevelopmental outcomes after neonatal surgery for major noncardiac anomalies. *Pediatrics.* 2016;**137**: e20151728.

6. Hansen TG, Pedersen JK, Henneberg SW, Morton NS, Christensen K. Neurosurgical conditions and procedures in infancy are associated with mortality and academic performances in adolescence: a nationwide cohort study. *Paediatr Anaesth.* 2015;**25**:186–92.

7. Holzman RS. Clinical management of latex-allergic children. *Anesth Analg.* 1997;**85**:529–33.

8. Vanderhaegen J, Naulaers G, Van Huffel S, Vanhole C, Allegaert K. Cerebral and systemic hemodynamic effects of intravenous bolus administration of propofol in neonates. *Neonatology.* 2010;**98**:57–63.

9. Jagannathan N, Sohn L, Fiadjoe JE. Paediatric difficult airway management: what every anaesthetist should know! *Br J Anaesth.* 2016;**117**(suppl 1): i3–i5.

10. Vutskits L. Cerebral blood flow in the neonate. *Paediatr Anaesth.* 2014;**24**:22–9.

11. McCann ME, Schouten AN. Beyond survival: influences of blood pressure, cerebral perfusion and anesthesia on neurodevelopment. *Paediatr Anaesth.* 2014;**24**:68–73.

12. Ward SL, Nickerson BG, van der Hal A, Rodriguez AM, Jacobs RA, Keens TG. Absent hypoxic and hypercapneic arousal responses in children with myelomeningocele and apnea. *Pediatrics.* 1986;**78**:44–50.

13. Kahle KT, Kulkarni AV, Limbrick DD Jr., Warf BC. Hydrocephalus in children. *Lancet.* 2016;**387**:788–99.

14. Rekate HL. A contemporary definition and classification of hydrocephalus. *Semin Pediatr Neurol.* 2009;**16**:9–15.

15. Leonard JR, Limbrick DD Jr. Intraventricular hemorrhage and post-hemorrhagic hydrocephelus. In: Albright AL, Pollack IF, Adelson PD, eds. *Principles and Practice of Pediatric Neurosurgery.* New York: Thieme; 2015:137–44.

16. Mazzola CA, Choudhri AF, Auguste KI, Limbrick DD Jr., Rogido M, Mitchell L, et al. Pediatric hydrocephalus: systematic literature review and evidence-based guidelines. Part 2: Management of posthemorrhagic hydrocephalus in premature infants. *J Neurosurg Pediatr.* 2014;**14**(suppl 1):8–23.

17. Stone SS, Warf BC. Combined endoscopic third ventriculostomy and choroid plexus cauterization as primary treatment for infant hydrocephalus: a prospective North American series. *J Neurosurg Pediatr.* 2014;**14**:439–46.

18. Limbrick DD Jr., Baird LC, Klimo P Jr., Riva-Cambrin J, Flannery AM, Pediatric Hydrocephalus Systematic Review and Evidence-Based Guidelines Task Force. Pediatric hydrocephalus: systematic literature review and evidence-based guidelines. Part 4: Cerebrospinal fluid shunt or endoscopic third ventriculostomy for the treatment of hydrocephalus in children. *J Neurosurg Pediatr.* 2014;**14**(suppl 1):30–4.

19. Meier PM, Guzman R, Erb TO. Endoscopic pediatric neurosurgery: implications for anesthesia. *Paediatr Anaesth.* 2014;**24**:668–77.

Anesthetic Considerations for Deep Brain Stimulator Placement

Eric Darrow

Introduction

Throughout history, literally since ancient times when the physician to Roman emperor Claudius, Scribonius Largo, in 46 AD wrote of applying electric rays (*Torpedo torpedo* and *Torpedo nobiliana*) to the cranial surface as a treatment of headaches, electrical stimulation has been used in the treatment of various neurological disorders.[1] Electroshock, introduced by Ugo Cerletti (1877–1963) in 1938 for the treatment of severe psychosis, was the first modern example of therapeutic application of brain stimulation.[2]

Functional neurosurgery has been a rapidly growing form of neurosurgical therapy. Traditionally, these have most commonly been performed for the treatment of medically refractory Parkinson's disease (PD), but expanded to include essential tremor, dystonia, and some neuropsychiatric diseases.[3] Surgical procedures such as pallidotomy and thalamotomy were performed to ameliorate the dystonic symptoms in patients with PD. However, over the past 30 years deep brain stimulation (DBS) has supplanted these irreversible surgical procedures. DBS evolved from observing the effects of electrical stimulation of deep brain loci when identifying the correct position of coagulant electrodes for these ablative procedures. Deep brain stimulators consist of the microelectrodes implanted in specific brain areas connected, with subcutaneously tunneled wires, to impulse generators located under the skin in the chest or abdomen. The impulse generators send electrical impulses to the microelectrodes, which alters the spontaneous neural discharges in these areas. The Food and Drug Administration (FDA) first approved thalamic DBS in 1997 for tremor, and globus pallidus internus (GPi) and subthalamic nucleus (STN) in 2003 for PD.[4] DBS has emerged as the treatment of choice in adults for the treatment of PD refractory to medical therapy. Fasano and Lozano reported that currently more than 100,000 patients have undergone DBS surgery.

As opposed to pallidotomy, DBS is less destructive of brain tissue, is associated with fewer cognitive and motor side effects, and is reversible and adjustable.[6]

More recently, DBS has also been found to be effective for the treatment of medically refractory dystonia, which frequently becomes symptomatic in childhood or early adolescence.[7] Dystonia is a syndrome of sustained muscle contractions producing twisting and repetitive movements or abnormal postures often resulting in simultaneous contraction of both agonist and antagonist muscles. Voluntary movement is often spastic and painful. Dystonias are classified as either primary (idiopathic) or secondary. Primary dystonia occurs without other neurological signs and without magnetic resonance imaging (MRI) evidence of brain abnormalities. Secondary dystonia is associated with a definable lesion in the CNS caused by stroke, cerebral palsy, encephalopathies, or neurodegenerative diseases. These are usually associated with abnormal brain images as seen on MRI or with a known history of major central nervous system (CNS) injury.[8] Primary dystonias can be generalized (primary generalized dystonia), segmental (affecting adjoining parts of the body), or focal (affecting one muscle or muscle group).[9] Primary dystonias are often hereditary. The best-known gene locus is the *DYT1* (also referred to as *TOR1A*), where a three-base pair deletion is responsible for approximately 30% of juvenile-onset primary generalized dystonias.[10] Medical management includes levodopa, trihexyphenidyl, baclofen, botulinum toxin injections, and others. Treatment of secondary dystonia with trihexyphenidyl has had mixed results. Irritability, sedation, and constipation have all been dose-limiting factors of trihexyphenidyl therapy. Botulinum toxin is useful for focal dystonias but has time-limited effectiveness, requiring repeated injections.[11]

Intrathecal baclofen (ITB) is a treatment option for both dystonia and spasticity in the pediatric population.[12] Baclofen is a gamma-aminobutyric acid (GABA) agonist that is thought to affect neurons in the spinal nerve roots and cortex. Oral baclofen does not adequately cross the blood-brain barrier and thus is often administered directly into cerebrospinal fluid (CSF), either as a bolus or as a continuous infusion, via a pump. Secondary dystonias tend to respond well to ITB therapy, while primary dystonias do not.[9] The incomplete efficacy of ITB and other drug regimens when treating dystonia and the successful use of DBS in PD led investigators to try DBS for the treatment of dystonia in the pediatric population.

In 2003, the Activa DBS (Medtronic, Minneapolis, MN) device was granted limited FDA approval in the United States for primary generalized and segmental dystonia, in patients ages 7 years or greater, under the humanitarian device exemption (HDE).[10] Both the GPi and STN targets were included in the HDE labeling.

The basal ganglia, specifically the globus pallidus, play an important role in dystonia. Electrophysiological recordings in the GPi of humans with primary dystonia show abnormal oscillatory discharge patterns.[10] This finding coupled with the successful reductions of dystonic muscle spasms with pallidotomy in PD patients has led to the targeting of the GPi for DBS microelectrode implantation. The GPi is by far the most targeted site for the placement of DBS with few studies targeting the STN.[3-14]

Most major surgical centers require patients to meet several criteria to be considered for DBS: (1) unequivocal diagnosis of primary or secondary dystonia; (2) failure to manage dystonia with anticholinergic, antiepileptic, benzodiazepines, baclofen, or, in patients with focal or segmental dystonia, treatment failure after injection of botulinum toxin; (3) significant disability, despite optimal medical management. Standardized rating scales are used to accurately assess clinical outcomes. The most commonly used rating scale for generalized dystonia is the Burke-Fahn-Marsden Dystonia Rating Scale (BFMDRS)[15,16] and for cervical dystonia is the Toronto Western Spasmodic Torticollis Rating Scale (TWSTRS).[17] Reviews and meta-analyses of several studies have examined the efficacy of DBS in the treatment of primary dystonia with and without the *DYT1* mutation.[18] Almost all studies have reported improvement with DBS, but the degree of improvement has varied widely across studies, ranging from 21% to 95% improvement in the BFMDRS movement score, with most studies showing 60% to 70% improvement.[3,5,10,11,14] For example, Vidailhet et al. studied 22 patients with primary generalized dystonia. The patients were evaluated preoperatively, and at 3, 6, and 12 months postoperatively. A mean improvement of 54% in the BFMDRS movement score was seen at 12 months with chronic stimulation. At 3 months, patients underwent videotaped double-blind evaluations in the presence and absence of neurostimulation on alternate days. When stimulated, patients showed a statistically significant mean improvement of 29% in the BFMDRS movement score, compared with the unstimulated condition.[19]

Several authors have reported long-term improvement of patients with primary dystonia who were treated with DBS of the GPi. Vidailhet et al. reported that in a 3-year follow-up study, their previously reported 22 patients continued to show mean improvement in BFMDRS movement scores of 58%.[20] Others have also reported long-term improvement for as long 10 years after surgery.[9,21-23] Goto et al. and Hebb et al. reported on cases where after several years of treatment the DBS was stopped without any deterioration in clinical benefit in cervical or cranial dystonia.[24,25]

The benefits of GPi DBS in primary dystonia are well documented, while the benefits in patients with secondary dystonia are less certain. Meta-analysis performed by Holloway et al. identified three factors associated with outcomes of DBS for dystonia: etiology of dystonia, duration of dystonia, and nucleus stimulated.[14] Several studies found significantly better outcomes in patients with primary dystonia than in those with secondary dystonia.[4,10,14] Patients with long-standing dystonia with fixed skeletal deformities can have limited functional improvement with DBS, even when dystonia symptoms are ameliorated.[26] Placement of DBS in the GPi showed overall better patient outcomes than those with DBS placed in the VLp of the thalamus.[27] In a more recent review, Fasano and Lozano expanded the list of predictors of surgical outcome to include etiology, brain MRI, body site, genetic status, phenomenology, duration of dystonia, implanted site, type of surgery, target, and energy delivered with stimulation.[5] Interestingly, Marks et al.[11] and Air et al.[7] noted that while patients with secondary dystonia (particularly cerebral palsy) showed less impressive responses to DBS, the caregivers reported meaningful benefits despite small absolute changes in rating scale scores. Traditional dystonia scales may not be able to distinguish small but meaningful improvements in levels of function that are important in this patient population.

The body of evidence has definitively demonstrated the value of DBS in the treatment of movement disorders as originally seen in adults with PD and more recently in patients of all ages with dystonia. As the duration of dystonia has been significantly correlated to outcomes, placing DBS in pediatric patients is becoming more commonplace. Surgical placement of DBS in the pediatric population presents substantial anesthetic challenges. The remainder of this chapter focuses on the techniques employed to overcome these challenges.

Anesthetic Considerations

There is currently no consistent agreement in the literature as to which anesthetic technique should be used for DBS surgery. The technique used varies according to institutional practices and has included monitored anesthesia care with nerve blocks or local anesthesia, conscious sedation, and general anesthesia. Currently, none of the anesthetic techniques for DBS insertion has produced significantly superior outcomes over the others.[7,10,14] However, several studies report that general anesthesia diminishes the microelectrode recordings (MERs) used to fine-tune the localization of the optimal site for placement of the DBS electrodes, as targeted using coordinates obtained with MRI.[28] Hutchinson found the firing rates in GPi were substantially decreased and long pauses were noted in patients with dystonia receiving general anesthesia, with propofol, compared to those mapped under local anesthesia.[29] The effect of propofol on GPi firing rates may be explained by the high density of GABA receptors in this region. Propofol has been reported to have a high affinity for GABA receptors in the GPi.[30–32] Several reports also recommend avoiding the use of benzodiazepines, due to their high affinity for GABA receptors and relatively long duration of action. They have been shown to significantly diminish MERs in the GPi.[32,33]

Conversely, Pinsker et al.[34] reported excellent results in a fairly large series where they implanted 86 DBS electrodes in 42 patients (reoperation in two patients) under general anesthesia with intravenous (IV) propofol and remifentanil. They did not report any diminution of MER due to general anesthesia. Further, they reported an average motor improvement from baseline of 64.72%

(range = 20.39–98.52%) as assessed by either the BFMDRS or the TWSTRS at the final patient follow-up greater than 1 year after implantation. These results compare well with the results noted by Holloway et al. in their meta-analysis.[14] Sanghera et al.[35] studied the effects of general anesthesia with desflurane in 11 pediatric patients with dystonia. They found no differences between awake and anesthetized patients with respect to GPi nuclei firing rates.

The previous studies notwithstanding, a substantially greater number of reports on DBS surgery employ monitored anesthetic care with local anesthesia. Of the drugs studied, dexmedetomidine has emerged as the drug of choice for awake craniotomies during DBS placement in both adult and pediatric populations.[3,6,11,14,28,29,31–33,36–38] Dexmedetomidine is a potent, highly selective α-2-adrenoreceptor agonist, acting at the subcortical regions of the brain, specifically within the locus ceruleus. Efferent neurons within the locus ceruleus release norepinephrine (NE), which stimulates wakefulness and arousal. The α-2-adrenoreceptors are present in the presynaptic membranes and inhibit the release of NE. By inhibiting the release of NE from the locus ceruleus, dexmedetomidine produces sedation that closely simulates natural sleep. While patients are well sedated, they can be easily aroused intraoperatively during DBS testing. Dexmedetomidine does not interact with GABA receptors and therefore doesn't alter MERs within the GPi. Koroglu et al.[38] compared the sedative, hemodynamic, and respiratory effects of dexmedetomidine to those of propofol in children undergoing MRI. Onset of sedation was significantly faster with propofol, but dexmedetomidine produced less hemodynamic changes and had significantly less respiratory depression. Propofol frequently produced brief periods of apnea and oxygen desaturation. This was very rare with dexmedetomidine. Respiratory effects seen with dexmedetomidine were usually due to the bolus being given too rapidly. Dexmedetomidine is therefore an excellent medication for use in "awake" anesthesia for DBS placement. With this in mind, the remainder of this chapter is devoted to the technique of "awake anesthesia" as practiced at my hospital (Cook Children's Medical Center [CCMC] in Fort Worth, TX).

Anesthesia for "Awake" DBS Placement: The CCMC Way

The overall surgical experience for the patient and their family can be divided into three basic time frames. These are (1) the preoperative evaluation and patient preparation; (2) day of surgery procedures including IV access, head frame placement and MRI scan, and DBS placement and testing; and (3) pulse generator implantation (typically occurs a few weeks after the electrode placement).

Patient Selection, Preoperative Evaluation, and Patient Preparation

Patient selection is critical to successful implantation. Risks and benefits should be weighed, and all alternatives, especially less invasive ones, must be considered. The use of DBS in primary genetic dystonias, especially *DYT1*, is now well accepted as a treatment option. There is now good experience with children in several institutions. Patients selected as candidates for DBS surgery undergo extensive neuropsychological assessment. The patients and their parents are provided with all the information necessary to making an informed decision about DBS placement.

The value of preoperative patient preparation and perioperative support is extremely important. Child life specialists or specially trained psychologists can teach the patients relaxation and stress management strategies. These include imagery, biofeedback, and distraction. Studies have found that child life preparation significantly reduced children's anxiety throughout the perioperative period. Further, anxiety scores were reportedly reduced for up to 1 month postoperatively.[39–41] At CCMC, a child life specialist meets with the patients and their families during the preoperative visit. The child life specialist then accompanies the patient throughout the surgery providing emotional support. This improves the likelihood that the patient can be successfully maintained under minimal anesthesia during the critical lead placement using MER, and allows for postplacement motor testing.

In addition to the preoperative preparation, the patient receives a thorough preanesthetic evaluation. Past medical and surgical histories are obtained and pertinent labs are drawn (typically complete blood count (CBC), basic metabolic panel, and coagulation studies). The anesthesiologist works closely with the child life specialist to help reduce the patient's (and the patient's family's) anxiety over the upcoming surgery. In institutions without child life services, the perioperative nursing staff and the anesthesia team can perform many of the preparation techniques.[39]

Day of Surgery

Induction, Head Frame Placement, and MRI Scan

On the day of surgery, the patient is met by the child life specialist and brought to a preoperative preparation room, where all the standard surgical paperwork and identification procedures are completed and surgical consents are signed. Older, cooperative patients have their IV started at this time. For younger or nervous patients, the IV is not started until they are in the operating room (OR). Typically, no preoperative medication is given and, as noted earlier, midazolam in particular is avoided owing to its significant inhibition of MERs in the GPi. However, if a patient is significantly upset intranasal dexmedetomidine (1 mcg/kg) can be given as a preoperative medication. Yuen et al.[42] compared the effects of intranasal dexmedetomidine and oral midazolam for premedication. They found no significant differences in parental separation acceptance, behavior scores at induction, and wake-up behavior scores. They noted that the dexmedetomidine treated patients were significantly more sedated at induction than the midazolam patients.

The patient is brought to the OR by the circulating nurse and the child life specialist. Here the IV is started (if needed) and head frame placed. All standard monitors are placed and the patient is initially sedated with inhalational N_2O for the IV placement. Once the IV is secured, the N_2O is discontinued and a bolus dose of dexmedetomidine (0.5–1 mcg/kg) is infused over 10 minutes, followed by a continuous infusion of 0.2–0.7 mcg/kg/hr. We avoid the use of anticholinergic drugs due to concerns their use combined with dexmedetomidine may cause significant hypertension and tachycardia. In addition, the first dose of vancomycin (10 mg/kg) is infused over 30 minutes. In order to reduce the discomfort associated with the placement of the head frame, a modified scalp block is performed (see Chapter 6). A complete scalp block involves regional anesthesia to the nerves that innervate the scalp, including the greater and lesser occipital nerves, the supraorbital and supratrochlear nerves, the zygomaticotemporal nerves, the auriculotemporal nerves, and the greater auricular nerves. Figure 9.1 is an anatomic representation of the nerve distribution in the scalp. Pinosky et al.[43] found that performing a scalp block significantly reduced the hemodynamic response to head

(a)

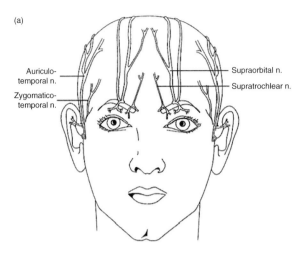

(b)

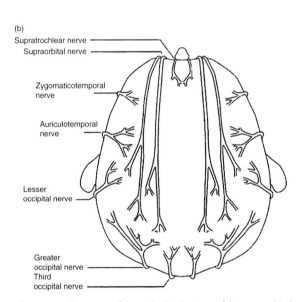

Figure 9.1. Illustration of the scalp distributions of the supraorbital, supratrochlear, and greater and lesser occipital nerves. Anterior view (a) and cephalad view (b). Performing a field block of these nerves provides for excellent anesthesia at the pin insertion areas of the stereotactic head frame. Source: Pinosky et al., The effect of bupivacaine skull block on the hemodynamic response to craniotomy, *Anesth Analg.* 1996;**83**:1256–61.

pinning in anesthetized patients. The modified scalp block involves the supraorbital and supratrochlear nerves anteriorly and the greater and lesser occipital nerves posteriorly. The supraorbital and supratrochlear nerves are blocked with 2 mL of 0.2% ropivicaine, on each side, as they emerge from the supraorbital notch. A 23-gauge needle is inserted approximately 1 cm lateral to the foramen and

advanced in a medial direction to avoid entering the foramen. The greater and lesser occipital nerves are blocked with a field block using 5 mL of 0.2% ropivicaine. A 22-gauge spinal needle is inserted approximately halfway between the occipital protuberance and the mastoid process and then advanced laterally along the nuchal line while injecting the ropivicaine. In our experience, this modified scalp block is very effective in reducing the discomfort associated with the head frame. In addition, our patients tend to report less postoperative headache associated with the head frame. As an added measure the scalp areas where the frame pins will be located are infiltrated locally with 2–3 mL of 0.5% bupivacaine. In fact, we use this as an indicator of the effectiveness of the scalp block. With an effective scalp block the patients do not respond to the needle stick or local injection. Because of its rapid onset and short duration of action, small boluses of propofol (0.5–1 mg/kg) can be given to more heavily sedate the patient during the scalp block and head frame placement. At CCMC we have found that preforming the scalp block and placing the head frame are more easily accomplished if the patient is propped up in a seated position. In fact, we routinely perform this part of the surgery in a wheelchair (Figure 9.2).

Prior to the placement of the head frame, a nasal cannula is placed on the patient in case supplemental O_2 is needed. Once the head frame is properly positioned and secured, the patient is placed on an MRI compatible stretcher and transported to the MRI scanner. Some institutions place a urinary catheter. We elect to not place urinary catheters in order to reduce the discomfort associated with them. Intravenous fluids are restricted to a standard maintenance infusion, trying to avoid the discomfort of bladder distension. At CCMC the above is performed on the surgical side of an intraoperative MRI suite and the patient is then taken to the diagnostic side where the MRI scan is performed to verify the GPi target coordinates in relation to the stereotactic head frame (Figure 9.3 shows the stealth MRI image of the DBS target coordinates). Our experience has led us to continue the dexmedetomidine infusion (0.2–0.7 µg/kg/hr) throughout the MRI scan and during the subsequent transport to the OR.

DBS Placement in the Operating Room

In the OR the patient is placed on the OR table in the recumbent position and made as comfortable as possible. The final target coordinates are calculated by the

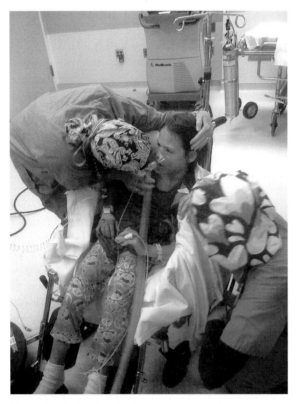

Figure 9.2. Patient breathing N₂O in preparation for IV start and scalp block. At our institution, the scalp blocks and head frame placement are routinely performed with the patient sitting in a wheelchair.

neurologist and the trajectory planned. During this time the child life specialist may employ strategies such as movies, music, books, and other distractions to keep the patient relaxed. During this time the dexmedetomidine can be continued at the same rate or can be reduced or turned off. This can be determined by how comfortable and calm the patient is. Figure 9.4 shows the patient watching a movie she had previously selected for the OR. However, for the majority of our patients, we prefer to continue the dexmedetomidine infusion until the optimal MERs are localized. At that time the infusion is discontinued so the patient will be alert enough for functional testing.

For dystonia cases, bilateral GPi are targeted, with careful attention to the planned entry point and trajectory. Major vessels and ventricles, as well as the eloquent brain areas are noted on the scan and avoided. Once the coordinates are verified, the head frame is attached to the bed, with the head slightly flexed. Care is taken to ensure the patient is comfortable and the shoulders are supported. Once the head frame is attached to the bed the patient has limited mobility. The patient is prepped and the scalp is injected with a combination of lidocaine/bupivacaine along the incision line. Again, this injection is supplemental to the previously performed scalp block. If the

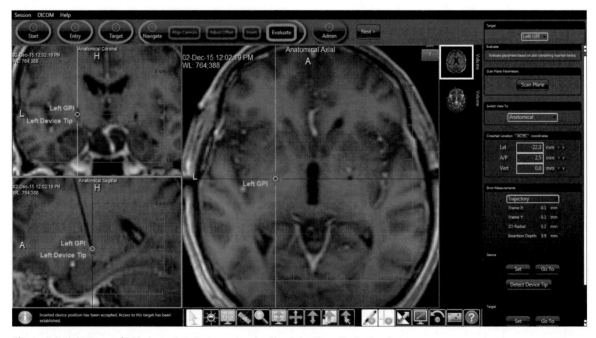

Figure 9.3. iMRI image of DBS electrode trajectory using the ClearPoint NeuroNavigation System.

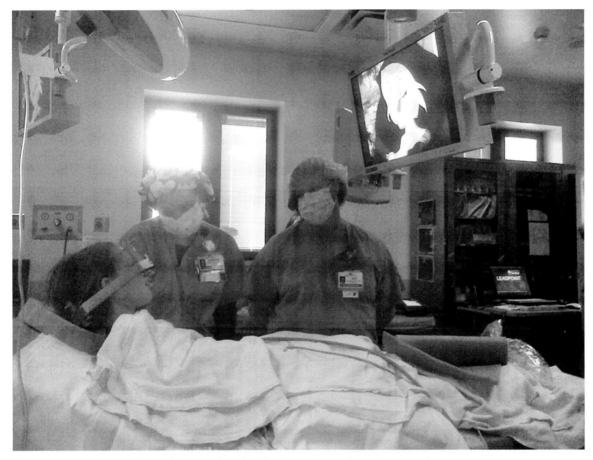

Figure 9.4. Patient comfortably watching a movie in the OR with the stereotactic head frame applied.

scalp block is adequate, the patient should have no response to the local infiltration of local anesthetic. Fluoroscopic x-ray is positioned. A transparent drape is used for the surgical field, so the surgeon can observe the patient while operating. The stereotactic arc is then attached to the head frame and all components are for proper fit. A large incision is made behind the hairline. The X, Y, and Z coordinates are then double checked to ensure the arc is accurate. Both burr holes are then made. At this time, an additional bolus of propofol (0.5–1.0 mg/kg) is given, in addition to the dexmedetomidine infusion, to diminish the patient's response to the drilling of the burr holes. This isn't particularly painful, but can be disturbingly loud for the patient. In addition, some authors suggest that opioid narcotics can reduce anxiety and discomfort during this time.[3] However, it has been our experience that opioids do not significantly improve the patients' comfort and, especially in CP

patients with secondary dystonia, can cause significant respiratory depression and desaturations. This often requires airway support consisting of measures ranging from simple chin lift to mask ventilation. Usually, the desaturations were short-lived and did not require endotracheal intubation or laryngeal mask airway (LMA) placement. In our initial trial of 18 surgeries on 16 patients we had to convert only one very young patient with dystonia secondary to CP to general anesthesia.[11]

Once the burr holes are made, no more propofol is given, until after the electrodes are secured, as it can attenuate the MERs. The dura is punctured and a microneedle is passed to the appropriate depth using a micro-driver system. The microneedle records the firing patterns of neurons in the GPi. When the correct location is found, the needle is removed, and the stimulating electrode is placed. If this is unsuccessful, we ensure the patient is not oversedated. If so,

71

the recordings improve with time by decreasing the dexmedetomidine infusion. If this is unsuccessful, a new pass with the microneedle is made, in a different trajectory, until satisfactory MERs are localized. In our series, Marks et al.[11] reported a maximum of 3 passed on one side, with an average of 1.6 passes on the right and 1.2 passes on the left. Usually, the right side was performed first, and adjustments were made on the trajectories, reducing the number of passes needed on the left. Once the electrode is placed it is then connected to an external generator, and the patient is tested for any improvement by checking tone in the leg or arm and watching for side effects (Figure 9.5). Once an acceptable response is obtained, the electrode is secured at the burr hole, and a fluoroscopic x-ray is performed to confirm that the electrode did not move while securing. The process is then repeated on the opposite side.

After the electrodes are secured the patient no longer needs to be conscious for the remainder of the surgery. General anesthesia is induced with propofol (2 mg/kg) and fentanyl (2 μg/kg) and an LMA is placed. Bilateral breath sounds are auscultated to ensure proper placement of the LMA. Because the patient's head is immobilized in the head frame and sterilely draped, the LMA is particularly well suited for airway management once the patient is under general anesthesia. The ends of the electrodes are then tunneled under the scalp galea to just above and behind the ear. Leads from both electrodes are tunneled down the same side of the neck, typically on the right side. After irrigation with antibiotic solution, the incision is closed. Early in our experience we would proceed with the implantation of the pulse generator immediately after placement of the electrodes. However, in order to reduce the risk of

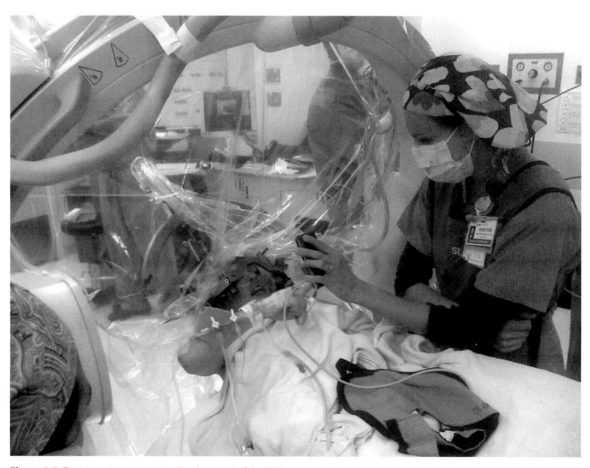

Figure 9.5. Testing motor response to the placement of the DBS.

postoperative infection, we now implant the pulse generator as a separate procedure a few weeks later.

Postoperatively, the patient has a computed tomography (CT) scan to ensure there is no intracranial bleeding or other complications. If no complications are found on CT, the patient is taken to the postanesthesia care unit to recover from the anesthetic. The patient is then admitted to the floor and discharged home less than 2 days later. Some patients experience improvement in their dystonic symptoms even without having the pulse generator implanted. This is thought to be a result of micro lesions created by the implanting of the DBS electrode and tends to be short-lived.[11]

Implantable Generator Placement

The implanting of the pulse generator (a few weeks later) does not involve craniotomy and requires no neuromonitoring. Therefore, this procedure can be performed effectively under standard general anesthesia, with no limitations as to the drugs used.

Potential Complications

The rate of intraoperative complications during DBS surgery varies widely with different studies. Overall, perioperative complications have been reported to occur in 12% to 16% of patients. Intraoperative respiratory complications have been reported to occur in 1.6% to 2.2% of patients.[30,32] Respiratory complications are usually related to sedation causing transient or significant hypoxemia, hypercarbia, or apnea. Stopping or decreasing the sedation, repositioning the head, or providing airway control is usually sufficient to alleviate most respiratory problems. Dexmedetomidine has been shown to produce significantly less respiratory depression than propofol.[38] It is imperative to have a means to control the airway readily available that can be used for airway access and ventilation in emergency situations. As the head is secured in a head frame that is fixed to the OR table, endotracheal intubation may prove extremely difficult. Therefore, an appropriately sized LMA should be available for emergency airway management.

Hypotension is also a potential problem, especially in the pediatric population, which may cause decreased cerebral perfusion. Dexmedetomidine can cause transient hypotension and bradycardia if given too rapidly. Fluid resuscitation will often improve the hypotension.

Venous air embolism (VAE) is a rare but dangerous complication with a reported incidence of 1.3% to 4.5%.[3] The classic sign of VAE is a sudden onset of coughing. Treatment of VAE is supportive and involves flooding the surgical field with saline, lowering the head of the bed to below the level of the heart, and applying bone wax to any exposed bone.

The most common neurological complications were intracranial hemorrhage (ICH) or seizure, having a reported incidence of 0.9% to 5%.[3,32] The severity of ICH can range from asymptomatic bleeds discovered on postoperative imaging to large hemorrhages requiring termination of surgery and causing permanent disabilities.[28] The number of MER passes and trajectories is positively related to the incidence of ICH.

Finally, postoperative infection had been the most prevalent complication having incidence rates of 5% to 33%. Pediatric patients had higher reported rates than their adult counterparts.[3,11] The higher incidence in children was primarily noted in children with significant neurological impairment. The reasoning for this is currently speculative. Infection management usually involves total or partial removal of the hardware and a regimen of antibiotics before reimplantation of the DBS. As mentioned earlier, infection concerns prompted our team to delay generator implantation for 2 to 3 weeks after electrode placement.

Advances in DBS Technology

Clinical outcome in DBS surgery is critically dependent on precise lead placement in the GPi. As discussed in this chapter, the most commonly used technique involves physiological localization while patients are "awake," with some reports of general anesthesia. "Awake" anesthesia is a very labor- and personnel-intensive process, especially with pediatric patients. To address these issues, Starr et al.[44] have developed methods for implanting DBS leads using real-time interventional MRI guidance in conjunction with a skull-mounted aiming device (ClearPoint NeuroNavigation System, MRI Interventions, Inc., Irvine, CA) (Figure 9.6). The precision afforded by this technique does not require input from an awake patient. The reported use of this device was associated with extremely high accuracy and excellent clinical outcomes. In addition, Martin et al.[45] reported that infection risk with this technique was comparable to

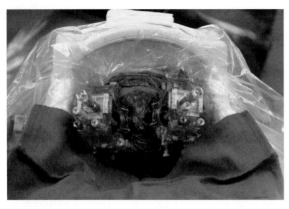

Figure 9.6. ClearPoint NeuroNavigation System with bilateral skull-mounted SmartFrame trajectory guides. Reprinted with permission from MRI Interventions, Inc., Wendelin Maners, VP.

that reported for large series of DBS electrodes implanted in a regular OR environment. At CCMC, we have placed DBS electrodes using the ClearPoint NeuroNavigation System with excellent outcomes. In addition, our postoperative infection rate has been noticeably less than seen with the "awake" technique in the regular OR.

From an anesthetic standpoint, since this technique uses real-time anatomical targeting and does not require any physiological testing, the procedure can be performed under general anesthesia without any restrictions to any medications normally used in pediatric anesthesia. Regardless of the anesthetic techniques used, the general principles of anesthesia care remain the same. The anesthesiologist needs to be aware of the unique requirements of these patients and of these procedures. Continuous monitoring and extreme vigilance are vital to early diagnosis and rapid treatment of complications in order to provide for a safe, comfortable surgical experience.

References

1. Rossi U. The history of electrical stimulation of the nervous system for the control of pain. In: Simpson BA, ed. *Electrical Stimulation and the Relief of Pain.* Amsterdam: Elsevier; 2003:5–16.

2. Sironi VA. Origin and evolution of deep brain stimulation. *Front Integr Neurosci.* 2011;8:42:1–5.

3. Osborn IP, Kurtis SD, Alterman RL. Functional neurosurgery: anesthetic considerations. *Int Anesthesiol Clin.* 2015;53(1):39–52.

4. Rekriwal A, Baltuch G. Deep brain stimulation: expanding applications. *Neurol Med Chir (Tokyo).* 2015;55:861–77.

5. Fasano A, Lozano A. Deep brain stimulation for movement disorders: 2015 and beyond. *Curr Opin Neurol.* 2015;28(4):423–36.

6. Sebeo J, Deiner SG, Alterman RL, Osborn IP. Anesthesia for pediatric deep brain stimulation. *Anesthesiol Res Pract.* 2010;2010:401419.

7. Air EI, Ostrem JA, Sanger TD, Starr PA. Deep brain stimulation in children: experience and technical pearls. *J Neurosurg Pediatrics.* 2011;8:566–74.

8. Fahn S, Bressman SB, Marsden CD. Classification of dystonia. *Adv Neurol.* 1998;78:1–10.

9. DiFrancesco MF, Halpern CH, Hurtig HH, Baltuch GH, Heur GG. Pediatric indications for deep brain simulation. *Childs Nerv Syst.* 2012;28:1701–14.

10. Ostrem JL, Starr PA. Treatment of dystonia with deep brain stimulation. *Neurotherapeutics.* 2008;5:320–30.

11. Marks WA, Honeycutt J, Acosta F, Reed M. Deep brain stimulation for pediatric movement disorders. *Semin Pediatr Neurol.* 2009;16:90–8.

12. Pin TW, McCartney L, Lewis L, Waugh MC. Use of intrathecal baclofen therapy in ambulant children and adolescents with spacity and dystonia of cerebral origin: a systematic review. *Dev Med Child Neurol.* 2011;53(11):1065.

13. Zhang JG, Zhang K, Wang ZC, Ge M, Ma Y. Deep brain stimulation in the treatment of secondary dystonia. *Chin Med J.* 2006;119:2069–74.

14. Holloway KL, Baron MS, Brown R, Cifu DX, Carne W, Ramakaishnan V. Stimulation for dystonia: a meta-analysis. *Neuromodulation.* 2006;4:253–61.

15. Burke RE, Fahn S, Marsden CD, Bressman SB, Maskowitz C, Friedman J. Validity and reliability of a rating scale for the primary torsion dystonias. *Neurology.* 1985;35:73–7.

16. Comella CL, Leurgans S, Wuu J, Stebbins GT, Chmura T. Dystonia Study Group. Rating scales for dystonia: a multicenter assessment. *Mov Disord.* 2003;18:303–12.

17. Comella CL, Stebbins GT, Chmura TA, Bressman SB, Lang AF. Teaching tape for the motor section of the Toronto Western Spasmotic Torticollis Scale. *Mov Disord.* 1997;12:570–5.

18. Lipsman N, Ellis M, Lozeno AM. Current and future indications for deep brain stimulation in pediatric populations. *Neurosurg Focus.* 2010;29(2):E2.

19. Vidailhet M, Vercueil L, Houeto JL, Krystkowiak P, Benabid AL, Cornu P, et al. Bilateral deep brain

stimulation of the globus pallidus in primary generalized dystonia. *N Engl J Med*. 2005;**352**:459–67.

20. Vidailhet M, Vercueil L, Houeto JL, Krystkowiak P, Lagrange C, Yelnik J, et al. Bilateral deep brain stimulation in primary generalized dystonia: a prospective 3 year follow-up study. *Lancet Neurol*. 2007;**6**:223–9.

21. Coubes P, Cif L, El Fertit H, Hemm S, Vayssiere N, Serrat S, et al. Electrical stimulation of the globus pallidus internus in patients with primary generalized dystonia: long-term results. *J. Neurosurg*. 2004;**101**: 189–94.

22. FitzGerald JJ, Rosendal F, de Pennington N, Joint C, Forrow B, Fletcher C, et al. Long-term outcome of deep brain stimulation in generalized dystonia: a series of 60 cases. *J Neurol Neurosurg Psychiatry*. 2014;**85**:1371–8.

23. Chang EF, Schrock LE, Starr PA, Ostrem JL. Long-term benefit sustained after bilateral pallidal deep brain stimulation in patients with refractory tardive dystonia. *Stereotact Funct Neurosurg*. 2010;**88**:304–10.

24. Goto S, Yamada K. Long-term continuous bilateral pallidal stimulation produces stimulation independent relief of cervical dystonia. *J Neurol Neurosurg Psychiatry*. 2004;**75**:1506–7.

25. Hebb MO, Chiasson P, Lang AE, Brownstone RM, Mendez I. Sustained relief of dystonia following cessation of deep brain stimulation. *Mov Disord*. 2007;**22**:1958–62.

26. Eltahawy HA, Saint-Cyr J, Giladi N, Lang AE, Lozano AM. Primary dystonia is more responsive than secondary dystonia to pallidal interventions: outcome after pallidotomy or pallidal deep brain stimulation. *Neurosurgery*. 2004;**54**:613–21.

27. Starr PA, Turner RS, Rau G, Lindsey N, Heath S, Volz M, et al. Microelectrode-guided implantation of deep brain stimulators into the globus pallidus internus for dystonia: techniques, locations and outcomes. *J Neurosurg*. 2006;**104**:488–501.

28. Venkatraghavan L, Manninen P. Anesthesia for deep brain stimulation. *Curr Opin Anaesthesiol*. 2011;**24**: 495–9.

29. Hutchinson WD, Lang AE, Dostrovsky JO, Lozano AM. Pallidal neuronal activity: implications for models of dystonia. *Ann Neurol*. 2003;**53**:480–8.

30. Venkatraghaven L, Luciano M, Manninen P. Anesthetic management of patients undergoing deep brain stimulator insertion. *Anesth Analg*. 2010;**110**(4): 1138–45.

31. Schapf DT, Sharma M, Deogaonkar M, Rezai A, Bergese SD. Practical considerations and nuances in

anesthesia for patients undergoing deep brain stimulation implantation surgery. *Korean J Anesthesiol*. 2015;**68**:332–9.

32. Poon CC, Irwin MG. Anaesthesia for deep brain stimulation and in patients with implanted neurostimulator devices. *Br J Anaesth*. 2009;**103**: 152–65.

33. Chakrabarti R, Ghazanwy M, Tewari A. Anesthetic challenges for deep brain stimulation: a systematic approach. *N Am J Med Sci*. 2014;**6**(8):359–69.

34. Pinsker MO, Volkmann J, Falk D, Herzog J, Steigerwald F, Denschl G, Mehdorn AM. Deep brain stimulation of the internal globus pallidus in dystonia: target localization under general anaesthesia. *Acta Neurochir*. 2009;**151**:751–8.

35. Sanghera MK, Grossman RG, Kahorn CG, Hamilton WL, Ondo WG, Jankovic J. Basal ganglia neuronal discharge in primary and secondary dystonia in patients undergoing pallidotomy. *Neurosurgery*. 2003;**52**:1358–73.

36. Rozet I. Anesthesia for functional neurosurgery: the role of dexmedetomidine. *Curr Opin Anaesthesiol*. 2008;**21**:537–43.

37. Maurtua MA, Cata JP, Martirena M, Deogaonkar M, Rezi A, Sung W, et al. Dexmedetomidine for deep brain stimulator placement in a child with primary generalized dystonia: case report and literature review. *J Clin Anesth*. 2009;**21**:213–16.

38. Koroglu A, Teksan H, Sagir O, Yucel A, Toprak H, Ersoy O. A comparison of the sedative, hemodynamic and respiratory effects of dexmedetomidine and propofol in children undergoing magnetic resonance imaging. *Anesth Analg*. 2006;**103**:63–7.

39. Brewer S, Gleditsch SL, Syblik D, Tietjens ME, Vacik HW. Pediatric anxiety: child life intervention in day surgery. *J Pediatr Nurs*. 2006;**21**(1):13–22.

40. Sorensen HL, Card CA, Malley MT, Strzelecki JM. Using a collaborative child life approach for continuous surgical preparation. *AORN J*. 2009;**90**(4): 557–66.

41. Justus R, Wilson J, Walther V, Wyles D, Rode D, Lim-Sulit N. Preparing children and families for surgery: Mount Sinai's multidisciplinary perspective. *Pediatr Nurs*. 2006;**32**(1):35–43.

42. Yuen VM, Hui V, Irwin MG, Yuen MK. A comparison of intranasal dexmedetomidine and oral midazolam for premedication in pediatric anesthesia: a double-blind randomized controlled trial. *Anesth Analg*. 2008;**106**:1715–21.

43. Pinosky ML, Dorman RL, Reeves ST, Harvey SC, Patel S, Palesch Y, Dorman BH. The effect of bupivacaine skull block on the hemodynamic response to craniotomy. *Anesth Analg.* 1996;**83**:1256–61.

44. Starr PA, Markun LC, Larson PS, Volz MM, Martin AJ, Ostrem JL. Interventional MRI-guided deep brain stimulation in pediatric dystonia: first experience with the ClearPoint system. *J Neurosurg Pediat.* 2014;**14**:400–8.

45. Martin AJ, Larson PS, Ziman N, Levesque N, Volz M, Ostrem JL, Starr PA. Deep brain stimulator implantation in a diagnostic MRI suite: infection history over a 10-year period. *J Neurosurg.* 2017;**126**:108–13.

Anesthesia for Fetal Neurosurgery

Elaina E. Lin and Kha M. Tran

Introduction

Fetal Therapy

Intrauterine fetal surgery is a new and rapidly evolving discipline. During fetal surgery the mother is an "innocent bystander" as her fetus is treated. However, the mother must also receive medical care in the course of the fetal therapy, and both she and the fetus are at risk for complications. Some fetal surgical procedures are performed in a minimally invasive fashion, with small sheaths introduced percutaneously through the maternal abdomen and uterus, while other fetal procedures require a full maternal laparotomy, exposure of the uterus, and a maternal hysterotomy. In some cases, the procedures are done in the middle of gestation, and the goal is for the fetus to continue to heal and develop in utero. In other cases, a near-term fetus is delivered at the end of the fetal procedure.[1] As these procedures involve two high-risk populations, frank discussions of the risk and benefit are required. These situations are complex, and as such, fetal therapy is often offered only when the fetus is at risk of death. A variety of processes often end in a final common pathway of hydrops fetalis. The fetal diseases that may cause hydrops and that may be treated in utero are wide-ranging. Some examples include twin-twin transfusion syndrome, massive lung tumors, and sacrococcygeal teratoma.[2] While many types of fetal neurological pathology may be detected with high-level fetal ultrasound and fetal magnetic resonance imaging, the only candidates for fetal neurosurgical therapy thus far have included fetal hydrocephalus and myelomeningocele (MMC). The fetal neurosurgical patient is different from other fetal surgical patients since the treatable fetal neurosurgical lesion is rarely life-threatening. Since the fetus is not at immediate risk of demise, the risks and benefits must be even more carefully considered before undertaking fetal neurosurgical therapy.

Hydrocephalus

Treatment of hydrocephalus in the postnatal period commonly involves diversion of the cerebrospinal fluid (CSF) from the cerebral ventricles into the peritoneal cavity. In the fetus, the CSF can be diverted into the amniotic fluid with a valved catheter that prevents retrograde flow of the amniotic fluid into the ventricles. Between 1982 and 1985, 41 fetuses with hydrocephalus secondary to a variety of conditions were treated with ventriculoamniotic shunts between 23 to 33 weeks of gestation. These shunts can be placed percutaneously, in a manner similar to intrauterine blood transfusion. While there were 34 survivors, the postnatal outcomes of the treated fetuses were not as encouraging as hoped, with more than half of the survivors left with serious neurologic handicaps. Only 35% of the survivors were found to be developing normally at follow-up.[3] Between 1999 and 2003, fetal ventriculoamniotic shunting was attempted in an additional four fetuses. These shunts were placed in an "open" fashion, via a maternal laparotomy and hysterotomy. Outcomes of these fetuses were not encouraging either, and the authors concluded that without new developments in the field, fetal ventriculoamniotic shunting would not be likely to offer any benefits.[4] The treatment of fetal MMC has seen much more success than that of hydrocephalus, and the remainder of this chapter focuses on fetal neurosurgical therapy for MMC.

Myelomeningocele

MMC is a neural tube defect that currently affects 5–10 pregnancies per 10,000 in the United States.[5] With routine prenatal screening, these defects can be detected in utero. Early studies in animal models showed that closure of these defects in utero improved neurological outcomes.[6] Since the conclusion of the Management of Myelomeningocele Study (MOMS) trial, which demonstrated the benefits of prenatal compared to postnatal repair of MMC,[7] fetal repair of

MMC is now being offered at centers around the world. Performing fetal neurosurgery has unique maternal and fetal considerations. As the number of fetal procedures increases, understanding these unique considerations will be important for the anesthesiologist.

MMC develops in the 3rd and 4th weeks of gestation when the embryonic neural plate fails to close along its length. This results in an open spinal canal and exposure of the spinal cord to the amniotic compartment. Babies born with MMC require closure within the first few days of life, and many are faced with lifelong disabilities including motor and sensory dysfunction, bowel and bladder dysfunction, sexual dysfunction, cognitive delay, Arnold-Chiari type II malformation, hydrocephalus, and tethered cord. The degree of neurological dysfunction is associated with the level of the vertebral defect. Higher anatomic defects are therefore more neurologically significant than lower defects.

Studies suggest that nerve damage is progressive over time. The two-hit theory of nerve damage has been postulated in which the first hit is the failure of the neural tube to form correctly, and the second hit is the damage caused by continued exposure of the nerves to the uterine environment. Early animal studies demonstrated that fetal closure of MMC resulted in improved neurological outcomes, presumably by decreasing the duration of exposure of the nerves to the uterine environment.[6] The MOMS trial was a multicenter randomized prospective clinical trial designed to evaluate the safety and efficacy of in utero repair of MMC. In order to be eligible for the trial, fetuses had to be between 19 and 26 weeks gestational age, have an upper MMC border of T1–S1, be a singleton pregnancy, and have normal karyotype. Maternal body mass index (BMI) had to be < 35 kg/m^2. The study was stopped early for efficacy. It demonstrated that in-utero repair decreased the need for ventriculoperitoneal (VP) shunt by 12 months of age and improved motor outcomes at 30 months of age when compared to postnatal repair.[7] Longer term follow-up (median follow-up time of 10 years) of non-MOMS trial fetal MMC repair patients showed that there is long-term improvement of functional status.[8] However, fetal surgery is not without risk to both the mother and fetus. Therefore, the anesthesiologist must understand the maternal and fetal physiology (summarized in Tables 10.1 and 10.2) and perioperative management unique to this type of surgery.

Table 10.1 Maternal Physiologic Changes during Pregnancy

Physiologic Change	Clinical Implication
Cardiovascular	
Increased cardiac output, decreased systemic vascular resistance	Supine hypotension from aortocaval compression
Respiratory/airway	
Engorgement of airway mucosa	Potential difficult intubation; use smaller endotracheal tube
Increased oxygen consumption and decreased functional residual capacity	Decreased reserve
Gastrointestinal	
Displacement of stomach, decreased lower esophageal sphincter tone, delayed gastric emptying	Increased aspiration risk
Neurological	
Increased nerve sensitivity, reduced protein levels, pH changes in CSF	Increased sensitivity to volatile agents, non-depolarizing neuromuscular blockade, and epidural anesthetics

Table 10.1 (cont.)

Physiologic Change	Clinical Implication
Hematologic	
Increase in coagulation factors and fibrinolysis	Increased risk of thrombosis and disseminated intravascular coagulation
Plasma volume increases more than red cell volume	Anemia

Table 10.2 Fetal Physiological Development

Physiologic State	Clinical Implication
Cardiovascular	
Myocardium higher proportion of noncontractile elements	Cardiac output very dependent on heart rate, minimally responsive to preload
Uteroplacental blood flow related to uterine perfusion pressure (the difference between uterine arterial and uterine venous pressure) and inversely related to uterine vascular resistance	Maternal hypotension, aortocaval compression, and uterine contractions decrease uterine blood flow; effects of vasopressors, vasodilators, and neuroaxial and volatile anesthetic agents on uterine blood flow can be variable because they affect both uterine arterial pressure and uterine vascular resistance
Fetal oxygen delivery dependent on ratio of maternal to fetal blood flow, oxygen partial pressure gradient, respective hemoglobin concentrations and affinities, placental diffusing capacity, and acid-base status of fetal and maternal blood (Bohr effect)	Many factors can disrupt fetal oxygenation
Hematologic	
Blood volume per kg of weight higher than in adult; 2/3 of blood volume on placental side of fetoplacental unit	Need greater blood volume for euvolemia
Fetus produces own coagulation factors, plasma concentrations of coagulation factors increase with gestational age	Fetus more prone to hemorrhage
Temperature regulation	
Dependent on maternal temperature, cannot thermoregulate on own	Maintaining euthermia during open fetal surgery can be difficult; need to infuse normothermic solution of lactated ringers into amniotic cavity
Neurologic	
Neurologic pathways for cortex are developing into the third trimester	Anesthetic requirements for fetus less than that for child

Preoperative Assessment and Preparation

Preparation for fetal neurosurgery is a multidisciplinary endeavor, involving maternal fetal medicine specialists, pediatric surgeons, pediatric neurosurgeons, radiologists, neonatologists, anesthesiologists, psychologists, social workers, and nurses. A complete maternal workup including history and physical exam with specific attention paid to symptoms such as dyspnea, syncope, and dizziness that may indicate undiagnosed underlying morbidity and labs including complete blood count, coagulation panel, and type and cross for blood are warranted. Particular attention should be paid to the airway and spine exams.

A complete fetal workup including diagnostic imaging (both ultrasound and magnetic resonance imaging (MRI)) to determine location and extent of fetal lesion, testing to exclude other anomalies, and preparation of O-negative, leukocyte depleted, irradiated, CMV negative blood cross matched to the mother is needed. The cross match is needed as maternal antibodies to red blood cells can cross the placenta. The inclusion criteria at the authors' institution have changed slightly since the MOMS trial, and currently, in order to be eligible for the surgery, the fetus must meet the following criteria: upper level of MMC must be between T1 and S1 with hindbrain herniation, gestational age at time of surgery between 23 weeks and 25 weeks 6 days, singleton pregnancy, normal karyotype, elevated amniotic fluid alpha fetoprotein, positive acetylcholinesterase, and lack of other significant anomaly such as cardiac disease. Maternal exclusion criteria include the following: age less than 18 years old, insulin-dependent pregestational diabetes, cerclage or incompetent cervix, placenta previa, placental abruption, short cervix < 20 mm, BMI > 40 kg/m^2, previous spontaneous delivery at < 37 weeks, maternal-fetal Rh isoimmunization, Kell sensitization, or history of neonatal alloimmune thrombocytopenia, maternal HIV or hepatitis B or C, uterine anomaly, hypertension that would increase risk of preterm delivery, other maternal condition that would contraindicate surgery, inability to comply with follow-up requirements after surgery, and lack of support or failure to meet other psychosocial criteria. It is imperative that the family be extensively counseled so that they understand all the potential risks and benefits.

Anesthetic Management

Anesthetic management of open fetal surgery requires an integration of cognitive and manual skills from the worlds of both pediatric and obstetric anesthesia. As with any anesthetic, communication and teamwork are crucial. Also crucial is a full understanding of the technical aspects of the surgical procedure and the infrastructure of the fetal care center. Many conflicting needs must be balanced. Some of the issues include finding a balance between providing adequate fetal perfusion and optimal operating conditions and balancing the needs of anesthetizing two patients at the same time. Measures to combat an increased risk of pulmonary edema also make the task of providing adequate fluid resuscitation harder. These issues are highlighted as a typical anesthetic for fetal MMC repair is described.

On the day of surgery, prior to induction, the mother should have a high lumbar/low thoracic epidural placed for postoperative analgesia. The abdominal incision for the surgery is higher than the incision performed for a cesarean section. The epidural should be tested to evaluate for intrathecal or intravascular placement, but it should not be fully dosed until the end of the surgical procedure. The patients often get either high-dose volatile anesthetic or nitroglycerin to relax the uterus, and the sympathectomy caused by an epidural block will exacerbate intraoperative hypotension. Indomethacin is given for tocolysis. H$_2$ receptor blockade and nonparticulate antacid are given for aspiration prophylaxis.

The patient is brought into the operating suite and positioned supine with left uterine displacement. Standard American Society of Anesthesiologists (ASA) monitors are placed. After preoxygenation, a rapid sequence induction is performed, followed by oral intubation. A second intravenous line and an arterial line are placed. While blood loss is often quite low, the gravid uterus can be a source of catastrophic bleeding. The invasive measurement of blood pressure is warranted as vasopressors must be titrated in a patient receiving high-dose volatile anesthetics or nitroglycerin. A Foley catheter is placed and ultrasonography is used to confirm fetal position. A manual version of the fetus may be necessary to get the MMC in the proper position.

Anesthesia is maintained with volatile agent. Desflurane is usually used for quicker titratability, but isoflurane and sevoflurane have also been used.

Administration of high doses of volatile anesthetic has been alluded to previously. The need for profound uterine atony is a unique consideration for open fetal surgical cases. The lower the uterine tone, the lower the resistance to blood flowing from the maternal circulation, and the better the operating conditions. It is also postulated that lower uterine tone will decrease the risk of placental abruption. Following maternal skin incision and exposure of the uterus, the volatile agent is increased until the uterine tone is (subjectively) judged to be low enough by the surgical team. Greater than 2 minimum alveolar concentration (MAC) of volatile agent is often required before uterine incision. If needed, nitroglycerin, either as bolus or infusion, can be used to further relax the uterus. The high levels of volatile anesthetic and potential use of nitroglycerin may cause significant vasodilation and hypotension in the mother. At the authors' institution, fluid administration is often kept to less than 500 mL to decrease chances of pulmonary edema. In the face of this fluid restriction, maternal blood pressure is augmented with a phenylephrine infusion. Additional boluses of ephedrine and phenylephrine are given as needed. Maternal blood pressure is typically maintained within 10% of maternal baseline blood pressure. Exposing a fetus to volatile anesthetic can cause myocardial depression.[9,10] There is evidence from some centers that use of supplemental intravenous anesthesia (propofol and remifentanil), in addition to a lower dose of volatile agent (about 1 MAC volatile agent), may decrease fetal cardiac dysfunction and fetal acidosis.[11,12]

The edges of the placenta must be clearly identified by ultrasound before any uterine incision is made. When an appropriate site on the uterus has been identified, a small uterine incision is made and a stapling device is used to extend the hysterotomy while preventing bleeding by sealing the membranes to the decidua and myometrium. There can be significant bleeding at this point if the device misfires, given the vascularity of the uterus and the uterine atony, or if venous sinuses are encountered. Small infusion catheters are placed into the now open amniotic space to infuse warmed, lactated ringers solution to replete amniotic leakage and maintain fetal and umbilical cord buoyancy. An intramuscular injection of opioid (fentanyl 20 mcg/kg) and muscle relaxant (vecuronium 0.2 mg/kg) is administered to the fetus by the surgeons. Although the fetus is being anesthetized by the halogenated agent via placental transfer from the mother, the additional fentanyl and vecuronium can further decrease fetal stimulation and ensure immobility, optimizing surgical conditions. After the hysterotomy is complete, the fetus is positioned so that the MMC is exposed in the hysterotomy window (Figure 10.1). The neurosurgeon then repairs the MMC by exposing and separating the neural structures, closing the native dura over the spinal cord when possible, closing the paraspinal myofascial flaps, and then closing the skin, either with a primary closure (Figure 10.2a) or with an acellular human dermis graft (Figure 10.2b).

To maximize fetal outcome, it is important that the fetus be monitored during the procedure. The fetal myocardium is less compliant than adult myocardium, and thus the fetus is much more dependent on heart rate than preload to maintain fetal cardiac output. Fetal bradycardia is an ominous sign of fetal distress.

At our institution, continuous fetal echocardiography by a pediatric cardiologist scrubbed into the procedure is preferred, as this provides real-time assessment of fetal heart rate, cardiac function, and cardiac filling.[10] Other methods of fetal monitoring may include intraoperative ultrasound to monitor uterine artery flow and fetal heart rate. Fetal pulse oximetry is possible, but technically challenging, since usually only the MMC is exposed. Blood gas assessment is also possible, but performed only in extremely rare circumstances.

Fetal well-being depends on adequate cardiac performance and adequate uterine blood flow through the placenta as the interface between mother and fetus. As mentioned, high doses of volatile anesthetic may cause fetal cardiac depression. If this is suspected, volatile anesthetic levels should be decreased, while monitoring uterine tone. Nitroglycerin can be given to aid in uterine relaxation if needed when the volatile anesthetic is decreased. The surgical manipulation of the fetus, uterus, and umbilical cord can decrease placental flow to the fetus. If this is suspected, the umbilical cord should be examined to ensure that it is not compressed or kinked. If fetal hypovolemia is suspected due to fetal blood loss, fetal transfusion through the umbilical vein or through a fetal peripheral intravenous (IV) can be considered. In some cases of fetal distress, fetal resuscitation with intramuscular or intravascular drugs may be necessary and, in extreme cases, fetal chest compressions may be required. A peripheral IV is not routinely placed in

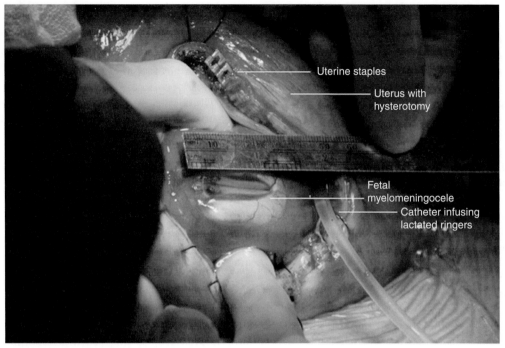

Figure 10.1. Fetal myelomeningocele is centered in the hysterotomy window. The defect is measured. Infusion catheters replace lost amniotic fluid with warmed lactated ringers solution.

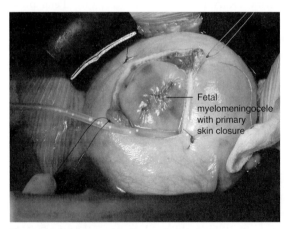

Figure 10.2a. Primary skin closure of myelomeningocele.

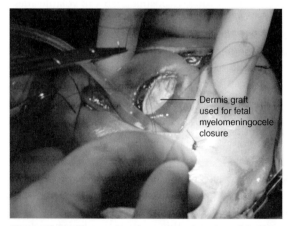

Figure 10.2b. Closure of myelomeningocele with acellular human dermis graft. Larger defects with insufficient skin for primary closure will require a graft.

the fetus, but an IV setup is primed and ready in the sterile field for use in the event of extreme fetal distress. If inadequate placental perfusion secondary to maternal hypotension or hypovolemia is suspected, increasing maternal blood pressure or maternal transfusion should be considered. The anesthesiologist must be vigilant in monitoring for fetal bradycardia, and fetal or maternal hemorrhage.

Once the MMC is repaired, the fetus is returned completely into the uterus and the uterus is closed. Magnesium sulfate is given intravenously for tocolysis with a 6-g load over 20 minutes followed by 4-g per hour infusion that is typically titrated off within 24 hours. Magnesium can cause muscle weakness and potentiate neuromuscular blockade, so special care must be taken to ensure that patients have sufficient strength to maintain respiratory effort postoperatively. Following closure of the hysterotomy, an omental flap is sewn over the hysterotomy to help prevent amniotic fluid leakage. As the magnesium bolus is nearing completion, the volatile agent can be decreased. Following maternal skin closure, neuromuscular blockade is reversed, and the mother is extubated once she is awake and protecting her airway. The epidural is dosed toward the end of the procedure to ensure adequate postoperative pain relief for the mother as well as decrease uterine irritability and contractility postoperatively.[13]

As previously mentioned, there is greater concern for maternal pulmonary edema following open fetal surgery than in other cases.[14] The use of tocolytics like magnesium sulfate and nitroglycerin can cause capillary leakage, thus increasing the risk of pulmonary edema. Some institutions opt to severely fluid restrict (<500 mL IV fluids intraoperatively), while other centers practice moderate fluid restriction (< 2 L IV fluids) in order to decrease incidence of pulmonary edema, but there are no clinical trials proving a benefit of fluid restriction. From an ethical standpoint, fetal surgery for MMC is unique in that the procedure offers no direct benefit to the mother while still carrying risk. Maternal safety is paramount. It is essential that the mothers understand the risks to themselves when providing informed consent.

The ability of a fetus to perceive pain is a controversial topic. It is clear that fetal procedures can elicit a stress response in fetuses as manifested by the release of stress hormones. A fetus can reflexively withdraw from a stimulus at 19 weeks. However, the perception of pain requires higher cortical activity, and it is unclear as to when the thalamic pain fiber pathways reach the cortex. Electroencephalographic studies show that cortical activities occur only 2% of the time in 24-week gestation fetuses. Therefore, it is unlikely that in the late second trimester, when these procedures take place, that fetuses experience pain in the way that adults perceive pain.[15,16]

Postoperative Concerns

For the first 24–48 hours following surgery, the mother and fetus are closely monitored. It is common for the uterus to have some contractions after the trauma of surgery, and tocodynamometry is used to monitor contractions. Tocolysis with IV magnesium is continued for 24 hours postoperatively. During magnesium tocolysis, the mother's level of consciousness, deep tendon reflexes, urine output, and serum magnesium concentrations are assessed. The mother is then transitioned to other tocolytics like nifedipine and/or indomethacin. Terbutaline has been used in the past. The mother is carefully monitored for symptoms of pulmonary edema in the first 48 hours. If this develops, the mother is treated with oxygen therapy, diuresis, and, if necessary, positive pressure ventilation. The mother is also monitored for any signs of infection, membrane separation, or wound dehiscence. Postoperative analgesia is managed with the epidural for the first 48 hours after surgery. Once the epidural is discontinued, and the patient is eating, the patient is transitioned to oral pain medications. Intravenous opioids can be used to supplement analgesia if needed.

Fetal well-being is monitored with ultrasound and fetal heart rate monitoring as needed. If there are signs of distress that cannot be alleviated in an otherwise viable fetus, an emergency cesarean section may be necessary. There should be an emergent delivery plan for all patients with the neonatology team immediately available to care for a very premature neonate.

If there are no complications in the immediate postoperative period, the mother can usually be discharged from the hospital in 3–5 days. After discharge, follow-up occurs at least weekly. In the first 3–4 weeks after discharge, the mother must remain on modified bed rest. After this period, the mother may gradually increase activity to a very light level. It is usually recommended that the patient remains in the area of the institution where the fetal surgery was performed for the duration of the pregnancy as the patient is considered high risk after open fetal surgery and few hospitals are experienced in management of these patients. Due to the large, often incompletely healed hysterotomy scar, the patient is at risk of uterine rupture, and if she goes into labor, the baby must be delivered by cesarean section. If the mother can stay pregnant until 37 weeks, the baby is delivered by a scheduled cesarean section. She should have blood typed and crossed for the procedure. Figure 10.3 depicts a child with a healed repair after delivery. Patients are counseled to not get pregnant again for at least 2 years after delivery of the child to decrease the chance of uterine rupture. All future deliveries will need to be by cesarean section.

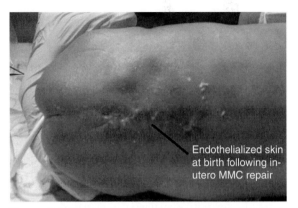

Endothelialized skin at birth following in-utero MMC repair

Figure 10.3. Near-term neonate after in utero myelomeningocele repair. Note-closed and endothelialized back at time of birth.

In the MOMS trial, the average gestational age at time of delivery after open fetal surgery was 34.1 weeks, with 13% of the patients delivering before 30 weeks' gestation. In contrast, the average gestational age at time of delivery of the postnatal repair group was 37.3 weeks, with none born before 30 weeks' gestation. In the prenatal repair group, there were two deaths, an intrauterine fetal demise detected at 26 weeks' gestation and a death at 23 weeks' gestation due to complications of extreme prematurity. In the postnatal repair group, there were also two deaths, both from complications of severe Arnold-Chiari II malformation. One-fifth of the prenatal repair group had symptoms of respiratory distress syndrome, secondary to premature birth. There were no maternal deaths, but complications included increased incidence of oligohydramnios, chorioamniotic separation, placental abruption, and spontaneous membrane rupture as compared to the control group. A third of the women were noted to have an area of dehiscence or area of very thin uterine scar at the time of the cesarean section.[7]

Fetal repair of MMC decreases the need for ventriculoperitoneal (VP) shunt placement by 1 year of age from 82% to 40%. Significant reversal of hindbrain herniation was also seen with no hindbrain herniation seen in 4% of the fetal repairs versus 36% of the postnatal repairs and 6% severe herniation seen in the fetal repair group versus 22% in the postnatal repair group. Of patients in the fetal repair group, 42% were able to walk independently at 30 months of life compared to 21% of postnatal repairs. Although these are certainly positive outcomes, neurological complications are also

possible after fetal surgery. In a patient population separate from the MOMS cohort, 30% of fetal MMC repair patients presented with symptomatic tethered cord syndrome at a median age of 27 months. Of those patients, 63% also had an associated intradural inclusion cyst. These patients required subsequent surgery to release the tethered cord and excise the cyst; however, some of these children did not regain bladder or lower extremity function despite surgery.[17,18] From clinical experience, the anesthetic considerations for subsequent neurosurgical procedures in the children who have had a prenatal repair are not significantly different from those for any other child undergoing similar procedures. The team should prepare for a potentially longer than usual surgery duration because of the scar tissue already present.

Future Directions

The future of fetal MMC repair will see growth in several areas, including surgical technique, patient selection criteria, and number of centers performing the procedure. Endoscopic fetal repair of MMC is being attempted on the premise that a minimally invasive approach may decrease recovery time and improve immediate and long-term morbidity for the mother.[19] However, one study reported that the endoscopic approach had higher rates of fetal mortality, premature rupture of membranes, chorioamnionitis, premature delivery, incomplete repair, and persistent hindbrain herniation when compared to the open fetal approach.[20] The minimally invasive approach continues to be studied in clinical trials, and the fetal therapy community continues to discuss the best options for mother and fetus.[21,22]

In addition, as more procedures are done, practitioners will become more comfortable relaxing patient eligibility criteria. This has already occurred with the change of the BMI exclusion cutoff from 35 to 40 kg/m^2. With relaxed criteria, the results of the MOMS trial may not be completely applicable, and outcomes for the newer populations must be evaluated.

For the time being, an open technique is the standard of care for fetal MMC repair. As additional centers begin to perform both open and endoscopic repair of MMC, they must develop the multidisciplinary expertise needed to keep mothers and fetuses safe. A MMC Maternal-Fetal Management Task Force has met to establish minimum criteria for centers performing fetal MMC repair to ensure optimal outcomes for both patients.[23]

References

1. Brusseau R, Mizrahi-Arnaud A. Fetal anesthesia and pain management for intrauterine therapy. *Clin Perinatol.* 2013;**40**(3):429–42.

2. Harrison MR. Fetal surgery. *Am J Obstet Gynecol.* 1996;**174**(4):1255–64.

3. Manning FA, Harrison MR, Rodeck C. Catheter shunts for fetal hydronephrosis and hydrocephalus. Report of the International Fetal Surgery Registry. *N Engl J Med.* 1986;**315**(5):336–40.

4. Bruner JP, Davis G, Tulipan N. Intrauterine shunt for obstructive hydrocephalus—still not ready. *Fetal Diagn Ther.* 2006;**21**(6):532–9.

5. Ferschl M, Ball R, Lee H, Rollins MD. Anesthesia for in utero repair of myelomeningocele. *Anesthesiology.* 2013;**118**(5):1211–23.

6. Meuli M, Meuli-Simmen C, Yingling CD, Hutchins GM, Timmel GB, Harrison MR, et al. In utero repair of experimental myelomeningocele saves neurological function at birth. *J Pediatr Surg.* 1996;**31**(3):397–402.

7. Adzick NS, Thom EA, Spong CY, Brock JW III, Burrows PK, Johnson MP, et al. A randomized trial of prenatal versus postnatal repair of myelomeningocele. *N Engl J Med.* 2011;**364**(11):993–1004.

8. Danzer E, Thomas NH, Thomas A, Friedman KB, Gerdes M, Koh J, et al. Long-term neurological outcome, executive functioning, and behavioral adaptive skills following fetal myelomeningocele surgery. *Am J Obstet Gynecol.* 2013;**208**(suppl 1):S183.

9. Rychik J, Tian Z, Cohen MS, Ewing SG, Cohen D, Howell LJ, et al. Acute cardiovascular effects of fetal surgery in the human. *Circulation.* 2004;**110**(12):1549–56.

10. Rychik J, Cohen D, Tran KM, Szwast A, Natarajan SS, Johnson MP, et al. The role of echocardiography in the intraoperative management of the fetus undergoing myelomeningocele repair. *Fetal Diagn Ther.* 2015;**37**(3):172–8.

11. Ngamprasertwong P, Michelfelder EC, Arbabi S, Choi YS, Statile C, Ding L, et al. Anesthetic techniques for fetal surgery: effects of maternal anesthesia on intraoperative fetal outcomes in a sheep model. *Anesthesiology.* 2013;**118**(4):796–808.

12. Boat A, Mahmoud M, Michelfelder EC, Lin E, Ngamprasertwong P, Schnell B, et al. Supplementing desflurane with intravenous anesthesia reduces fetal cardiac dysfunction during open fetal surgery. *Paediatr Anaesth.* 2010;**20**(8):748–56.

13. Lin EE, Tran KM. Anesthesia for fetal surgery. *Semin Pediatr Surg.* 2013;**22**(1):50–5.

14. DiFederico EM, Burlingame JM, Kilpatrick SJ, Harrison M, Matthay MA. Pulmonary edema in obstetric patients is rapidly resolved except in the presence of infection or of nitroglycerin tocolysis after open fetal surgery. *Am J Obstet Gynecol.* 1998;**179**(4):925–33.

15. Fisk NM, Gitau R, Teixeira JM, Giannakoulopoulos X, Cameron AD, Glover VA. Effect of direct fetal opioid analgesia on fetal hormonal and hemodynamic stress response to intrauterine needling. *Anesthesiology.* 2001;**95**(4):828–35.

16. Lee SJ, Ralston HJP, Drey EA, Partridge JC, Rosen MA. Fetal pain. *JAMA.* 2005;**294**(8):947–54.

17. Danzer E, Adzick NS, Rintoul NE, Zarnow DM, Schwartz ES, Melchionni J, et al. Intradural inclusion cysts following in utero closure of myelomeningocele: clinical implications and follow-up findings. *J Neurosurg Pediatr.* 2008;**2**(6):406–13.

18. Moldenhauer JS, Soni S, Rintoul NE, Spinner SS, Khalek N, Martinez-Poyer J, et al. Fetal myelomeningocele repair: the post-MOMS experience at the Children's Hospital of Philadelphia. *Fetal Diagn Ther.* 2015;**37**(3):235–40.

19. Belfort MA, Whitehead WE, Shamshirsaz AA, Ruano R, Cass DL, Olutoye OO. Fetoscopic repair of meningomyelocele. *Obstet Gynecol.* 2015;**126**(4):881–4.

20. Verbeek RJ, Heep A, Maurits NM, Cremer R, Hoving EW, Brouwer OF, et al. Fetal endoscopic myelomeningocele closure preserves segmental neurological function. *Dev Med Child Neurol.* 2012;**54**(1):15–22.

21. Pedreira DAL, Zanon N, Nishikuni K, De Sá RAM, Acacio GL, Chmait RH, et al. Endoscopic surgery for the antenatal treatment of myelomeningocele: the CECAM trial. *Am J Obstet Gynecol.* 2015;**214**(1):111.e1.

22. Flake A. Percutaneous minimal-access fetoscopic surgery for myelomeningocele—not so minimal! *Ultrasound Obstet Gynecol.* 2014;**44**(5):499–500.

23. Cohen AR, Couto J, Cummings JJ, Johnson A, Joseph G, Kaufman BA, et al. Position statement on fetal myelomeningocele repair. *Am J Obstet Gynecol.* 2014;**210**(2):107–11.

Anesthesia for Craniofacial Surgery

Elaina E. Lin and Paul A. Stricker

Introduction

Anesthetic management of children undergoing craniofacial reconstruction surgery represents an important domain of neuroanesthesia that is specific to the pediatric anesthesiologist. Craniofacial surgical procedures as discussed herein refer to reconstructive surgical procedures of the bones of the head and face most commonly performed to treat craniofacial deformity secondary to craniosynostosis. These procedures are generally performed at tertiary pediatric medical centers, as the incidence of craniosynostosis is only approximately 1 in 2,000 live births. The goals of these operations are twofold: to normalize skull shape and appearance and to prevent neurocognitive sequelae that can occur secondary to increased intracranial pressure (ICP) associated with craniosynostosis.

In those children at risk for neurodevelopmental disturbances arising from elevated ICP due to craniosynostosis, the benefit of cranial vault remodeling and expansion is easily appreciated. However, what is often underappreciated is the profound, positive, lifelong effect normalization of appearance can have for all children with skull deformities from craniosynostosis. Taken together with the myriad challenges of providing safe anesthetic care, it is unsurprising that many pediatric anesthesiologists derive great satisfaction in ensuring a safe perioperative course for children undergoing these surgeries.

Preoperative Assessment and Preparation

Patients undergoing craniofacial surgery require a thorough history and physical as well as laboratory testing prior to their procedure. The majority of infants presenting with craniosynostosis (80–95%) present with isolated forms of craniosynostosis; that is, they present as a premature fusion of one or more sutures not in association with a constellation of other abnormalities. Most of these children with isolated craniosynostosis are otherwise healthy.

In the remaining cases, craniosynostosis occurs as syndromic craniosynostosis. These forms of craniosynostosis are less common and are associated with typical associated physical features depending on the syndrome. Syndromic forms of craniosynostosis (and their associated incidence) include but are not limited to Apert syndrome (1 per 65,000), Crouzon syndrome (1 per 60,000), Pfeiffer syndrome (1 per 100,000), Saethre-Chotzen syndrome (1 per 25,000–50,000), and Muenke syndrome (1 per 10,000). Syndromic forms of craniosynostosis may have associated abnormalities such as midface hypoplasia and retrusion. These children may occasionally be difficult to intubate, and appropriate difficult airway preparation may be required. The more common respiratory challenge in children with syndromic forms of craniosynostosis is upper airway obstruction and obstructive sleep apnea. Preexisting upper airway obstruction and sleep apnea may necessitate postoperative tracheal intubation and mechanical ventilation in some children. In severe cases, some children require tracheostomy in infancy, which may ultimately be removed following midface advancement procedures performed when these children reach school age.

Preoperative laboratory evaluation should include a complete blood count (hemoglobin, hematocrit, platelet count) and a specimen for type and screen at a minimum. In most cases, cross matching of blood is warranted. Young infants tolerate only small volumes of blood loss and may be present for surgery at their physiologic red blood cell nadir. Even in procedures associated with low rates of transfusion, there is often the potential for unanticipated significant hemorrhage. Many centers routinely obtain a preoperative coagulation profile (prothrombin time [PT], international normalized ratio [INR], partial thromboplastin time [PTT]). Other centers reserve such testing for patients with a history or family history of bleeding disorders.

Patients with craniosynostosis may have elevated ICP. Elevated ICP may be diagnosed by ophthalmic exam or computed tomography (CT) scan or inferred from nonspecific findings like headaches in older children. However, many children with elevated ICP are asymptomatic. The incidence of elevated ICP in multiple suture craniosynostosis was 47% and in isolated single-suture craniosynostosis was 14%.[1] Although there is a relatively high incidence of elevated ICP, most children can safely be induced with an inhalational induction.

Surgical Procedures

Modified Pi Procedure

The modified pi procedure (so named for the similarity of the shape of the cut bone to the Greek letter pi) and its variants are open surgical procedures most commonly performed for sagittal craniosynostosis in infants 2–4 months old. These procedures do not involve bone grafting or complex reconstruction and are much shorter in duration as compared to complex cranial vault reconstruction procedures. Owing to the large scalp incision, extensive calvarial osteotomies, small size of patients, and time of surgery coincident with the nadir physiologic anemia of infancy, these surgeries carry risks of significant blood loss and transfusion is common. Open surgical techniques represent the traditional surgical approach to sagittal synostosis and remain the primary procedure at many centers. The principal advantage of the open approach is that the procedure is completed in a single operation and postoperative helmeting is not required.

Neuroendoscopic Surgery

The surgical technique of neuroendoscopically resecting a strip of the synostotic sagittal suture through two small scalp incisions followed by parietal barrel stave osteotomies was pioneered by Drs. Jimenez and Barone between 1996 and 1998.[2] The limited scalp incisions and reduced extent of cranial osteotomies allow for these procedures to commonly be performed without blood transfusion. However, owing to the difference in surgical technique, postoperative helmeting is required for up to 6 months to achieve the desired remodeling of skull shape.

Spring-Mediated Cranioplasty

Spring-mediated cranioplasty was first performed in infants during the same time period that neuroendoscopic approaches to craniosynostosis were developed. In spring-mediated cranioplasty, a more limited scalp incision is performed than with an open procedure, and the synostotic suture is cut free along its length and calibrated pretensioned springs are positioned between the cut edges of bone on either side of the released suture. The incision is then closed, and over the ensuing months the springs cause cranial expansion perpendicular to the affected suture and remodel skull shape. Once the desired remodeling is achieved, the springs are removed in a brief procedure a few months following the initial surgery. Like neuroendoscopic procedures, spring-mediated cranioplasty has the advantage of significantly reduced blood loss and transfusion compared to open procedures. Postoperative helmet therapy is also not required. The main drawback of this approach is the need for a second operation to remove the springs.

Complex Cranial Vault Reconstruction

Complex cranial vault reconstruction (CCVR) is typically performed in infants 6–12 months old to treat a wider array of cranial vault deformities, including those arising from metopic synostosis, unicoronal synostosis, multisuture craniosysnostosis, and syndromic craniosynostosis (Figure 11.1). These are open surgical procedures that involve wide scalp incisions, extensive craniotomies, and reconstruction of large areas of the cranial vault, often with bone grafting. Consequently, these are longer operations with greater amounts of blood loss and transfusion. Broadly, these procedures fall into three categories: fronto-orbital advancement/anterior cranial vault reconstruction, mid- and posterior cranial vault reconstruction, and total cranial vault reconstruction. In contrast to the other surgical procedures outlined above, CCVR is performed in older children as well as in infants.

LeFort III Osteotomy with Distraction Osteogenesis

Midface hypoplasia is a phenotypic component of most forms of syndromic craniosynostosis. Hypoplasia of the midface results in proptosis and abnormalities of the ocular axis. In some children, complete closure of the eyelids is difficult and corneal damage ensues from chronic corneal exposure. Midface retrusion also causes obstructive sleep apnea, which can be severe. Modern surgical correction of midface hypoplasia is achieved by performing LeFort III osteotomies and application of a

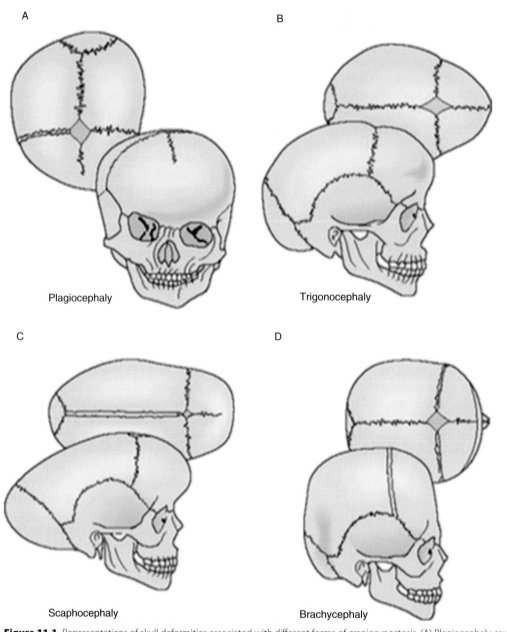

A

Plagiocephaly

B

Trigonocephaly

C

Scaphocephaly

D

Brachycephaly

Figure 11.1. Representations of skull deformities associated with different forms of craniosynostosis. (A) Plagiocephaly caused by unicoronal synostosis; (B) trigonocephaly caused by metopic synostosis; (C) scaphocephaly caused by sagittal synostosis; (D) brachycephaly caused by bicoronal synostosis. Source: Seruya M, Magge S, Keating R, Diagnosis and surgical options for craniosynostosis, in: Ellenbogo RG, Abdulrauf S, Sekhar L, eds., *Principles of Neurologic Surgery*, 3rd ed., St Louis, MO: Saunders; 2012:138.

halo to facilitate distraction osteogenesis. In those children with coexistent forehead retrusion, a LeFort III monobloc procedure is performed, where a bifrontal craniotomy is performed together with the LeFort III osteotomies, and the bones of the midface and the anterior vault are advanced together.

Intraoperative Management

Premedication may be warranted in order to decrease anxiety, especially in patients with syndromic craniosynostosis that may require multiple surgeries. In the patient presenting without intravenous access, an inhalational induction is usually safe. However, patients with signs of significantly elevated ICP may require intravenous induction for a more controlled induction. If difficult airway management is anticipated, the necessary airway equipment should be prepared accordingly. In general, orotracheal intubation with a standard (straight) endotracheal tube is preferred. Nasotracheal intubation is preferred by some to improve tube stability in infants in the prone position, the position for modified pi and posterior cranial vault reconstruction.

Neuromuscular blockade is especially useful to facilitate tracheal intubation and in preventing coughing and movement during laryngoscopy and patient positioning. Spontaneous ventilation should be avoided to minimize the likelihood and extent of venous air embolism, which occurs commonly in children undergoing these procedures.[3,4] Nitrous oxide is also usually avoided for the same reasons. A precordial Doppler may be used to help detect air embolism. However, because the Doppler is so sensitive to any turbulence in the venous system, many anesthesiologists do not use a precordial Doppler. Because of the potential for significant blood loss, at least two "large bore" (preferably 22 gauge or larger) intravenous catheters should be placed. An arterial catheter is recommended to continuously monitor blood pressure and rapidly detect hypotension, as well as for frequent blood sampling. The data suggest that central venous pressure monitoring is not useful;[5] however, placement of a central venous catheter may be warranted if it is not possible to obtain sufficient peripheral venous access or if there is an anticipated need for prolonged vascular access.

The most challenging aspect of intraoperative management is assessment of blood loss and keeping up with replacement of volume losses. Neither heart rate nor central venous pressure is a reliable indicator of hypovolemia.[5,6] Arterial blood pressure monitoring in combination with qualitative arterial waveform assessment and hemodynamic response to fluid challenges has traditionally been used to gauge intravascular volume status. More recently, continuous automated quantitative measurement of arterial waveform variability has been developed, but there are minimal data to date to support the utility of these devices in infants. Vigilant monitoring of the surgical field for blood loss is important; however, accurate blood loss estimation can be difficult given that most

of the blood is on the surgical drapes and is mixed with irrigation fluid (Figure 11.2).

Several strategies have been utilized to minimize blood loss. The greatest reductions result from surgical technique. Endoscopic strip craniectomy and spring-mediated cranioplasty are surgical techniques that result in less blood loss due to smaller incisions. Other surgical techniques such as use of plasma radiofrequency dissection tools, scalp clips, temporary scalp blocking sutures, and infiltration of the scalp with epinephrine aid in obtaining hemostasis. Meticulous attention to hemostasis is likely the most important modifiable variable affecting blood loss.

Since the restriction of aprotinin use in 2008, the most commonly used antifibrinolytics for craniofacial surgery are tranexamic acid (TXA) and ε-aminocaproic acid (EACA). There is evidence that both TXA and EACA reduce blood loss and decrease the need for blood transfusion in children undergoing craniofacial surgery.[7–9]

Various approaches to replacement of blood loss have been used in craniofacial surgery. The most common approach is replacement of initial losses with crystalloid, with the addition of packed red blood cells (PRBCs) once a threshold of loss has been reached. Fresh frozen plasma (FFP) and platelets are transfused once enough loss and replacement has occurred for dilutional coagulopathy to develop, typically starting after a blood volume has been lost. Some centers employ a hemostatic approach to resuscitation, where FFP is administered with PRBCs prophylactically in a 1:1 ratio. Some centers replace blood loss with whole blood, which has the additional advantage of replacing platelets. With massive hemorrhage, fibrinogen replacement may be necessary; in the United States this is currently replaced with cryoprecipitate. Another option is fibrinogen concentrate, which may carry additional expense. With uncontrolled massive hemorrhage that persists despite optimal component therapy, administration of recombinant activated factor VII may be an option, although its high cost and the risk of thrombotic complications should be weighed against the potential benefits.

A number of techniques have been employed to decrease transfusion risks. To mitigate the risk of hyperkalemia and hyperkalemic cardiac arrest from the rapid infusion of stored PRBCs, many centers transfuse PRBCs that have been in storage less than

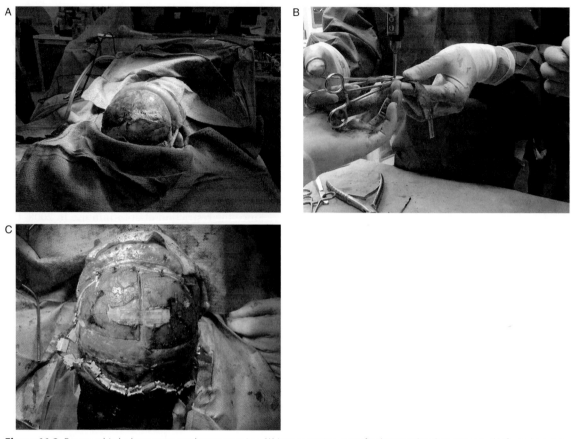

Figure 11.2. Fronto-orbital advancement and reconstruction. (A) Intraoperative view after bicoronal scalp incision and bifrontal craniotomy. (B) The excised bones are cut, shaped, and repositioned using plates and screws to achieve the desired appearance at the surgical side table. (C) Replacement of reshaped cranial bones. Note the use of temporary scalp blocking sutures, which help with surgical hemostasis.

7 days from collection or have been washed and resuspended in saline prior to transfusion. Infectious risk may be decreased by obtaining donor matched PRBCs and FFP. Transfusion of allogenic blood is minimized by the use of cell salvage and adoption of transfusion protocols that establish transfusion thresholds.

Postoperative Concerns

The primary concerns during and immediately after emergence from anesthesia include ensuring adequate analgesia, a patent airway with satisfactory ventilation, and continued satisfactory hemostasis. It is routine practice at many institutions for these children to be admitted to the intensive care unit, primarily for frequent neurologic examinations.

Postoperative analgesia is achieved with intermittent intravenous opioids and acetaminophen. Serial hemoglobin measurements may be indicated based on the last hemoglobin result and the amount of ongoing losses through surgical drains. Coagulation testing may be indicated depending on the extent of intraoperative hemorrhage and the conduct of its replacement. Serum electrolytes may be followed; mild postoperative hyponatremia is not uncommon following craniofacial surgery.

Children who sustain intraoperative dural rents may develop cerebrospinal fluid leaks, which may present as persistent voluminous surgical drain output. Neurologic events including seizures may also occur. Later complications may include surgical site infections.

References

1. Renier D, Sainte-Rose C, Marchac D, Hirsch JF. Intracranial pressure in craniostenosis. *J Neurosurg.* 1982;**57**(3):370–7.

2. Jimenez DF, Barone CM. Endoscopic craniectomy for early surgical correction of sagittal craniosynostosis. *J Neurosurg*. 1998;**88**(1):77–81.

3. Faberowski LW, Black S, Mickle JP. Incidence of venous air embolism during craniectomy for craniosynostosis repair. *Anesthesiology*. 2000;**92**(1):20–3.

4. Tobias JD, Johnson JO, Jimenez DF, Barone CM, McBride DS. Venous air embolism during endoscopic strip craniectomy for repair of craniosynostosis in infants. *Anesthesiology*. 2001;**95**(2):340–2.

5. Stricker PA, Lin EE, Fiadjoe JE, et al. Evaluation of central venous pressure monitoring in children undergoing craniofacial reconstruction surgery. *Anesth Analg*. 2013;**116**(2):411–19.

6. Stricker P, Lin E, Fiadjoe J, Sussman E, Jobes D. Absence of tachycardia during hypotension in infants and children undergoing craniofacial reconstruction surgery. *Anesth Analg*. 2012;**115**(1):139–46.

7. Dadure C, Sauter M, Bringuier S, et al. Intraoperative tranexamic acid reduces blood transfusion in children undergoing craniosynostosis surgery: a randomized double-blind study. *Anesthesiology*. 2011;**114**(4):856–61.

8. Goobie SM, Meier PM, Pereira LM, et al. Efficacy of tranexamic acid in pediatric craniosynostosis surgery: a double-blind, placebo-controlled trial. *Anesthesiology*. 2011;**114**(4):862–71.

9. Hsu G, Taylor JA, Fiadjoe JE, et al. Aminocaproic acid administration is associated with reduced perioperative blood loss and transfusion in pediatric craniofacial surgery. *Acta Anaesthesiol Scand*. 2016;**60**(2):158–65.

Anesthesia for Cerebrovascular Disease in Children

Laura C. Rhee and Craig D. McClain

Introduction

Pediatric cerebrovascular disease is rare. When it does present in children, it usually manifests as either hemorrhagic or ischemic stroke. The underlying structural problems that cause these events can be categorized as (1) structural changes in preexisting blood vessels (e.g., aneurysms, dissections in arteries), (2) pathologic vascular structures (e.g., arteriovenous malformations, cavernous malformations), and (3) progressive arteriopathies (e.g., moyamoya disease). Anesthetic management for patients presenting for surgical management of these disorders primarily involves maintaining optimal cerebral perfusion and oxygen delivery. The procedures may be quite lengthy and can involve significant blood loss. Further, various perioperative management approaches to these procedures involve the logistical challenges of integration of multiple services and anesthetizing locations, often under the same anesthetic. Practitioners must be familiar with not only the basics of cerebral physiology and factors that affect cerebral blood flow, but also how these various pathologies affect normal physiology. Maintaining a safe anesthetic for these children is a complicated dance between hemodynamic stability, adequate ventilation and oxygenation, pharmacology, sound fluid management, and neuromonitoring. This chapter focuses on discussing relatively common cerebrovascular pathologies in children. Pathophysiology and anesthetic management will be highlighted.

Pediatric Stroke

Stroke is a common and potentially debilitating manifestation of cerebrovascular disease, potentially causing possible lifelong disability. Mechanistically, stroke may be classified as either ischemic or hemorrhagic. Ischemic stroke is the result of compromised blood flow to the brain. It can be a consequence of arterial occlusion or venous occlusion of intracranial veins or sinuses. Hemorrhagic stroke occurs secondary to vascular rupture, which can be the result of pathologic vessels or a secondary consequence of an ischemic stroke.[1]

Strokes in pediatric patients affect up to 1 in 1,600 neonates, with older children having a stroke rate of 2.3–13 per 100,000 per year.[2] Survival rates from stroke in children far exceed those of adults, however this is not without significant morbidity; over half will live with permanent neurological sequelae.[3] The incidence of both ischemic and hemorrhagic stroke appears to be increasing. The greater availability of diagnostic imaging has led to an increase in the diagnoses of stroke, while advances in the treatment of diseases that predispose to stroke have allowed for greater survival in these patient populations. The annual incidence of pediatric stroke ranges from 4.6 to 13 in 100,000 across children of all ages.[4,5]

Coexisting disorders that have been identified as risk factors for *ischemic* stroke are congenital heart disease, head trauma, infection (meningitis/encephalitis), sepsis, and sickle cell disease. There is some overlap in the risk factors identified for *hemorrhagic* stroke, including congenital heart disease and sepsis in addition to arteriovenous malformations (AVMs).[6] Male children have been identified as being at greater risk of experiencing stroke, as have African American children, even after accounting for sickle cell disease.[7,8]

Pathologies Related to Structural Changes in Blood Vessels

Aneurysms

Intracranial aneurysms are focal enlargements of an arterial wall due to disruption of arterial wall integrity. They can form secondary to trauma (5–10%), infection (15%), or, most commonly, dissection (50%).[9] Aneurysms may be associated with a predisposing genetic disorder. For example, patients with coarctation of the aorta or polycystic kidney disease have an increased incidence of aneurysms, which usually remain asymptomatic during childhood. While less than 2% of aneurysms are found in pediatric patients,[10] those that do rupture during childhood are most often fatal. Subarachnoid hemorrhage from spontaneous dissection is the most common presenting symptom.

Intracranial aneurysms account for about 10–15% of hemorrhagic strokes in patients younger than 20 years.[11] Saccular, or "berry," aneurysms, which are classically seen in adults, are less common in children. The most common type of aneurysm found in the pediatric population is complex aneurysms including giant, mycotic, traumatic, multiple, or dissecting aneurysms.[12] These types of lesions have significant treatment implications, as their endovascular occlusion and surgical clipping can be more challenging. Endovascular occlusion is considered the first choice and can be utilized for most aneurysms, but microvascular treatment must still be used in some instances, such as when clip reconstruction or bypass is needed.

Preoperative blood pressure control is typically instituted prior to the procedure. This may be achieved with antihypertensive drugs such as labetalol, hydralazine, nicardipine, or even sodium nipride. The use of nimodipine (typical in the adult patient) is controversial in children. Patients may also be on antiepileptic medications as well. If elevated intracranial pressure from a subarachnoid hemorrhage is of concern, an external ventricular drain may be placed to prevent hydrocephalus. Approximately one-third of all subarachnoid hemorrhage (SAH) patients will ultimately require treatment of hydrocephalus, often involving placement of a ventricular shunt.

Anesthetic management again depends on the planned intervention. For aneurysm resection via craniotomy, the usual anesthetic concerns for a craniotomy apply. As expected, adequate intravenous (IV) access should be obtained and arterial waveform monitoring is essential. Preparation for potential sudden and massive blood loss is crucial; blood products should be on hand in the operating room (OR) and ready to administer. Perioperative hemodynamic stability is of utmost importance. Deep preoperative sedation may be preferable to facilitate a smooth induction and avoidance of sudden hypertensive episodes. Adequate depth of anesthesia prior to invasive procedures such as endotracheal intubation or placement of head pins is necessary to prevent precipitous hypertension.

The utility of a skull block to attenuate blood pressure swings during head pinning and incision has been demonstrated in the adult population, although its usefulness in smaller children may be limited by threshold of local anesthetic toxicity.[13] Care should be taken by the surgical team on injection of local anesthetic into the surgical field to avoid excessive use of epinephrine and consequent tachycardia and hypertension. Excessive hypertension during emergence must also be avoided to prevent postoperative bleeding. However, in most cases of aneurysm clipping, a slightly elevated blood pressure may be desirable postoperatively to minimize the risk of vasospasm.

Immediate awakening after aneurysm clipping is particularly important to allow for a neurologic examination. Postclipping, vasogenic cerebral edema with increased intracranial pressure (ICP) or hemorrhage may occur secondary to normal perfusion pressure breakthrough (NPPB). NPPB occurs when vessels surrounding the aneurysm that were chronically maximally dilated are unable to autoregulate (and vasoconstrict) after clipping. Hyperemia then ensues at normal perfusion pressures (or normotension). Thus, moderate hypotension postoperatively (while maintaining CPP) may be desired. Treatment for NPPB may also involve moderate hypothermia and therapy for increased ICP, including diuretics, or head elevation.

Postoperative concerns following aneurysm resection or embolization include vasospasm, serum sodium disturbances, and rehemorrhage. Vasospasm is extremely rare in children, but when it does occur it is typically 4 to 14 days postoperatively. The treatment strategy for vasospasm—which has been extrapolated from the adult literature—includes the calcium channel blocker nimodipine (though controversial in children), "triple-H" therapy (hydration, hemodilution, and hypertension), and angioplasty or intra-arterial vasodilators. If hyponatremia occurs, its exact cause must be identified in order to determine the appropriate treatment. If it is due to cerebral salt wasting syndrome (hypovolemic hyponatremia), treatment is with IV replacement of isotonic fluids. If syndrome of inappropriate antidiuretic hormone (SIADH) is diagnosed (hypervolemic hyponatremia), water restriction should be instituted. Very rarely, rehemorrhage or stroke can occur from faulty clip placement. If this occurs, surgical exploration and evacuation may be necessary. This may involve a reopening of the craniotomy to adjust, reposition, or replace the clip.

Vascular Effects of Trauma and Infection: Carotid Dissection and Cerebral Venous Sinus Thrombosis

Carotid artery dissection (CAD), though rare, is an important cause of acute ischemic stroke in children. The estimated incidence of CAD in children is low at 0.03% after blunt head/neck trauma. However, in children, CAD can be clinically silent, and this frequency may be underestimated.[14] The location of carotid dissections may be extracranial or intracranial. These children will often require an anesthetic for magnetic resonance imaging (MRI) and MRA evaluation of the injury. Extracranial CADs are, overall, the most common location of traumatic vascular dissections of the head and neck in all patients (adults and children).[14] Extracranial CAD is typically a result of trauma to the neck or spine, due to blunt trauma, hyperextension, or rotational injury. Arterial dissection has been associated with a number of other comorbidities including connective tissue diseases (e.g., Ehlers-Danlos syndrome), substance abuse, use of oral contraceptives, and fibromuscular dysplasia. However, CAD can occur in otherwise healthy patients as well. Importantly, dissection may go unnoticed at the time of injury and symptoms of TIA or stroke may be delayed several days after the inciting event. Although intracranial CAD is rare in adults, it is relatively common in children, accounting for 60% of carotid dissections, which are usually spontaneous in nature with no identifiable predisposing risk factors.[14] However, traumatic intracranial CAD may be caused by penetrating soft palate injuries with objects such as pens or sticks and is associated with high morbidity and mortality. Patients presenting with intracranial CAD are also at risk of SAH in addition to embolic stroke.

Treatment of symptomatic extracranial CAD typically involves anticoagulation (in patients without concurrent intracranial dissections). For extracranial CAD, surgical intervention, such as endarterectomy and thrombectomy or carotid ligation, is usually reserved for patients with recurrent transient ischemic attacks (TIAs) or progressive neurologic deficits. In contrast, aggressive surgical intervention such as clipping or resection is typical for most patients with intracranial CAD (though endovascular techniques have been employed successfully).[14]

Cerebral venous sinus thrombosis (CVST) is rare, affecting 0.67 per 100,000 children per year, however it accounts for a significant proportion of ischemic strokes in the pediatric population.[15] At approximately 50% of children with CVST, neonates and young infants are among the most commonly affected. The etiology of CVST is often multifactorial and there are many comorbid conditions that have been identified as risk factors. Perinatal complications tend to dominate in the neonatal population. For children outside of the neonatal period, infection is the most commonly associated condition with CVST and prothrombotic disorders are also very frequently encountered. Other common systemic risk factors in toddlers and older children include fever, dehydration, anemia, and various acute and chronic medical conditions (congenital heart disease, autoimmune disease, malignancy, renal disease). Many children have *coincident* local head or neck pathology, such as head trauma, CNS tumors, recent intracranial surgery, or infections such as otitis media or mastoiditis.[16]

Clinical presentation of CVST is highly variable and may be very nonspecific. Presenting symptoms may be subtle and overlap with those of coexisting conditions. Neurologic symptoms may include headache, seizures, altered level of consciousness, encephalopathy, and focal and/or diffuse neurologic deficits.[15]

Treatment of CVST first includes supportive care to correct underlying disturbances from coexisting conditions (hydration, antibiotics). Symptomatic measures, such as anticonvulsants to control seizures and surgical or medical therapies to decrease intracranial pressure, are often necessary. Anticoagulation for at least several months with unfractionated heparin, low molecular weight heparin, or warfarin is also often employed—more so in older infants and toddlers—and does not appear to be associated with increased risk of hemorrhage. While thrombolysis, thrombectomy, and surgical decompression have been used successfully, these therapies are poorly studied in the pediatric population. Even with aggressive treatment, many survivors will suffer from long-term motor and cognitive deficits or chronic neurologic symptoms secondary to CVST.[15]

Anesthetic management of patients with CAD and CVST includes bearing in mind that these patients are likely to be anticoagulated, and so are at risk for extracranial bleeding complications. If trauma is a suspected or known etiology for either CAD or CVST, appropriate evaluation of the patient should be made and airway precautions should be taken. If CVST occurs in the setting of infection or sepsis, patients may require more aggressive fluid resuscitation or invasive hemodynamic monitoring. Many patients with CVST will show signs of increased ICP and may develop vasogenic edema, both of which may require treatment with diuretics, head elevation, or other measures to lower the ICP.[16]

Pathologic Vascular Structures

Arteriovenous Malformations

AVMs result from abnormal development of the intervening capillary bed between cerebral arteries and veins, leading to a direct arteriovenous connection. Without the normal capillary bed to slow blood flow, a low resistance vascular interface is created, which leads to a high-flow shunt. This direct arteriovenous (AV) connection also leads to hypertrophy and dilation of the arterial and venous components of the AVM.[17] Over time, the surrounding tissues are deprived of blood supply and nutrients. The surrounding brain parenchyma may atrophy secondary to ischemia as a result of the steal phenomenon.[18] The precise mechanism by which these malformations occur is unclear, however they are thought to form during the third week of embryogenesis.

AVMs are the most common cause of spontaneous intraparenchymal hemorrhage and hemorrhagic stroke in children.[2] While AVMs are less common in children than in adults, mortality secondary to hemorrhagic events in children is much higher than in adults (20% vs. 6–10%).[19] It is hypothesized that this is related to a higher incidence of posterior fossa and deep-seated (basal ganglia, thalamus) AVMs in children; not only are malformations in these locations more prone to bleeding, but hemorrhage also more frequently results in a catastrophic outcome.[20] Nonetheless, most (82%) of AVMs in the pediatric population are supratentorial in location, typically in the distribution of the middle cerebral artery.[19]

Malformations that are diagnosed prior to rupture may cause epilepsy, hydrocephalus, or (rarely) congestive heart failure (CHF) in the neonatal period. Unless a malformation is large enough to cause CHF, most remain clinically silent until a stroke or

seizure occurs. Unfortunately, the initial presentation in children is typically hemorrhage (80–85%), which may produce symptoms of sudden headache, seizures, nausea/vomiting, or focal neurologic deficits.

Treatment modality depends on the size, complexity, and location of the lesion; options include observation, embolization, radiation, or surgical resection. Surgical resection is the gold standard for smaller, less complex, and accessible malformations. For those located in surgically inaccessible (deep-seated) or eloquent areas, radiation (radiosurgery) with proton beam or gamma knife may be indicated. The evolution of 3D printing has allowed these lesions to be printed preoperatively to help the surgeon better understand the vascular anatomy and hopefully improve ability to facilitate a complete resection. With advances in endovascular technology, embolization has become more useful as an adjuvant therapy, but alone is rarely curative. The intent of embolization is to decrease size and blood flow to the lesion, creating a solid brittle mass that is later surgically resected with less blood loss. After embolization the tissue surrounding the AVM will gradually adjust to changes in perfusion. Occasionally the risk of treatment will outweigh benefit, in which cases observation is the best option. Many AVMs will require multimodality therapy, which has been shown to be an effective strategy for successful obliteration.[19,20] Posttreatment, the risk of rebleeding during the first 6 months is approximately 6% and then 3% per subsequent year.

Anesthetic management for AVMs depends on the treatment modality. Embolic procedures in the interventional radiology (IR) suite are typically performed under a standard general anesthetic with appropriate neuromuscular blockade as avoidance of patient movement is crucial. Adequate IV access should be obtained prior to the procedure and blood products should be immediately available. The potential for bleeding from the femoral sheath site should be considered, especially in smaller patients, given that heparinization is required and these procedures may last hours. Euvolemia or slight hypervolemia are recommended, however the potential for fluid overload also exists, given the large volume of heparinized saline that may be administered by the neurointerventionalist.[21] Large quantities of contrast are often injected, which may contribute to volume overload. These agents may have a high osmolality contributing to a tremendous shift of fluid into the intravascular space. This may result in heart failure or pulmonary edema. Care must be taken to use contrast judiciously and not overadminister. Excessive contrast can precipitate a nephropathy, which can be treated with cessation of contrast, alkalization of urine, and administration of IV fluids. Special attention to volume status is necessary in infants who may already be in high-output CHF and are receiving multiple inotropic agents. Invasive blood pressure monitoring via an arterial line is recommended to facilitate close monitoring and fine control of blood pressure. Should an occlusion occur during embolization, blood pressure should be augmented to maintain perfusion distally. Postprocedurally after partial embolization, abrupt increases in blood pressure should be avoided.[19] Last, in case of a possible rupture, induced hypotension may be required in order to minimize blood loss. One should always be prepared for a possible emergency craniotomy should this occur.

If a surgical resection via craniotomy is performed in the OR, anesthetic goals are in line with those for similar craniotomies: optimize cerebral perfusion pressure (CPP) and oxygen delivery via maintenance of adequate mean arterial pressure and appropriate ventilator parameters. Avoidance of hemodynamic lability is crucial to avoid rupturing the AVM. As with embolization, being prepared for sudden blood loss is essential. As such, adequate IV access and arterial line are helpful. Brain relaxation techniques such as moderate hyperventilation or osmotic diuresis may aid in enhancing surgical exposure.

More modern approaches to interventional treatment of AVMs often involve a combination of embolization in the neurointerventional suite followed by surgical resection. In our institution, we routinely will combine these procedures over two anesthetics (first day is embolization followed by the next day of surgical resection and confirmatory angiography) or under a single anesthetic. The surgical resection can be followed by immediately cerebral angiography to confirm total resection of the AVM. This can then be followed by emergence from anesthesia and transfer to the intensive care unit (ICU).[19]

Both inhalational and IV agents have been used safely for the anesthetic for these lesions. Inhalational agents (except N_2O) decrease cerebral metabolic rate and increase cerebral blood flow (vasodilate), while IV agents (except ketamine) decrease cerebral metabolic rate and decrease cerebral blood flow in a dose-dependent manner. It is thought that vasodilating agents may induce a steal phenomenon while vasoconstrictors result in inverse steal. No evidence exists favoring one technique over another in terms of outcome for these patients. As with many aspects of anesthesia and critical care, it is likely that the most important thing is an engaged practitioner who understands both normal and pathological physiology and is able to quickly intervene. Certainly, maintenance of normotension and avoidance of large swings in blood pressure are crucial.

As many patients with AVMs may present with seizures, the patient's anticonvulsant regimen must be considered when redosing narcotics and muscle relaxants. Because of the upregulation of the cytochrome p450 system induced by many anticonvulsants, these types of drugs (benzodiazepines, some opioids, and muscle relaxants) will likely need to be redosed sooner as they are undergoing accelerated metabolism.[22] Anticonvulsants should be continued into the perioperative period. A smooth emergence that avoids significant hypertension is ideal. Often, a technique utilizing higher dose opioid drugs intraoperatively can aid in facilitating a neurologic exam shortly after surgery and prior to extubation.

Perioperative complications may include hydrocephalus, stroke, or rehemorrhage. SAH may result in hydrocephalus and may initially require an external drain to lower CSF volume and monitor ICP. Approximately one-third of all SAH patients will ultimately require a ventricular shunt. Faulty clip placement or a residual AVM may result in rehemorrhage or stroke. Residual lesions should be investigated with postoperative vascular imaging if possible and treated with evacuation of a clot if necessary and/or reopening of the craniotomy and further resection.

Vein of Galen Malformation

Of particular interest to pediatric neuroanesthesiologists is the vein of Galen malformation (VOGM). This is a rare (1/25,000 live births) AVM that presents most often in the neonatal period.[23] Up until the advent of endovascular approaches to treatment in the late 1980s, the mortality was exceptionally high with open surgical treatment of these lesions (37.4%). Neonates had the worst prognosis with mortality in excess of 90%.[24] Subsequently, the development of endovascular techniques has offered substantial advantage with a 2006 series reporting a mortality rate of 10.6% with 74% of those that survived having no significant neurologic morbidity.[25]

Depending on the period of development during which the VOGM manifests, presentation and pathology will vary. Prenatally, loss of brain parenchyma and calcification may occur. Postnatally, several other problems may occur including hydrocephalus with facial and scalp vein prominence. Further, the presence of a low resistance circuit in the brain can predispose the patient to high-output cardiac failure in the neonatal period, often accompanied by pulmonary hypertension.[26] Occasionally, children with lesions that don't result in hemodynamic collapse will not present until later childhood or even adulthood. These patients often present with headaches or hemorrhage.

The anesthetic management of these children is most often complicated by the cardiovascular problems inherent to the low resistance circuit of the VOGM. These patients are often already on inotropic and pressor support by the time the anesthesiologist gets involved. Extreme caution must be taken with these patients, as their cardiovascular status can be quite tenuous. It is not uncommon for these patients to have a series of endovascular treatment procedures in the neuroradiologic suite. The degree of ventilatory and hemodynamic support can change rapidly, and anesthesiologists should be prepared to titrate to pre-defined goals. Certainly, invasive monitoring and central venous access are necessary in these patients, as is a reliable way of administering large amounts of intra-vascular volume support if needed.

Cavernous Malformations

Cavernous malformations (CMs) are vascular lesions found throughout the central nervous system. They are composed of a dense mass of thin sinusoidal vessels, often encapsulated and multilobar, without intervening brain parenchyma. These lesions may grow and shrink in a dynamic manner, as they are prone to repeated microhemorrhage and thrombosis. This creates a hemosiderin-laden ring and often cal-cifications surrounding the lesion.[27] Most cases of CMs are sporadic, and a unifying cause has yet to be determined. However, three genes have been identi-fied in association with CM formation and patients with familial CMs may develop multiple lesions

throughout life.[28] Cerebral CMs are known to appear de novo after radiation therapy.[29]

Clinical presentation of CMs is highly variable; incidental lesions may be found in asymptomatic patients or patients may present with a variety of neurologic symptoms such as headache, seizure, or focal neurologic deficits.[29] In contrast to lesions in adults, pediatric CMs are typically larger, more prone to bleeding, and more likely associated with other vascular anomalies. However, compared to higher flow lesions such as AVMs or aneurysms, risk of hemorrhage from CMs is lower, and bleeding is generally less often fatal unless its location confers a higher risk, such as the brainstem or posterior fossa.[29]

Treatment for asymptomatic lesions is typically observation with serial imaging. For symptomatic CMs, those that hemorrhage, or demonstrate radio-graphic evidence of enlargement, surgical resection is undertaken. CMs in the eloquent cortex or brainstem should be approached with caution; lesions with recurrent hemorrhage may justify surgical excision. Ideally, resection takes place a minimum of 4–6 weeks after hemorrhage to allow swelling to subside. Outcomes from resection are generally very good in terms of morbidity and mortality; however if not excised completely, CMs can recur.[29]

Anesthetic management for resection of caver-nous hemangioma is similar to that for craniotomies for other vascular lesions. Optimizing CPP and main-taining hemodynamic stability are important. However, in contrast to resection of high-flow lesions such as aneurysms and AVMs, the risk of intraopera-tive and postoperative complications, such as rapid hemorrhage, is much lower with the low-pressure bleeding that typifies CMs.

Progressive Arteriopathies: Moyamoya

Moyamoya is a rare chronic vascular disorder defined by progressive stenosis and potential occlusion of the internal carotid arteries with development of an abnormal vascular network of collaterals in the cere-bral cortex, which gives rise to a "puff of smoke" appearance during cerebral angiography (Figure 12.1). The clinical presentation of moyamoya in children includes TIAs, which may progress to strokes and eventual fixed neurologic deficits. These ischemic attacks are typically precipitated by decreased cerebral blood flow, often as a result of

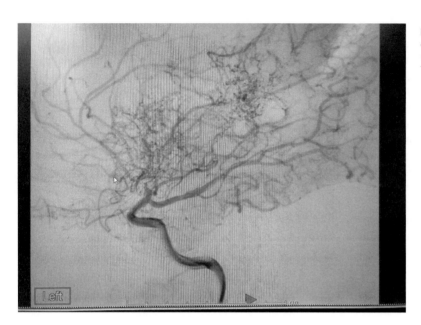

Figure 12.1. This angiogram displays the classic "puff of smoke" appearance of the moyamoya vessels in the distribution of the left internal carotid.

hyperventilation, but may also be triggered by stress, fatigue, dehydration, and infection.[30] If left untreated, there is a high rate of morbidity and mortality. While moyamoya disease is the idiopathic form of the disorder, moyamoya syndrome is the arteriopathy that is found in conjunction with another associated condition. These associated pathologies may include prior radiotherapy to the head or neck; genetic disorders such as Down syndrome, neurofibromatosis type I, large facial hemangiomas, sickle cell anemia, and other hemoglobinopathies; autoimmune disorders such as Graves's disease; congenital cardiac disease; or renal artery stenosis.

There appear to be bimodal peaks of incidence in the age distribution of patients who present with moyamoya. The first peak occurs in the first decade of life, while the second peak occurs in the fourth decade. For unknown reasons, this disorder more commonly affects children of East Asian ancestry.

Medical management for moyamoya disease includes antiplatelet therapy such as aspirin and occasionally calcium channel blockers. However, given the progressive nature of the disease, surgical revascularization has been shown to be far superior as a primary treatment, even in asymptomatic children.[1] Surgery is performed to prevent cerebral infarction by improving cerebral perfusion distal to the lesion.

Surgical management can be broadly divided into direct and indirect approaches. Direct approaches involve vascular techniques that bypass the stenotic section of the internal carotid artery (ICA). This involves placement of grafts that allow blood from the external carotid system to perfuse the cerebral cortex in the ICA distribution distal to the stenosis. While this technique is commonly used in adults, the technical challenges inherent to this approach make it more risky for pediatric patients, particularly smaller children. Alternatively, indirect approaches have been utilized extensively with great success. The indirect approach takes advantage of angiogenic factors that are expressed in the cerebrospinal fluid (CSF) of chronically ischemic brains. These factors can be activated when blood flow is provided in close approximation to the subarachnoid space. Thus, a new network of vessels to perfuse the cerebral cortex can grow. Of note to the anesthesiologist, the care for patients postoperatively will be directly related to the type of surgical approach employed. The anesthesiologist needs to be intimately familiar with the technique. For patients undergoing a direct approach, blood flow is ideally immediately improved. However, with the indirect approach, patients are essentially no better at the conclusion of the surgical procedure than they were preoperatively. They are indeed set up for success, but ingrowth of new vessels takes weeks to months to occur. Thus, the same considerations apply postoperatively as existed preoperatively.

While direct techniques to bypass the stenosis of the ICA and the middle cerebral artery (MCA) have been successful in selected patients, the most common surgical operation for palliation in the pediatric population are indirect techniques. Pial synangiosis is the most commonly employed technique currently. This procedure involves suturing a branch of the external carotid artery (usually the superficial temporal artery) on to the pial surface of the brain to encourage angiogenesis. The artery is first mapped out using Doppler ultrasound. The artery is then dissected free from the surrounding tissue. It should be noted it is *not* ligated. Following the arterial dissection, a craniotomy is turned under the dissected artery and the arachnoid is opened (Figure 12.2). The artery is then sutured directly on to the pia mater and the wound is closed. This technique utilizes the ischemic brain's tendency to attempt to augment blood flow through the development of collateral vessels: the placement of a pedicle of vascularized tissue provides the chronically ischemic cortex with a source from which to develop such collateral blood flow. Surgical revascularization performed at experienced pediatric centers significantly reduces the risk of future stroke in the subsequent decades.[32] Anesthetic management of these patients should focus on preoperative optimization as well as intra- and postoperative preservation of CPP and cerebral blood flow (CBF). It is important to understand that patients with moyamoya do not, at baseline, have a normal relationship between CBF and cerebral metabolic rate for oxygen ($CMRO_2$). In fact, patients with moyamoya already have maximally dilated cerebral vasculature, so there is very little way to increase CBF. This results in a situation where any decrease in CBF results in inadequate

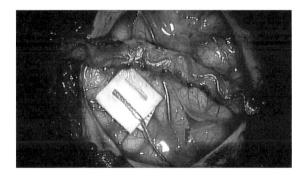

Figure 12.2. The target artery can be seen in this photograph. At this point of the pial synangiosis, the target artery has been dissected out and the bone flap has been removed, dura opened, and arachnoid opened. The artery is now ready to be directly sutured on to the pia mater. This will provide a blood source to encourage angiogenesis in the ischemic cortex and ultimately improve cerebral blood flow.

delivery of oxygen. Further, it is believed that while these patients do possess some ability to autoregulate, the limits of a given patient's autoregulation are quite narrow and can vary from patient to patient.

Because maintenance of CBF is crucial in these patients, normotension and normocapnia are the two fundamental anesthetic goals.[33] Generally speaking, these patients will tolerate mild hypertension and hypercapnea much better than hypotension and hypocapnia. However, excessively high blood pressure or carbon dioxide tensions should be avoided as well. In order to achieve normotension, most patients are preadmitted to the hospital the night prior to surgery and receive IV hydration (often 1.5× maintenance) to avoid dehydration that may occur with fasting. This minimizes the cardiovascular effects that vasodilating anesthetic agents can have. It is critical to maintain normotension intraoperatively and postoperatively in order to preserve blood flow to spontaneous collateral vessels from the external carotid system. Because patients with moyamoya disease have reduced hemispheric blood flow, cerebral vasoconstriction secondary to hypocapnia must be avoided. Excessive hypercapnia may also result in a steal phenomenon from ischemic areas. This reduced regional blood flow may cause significant electroencephalography (EEG) and neurologic changes. Thus, maintenance of intraoperative normocapnia is critical.

Intraoperative monitoring of these patients typically consists of standard American Society of Anesthesiologists (ASA) monitors, invasive blood pressure monitoring, and a modified EEG. Continuous end-tidal CO_2 monitoring is essential and even mild hyperventilation should be avoided. Since there is no readily available simple way of assessing real-time global CBF, intraoperative EEG monitoring is utilized to detect and potentially treat cerebral ischemia.[34] If slowing is noted on the EEG, it may be indicative of inadequate CBF and oxygen delivery. The anesthesiologist must immediately address the factors that affect CBF including adjustments to the patient's blood pressure and partial pressure of carbon dioxide (ventilation); anesthetic agents may be necessary to ensure an adequate match of CBF to $CMRO_2$.

Postoperatively, patients who have undergone indirect approaches must be appropriately managed. In the immediate postoperative period, these patients will still be at high risk for stroke. Thus, care must be taken to emerge quickly, but smoothly from general anesthesia. Providing appropriate analgesia is essential in order to facilitate a smooth extubation without hypertension or hyperventilation induced by pain and crying. Patients will need to continue to be hydrated until they achieve adequate oral intake of fluids. If patients manifest any crying or distress despite adequate analgesia, small doses of dexmedetomidine (0.5–1 ug/kg IV) after the initial exam are often helpful without compromising either hemodynamics or future neurologic exam.

References

1. Freundlich CL, Cervantes-Arslanian AM, Dorfman DH. Pediatric stroke. *Emerg Med Clin North Am*. 2012;**30**:805–28.

2. Bernson-Leung ME, Rivkin MJ. Stroke in neonates and children. *Pediatr Rev*. 2016;**37**:463–77.

3. Cardenas JF, Rho JM, Kirton A. Pediatric stroke. *Childs Nerv Syst*. 2011;**27**:1375–90.

4. Wintermark M, Hills NK, deVeber GA, Barkovich AJ, Elkind MS, Sear K, et al. Arteriopathy diagnosis in childhood arterial ischemic stroke: results of the vascular effects of infection in pediatric stroke study. *Stroke*. 2014;**45**:3597–605.

5. Agrawal N, Johnston SC, Wu YW, Sidney S, Fullerton HJ. Imaging data reveal a higher pediatric stroke incidence than prior US estimates. *Stroke*. 2009;**40**:3415–21.

6. Lo W, Stephens J, Fernandez S. Pediatric stroke in the United States and the impact of risk factors. *J Child Neurol*. 2009;**24**:194–203.

7. Smith ER, McClain CD, Heeney M, Scott RM. Pial synangiosis in patients with moyamoya syndrome and sickle cell anemia: perioperative management and surgical outcome. *Neurosurg Focus*. 2009;**26**:E10.

8. Roach ES, Golomb MR, Adams R, Biller J, Daniels S, Deveber G, et al. Management of stroke in infants and children: a scientific statement from a Special Writing Group of the American Heart Association Stroke Council and the Council on Cardiovascular Disease in the Young. *Stroke*. 2008;**39**:2644–91.

9. Krings T, Geibprasert S, terBrugge KG. Pathomechanisms and treatment of pediatric aneurysms. *Childs Nerv Syst*. 2010;**26**:1309–18.

10. Gross BA, Smith ER, Scott RM, Orbach DB. Intracranial aneurysms in the youngest patients: characteristics and treatment challenges. *Pediatr Neurosurg*. 2015;**50**:18–25.

11. Jordan LC, Johnston SC, Wu YW, Sidney S, Fullerton HJ. The importance of cerebral aneurysms in childhood hemorrhagic stroke: a population-based study. *Stroke*. 2009;**40**:400–5.

12. Garg K, Singh PK, Sharma BS, Chandra PS, Suri A, Singh M, et al. Pediatric intracranial aneurysms—our experience and review of literature. *Childs Nerv Syst*. 2014;**30**:873–83.

13. Geze S, Yilmaz AA, Tuzuner F. The effect of scalp block and local infiltration on the haemodynamic and stress response to skull-pin placement for craniotomy. *Eur J Anaesthesiol*. 2009;**26**:298–303.

14. Chamoun RB, Jea A. Traumatic intracranial and extracranial vascular injuries in children. *Neurosurg Clin N Am*. 2010;**21**:529–42.

15. deVeber G, Andrew M, Adams C, Bjornson B, Booth F, Buckley DJ, et al. Cerebral sinovenous thrombosis in children. *N Engl J Med*. 2001;**345**:417–23.

16. Dlamini N, Billinghurst L, Kirkham FJ. Cerebral venous sinus (sinovenous) thrombosis in children. *Neurosurg Clin N Am*. 2010;**21**:511–27.

17. El-Ghanem M, Kass-Hout T, Kass-Hout O, Alderazi YJ, Amuluru K, Al-Mufti F, et al. Arteriovenous malformations in the pediatric population: review of the existing literature. *Interv Neurol*. 2016;**5**:218–25.

18. Niazi TN, Klimo P Jr., Anderson RC, Raffel C. Diagnosis and management of arteriovenous malformations in children. *Neurosurg Clin N Am*. 2010;**21**:443–56.

19. Gross BA, Storey A, Orbach DB, Scott RM, Smith ER. Microsurgical treatment of arteriovenous malformations in pediatric patients: the Boston Children's Hospital experience. *J Neurosurg Pediatr*. 2015;**15**:71–7.

20. Di Rocco C, Tamburrini G, Rollo M. Cerebral arteriovenous malformations in children. *Acta Neurochir (Wien)*. 2000;**142**:145–56; discussion 156–8.

21. Darsaut TE, Guzman R, Marcellus ML, Edwards MS, Tian L, Do HM, et al. Management of pediatric intracranial arteriovenous malformations: experience with multimodality therapy. *Neurosurgery*. 2011;**69**: 540–56; discussion 556.

22. Soriano SG, Martyn JA. Antiepileptic-induced resistance to neuromuscular blockers: mechanisms and clinical significance. *Clin Pharmacokinet*. 2004;**43**:71–81.

23. Hrishi AP, Lionel KR. Periprocedural management of vein of Galen aneurysmal malformation patients: an 11-year experience. *Anesth Essays Res*. 2017;**11**:630–5.

24. Johnston IH, Whittle IR, Besser M, Morgan MK. Vein of Galen malformation: diagnosis and management. *Neurosurgery*. 1987;**20**:747–58.

25. Lasjaunias PL, Chng SM, Sachet M, Alvarez H, Rodesch G, Garcia-Monaco R. The management of vein of Galen aneurysmal malformations. *Neurosurgery.* 2006;**59**:S184–94; discussion S3–13.

26. Burch EA, Orbach DB. Pediatric central nervous system vascular malformations. *Pediatr Radiol.* 2015;**45**(suppl 3):S463–72.

27. Landrigan-Ossar M, McClain CD. Anesthesia for interventional radiology. *Paediatr Anaesth.* 2014;**24**:698–702.

28. Raychaudhuri R, Batjer HH, Awad IA. Intracranial cavernous angioma: a practical review of clinical and biological aspects. *Surg Neurol.* 2005;**63**:319–28; discussion 328.

29. Gross BA, Du R, Orbach DB, Scott RM, Smith ER. The natural history of cerebral cavernous malformations in children. *J Neurosurg Pediatr.* 2016;**17**:123–8.

30. Smith ER, Scott RM. Cavernous malformations. *Neurosurg Clin N Am.* 2010;**21**:483–90.

31. Kim JS. Moyamoya disease: epidemiology, clinical features, and diagnosis. *J Stroke.* 2016;**18**:2–11.

32. Titsworth WL, Scott RM, Smith ER. National analysis of 2454 pediatric moyamoya admissions and the effect of hospital volume on outcomes. *Stroke.* 2016;**47**: 1303–11.

33. Soriano SG, Sethna NF, Scott RM. Anesthetic management of children with moyamoya syndrome. *Anesth Analg.* 1993;**77**:1066–70.

34. Vendrame M, Kaleyias J, Loddenkemper T, Smith E, McClain C, Rockoff M, et al. Electroencephalogram monitoring during intracranial surgery for moyamoya disease. *Pediatr Neurol.* 2011;**44**:427–32.

Chapter 13

Epilepsy Surgery

Hubert A. Benzon, Douglas Hale McMichael, and Craig D. McClain

Introduction

Epilepsy is one of the most common neurologic disorders. There has been significant improvement in the medical management of epilepsy. Despite the development of new drugs and treatment regimens, the prevalence of pharmacologically intractable seizures is still high, leading to significant developmental delays. Intractable epilepsy is defined as failure of more than two antiepileptic drugs and having more than one seizure per month over a period of 18 months. Advances in neuroimaging techniques and electroencephalography (EEG) have provided epileptologists with surgically resectable anatomic targets that mediate some of these medically intractable seizure disorders.[1] Neurosurgeons have utilized these technologies to dramatically improve outcomes in these patients.

Within this population, there are a few notable differences between children and adults. The developing brain has a lower seizure threshold, which results in a more frequent occurrence of catastrophic epilepsy in young children. Cerebrovascular physiology is different in children. Compared to adults, infants have more of their cardiac output directed toward the brain, resulting in a greater cerebral blood volume. That distinction, coupled with the fact that children have a lower baseline mean arterial pressure than adults, puts infants at greater risk of hemodynamic instability during neurosurgical procedures. Neonates have decreased hepatic function—leading to delayed metabolism of drugs—and decreased renal function, which limits their ability to compensate for changes in fluid and solute loads. Combined, these may alter the clearance of medications administered to neonates.

Perioperative Considerations

Basics of Epilepsy Terminology

Prior to embarking on the workup and treatment of epilepsy, it is necessary to understand the basic anatomy and physiology used to describe these phenomena. The *ictal onset zone* refers to the region where clinical seizures originate. The *epileptogenic lesion* refers to the structural lesion that is causally related to the epilepsy. *The epileptogenic zone* refers to the region of cortex that actually generates epileptic seizures. Last, the *irritation zone* refers to the cortex that generates abnormal EEG discharges between seizures known as *interictal spikes*

Preoperative Evaluation

1. A thorough preoperative evaluation is necessary for any patient presenting to the operating suite. A history and physical examination must be carefully performed as many of these patients have significant comorbidities. One should pay careful attention to the respiratory and cardiac systems. Cardiac function should be optimized prior to surgery. A complete airway examination should be performed as some craniofacial anomalies may require special techniques to secure the airway. The evaluation should also attempt to detect underlying conditions that are leading to the seizures and to describe disabilities resulting from progressive neurologic dysfunction.[2]

2. Preoperative laboratory testing should include a complete blood count to assess for a baseline hematocrit level and coagulation studies to look for any unknown coagulation disorders. Given the significant blood loss that can occur during the procedure, underlying coagulopathies should be corrected preoperatively. Typed and screened or cross-matched blood should be available.

3. Serum anticonvulsant levels should be determined preoperatively to detect subtherapeutic or toxic concentrations. The anticonvulsant medications that most of these patients require often have notable side effects:

a. Valproic acid is known to cause abnormalities of hematologic function—such as abnormal coagulation, depression of red or white blood cell production, or decreased platelet counts—that can be especially concerning during intracranial surgery.[3]

b. Many anticonvulsants enhance the metabolism of non-depolarizing muscle relaxants and opioids via upregulation of the cytochrome P450 system. Hence, an increased amount of these drugs may be a necessary component of the anesthetic plan (Figure 13.1). Newer anticonvulsants seem to have less of an effect on the metabolism of anesthetic drugs.[4]

4. Special consideration should be given to patients with a history of tuberous sclerosis. This hamartomatous disease presents with cutaneous and intracranial lesions, with lesions infiltrating the cardiac, renal, and pulmonary systems. Preoperative electrocardiograph (EKG) and echocardiogram should be performed to assess for functional defects from the possible cardiac rhabdomyomas leading to obstruction of intracardiac blood flow, dysrhythmias, or abnormal conduction pathways. Renal lesions can lead to hypertension or decreased renal function.[5]

5. A ketogenic diet is a high-fat, low-carbohydrate diet that promotes ketosis; this has been used as an adjuvant for intractable epilepsy. However, ketosis can promote a metabolic acidosis, which can be exacerbated with the use of carbohydrate-containing solutions. Therefore, these patients should be given normal saline instead of lactated Ringer's solution. Intraoperatively, these patients should have their acid base status and plasma glucose levels measured frequently.[6]

Imaging Techniques

All these patients will have an imaging study prior to surgical resection in the operating room (OR). Various imaging techniques are utilized to assess structural or functional epileptogenic zones. Magnetic resonance imaging (MRI) is the modality of choice for structural imaging and is particularly effective for focal epilepsy. That being said, no pathology is found on MRI in up to 20% of patients, necessitating other modalities.

Single photon emission computed tomography (SPECT) is the only modality able to reliably identify the ictal onset zone. In order to obtain an image, a radioactive tracer is injected during a seizure; epileptogenic areas have increased cerebral blood flow (CBF), leading to increased uptake and subsequently increased intensity on SPECT.

Positron emission tomography (PET) utilizes 18-fluorodeoxyglucose (18-FDG) as a measure of neuronal uptake of glucose, which allows the radiologist to visualize cellular metabolism; with this modality, an epileptogenic zone is indicated by a hypometabolic area. PET is best utilized during the interictal period.

Other imaging modalities include MR spectroscopy (MRS), functional MRI (fMRI), and diffusion tensor imaging (DTI). In general, the imaging modality chosen should be tailored to the clinical situation, and the number of imaging studies (and attendant general anesthetics) should be apportioned judiciously.

Magnetoencephalography (MEG) provides direct information about evoked and spontaneous neural activity; it resembles EEG, but focuses on different anatomic areas and electrochemical processes. Whereas EEG measures extracellular currents at gyral crests, MEG measures intracellular currents at fissures and sulci.

Most adults will be able to tolerate these imaging modalities without sedation. However, infants and

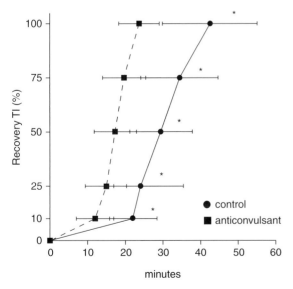

Figure 13.1. Long-term anticonvulsant therapy decreased the half-life of phenytoin and carbamazepine and their derivatives. This leads to rapid recovery of neuromuscular blockade.[4]

some adolescents are uncooperative, and therefore require sedation or anesthesia in order to obtain optimal imaging. In order to take advantage of the increasingly fine resolution of the above modalities, general anesthesia is increasingly becoming the preferred technique.

Anesthesia for Diagnostic Studies

When administering a general anesthetic for the purposes of diagnostic studies, it is important to be mindful of how different medications can affect the results. Most static imaging—e.g., MRI—is not affected by the anesthetic technique, whereas dynamic studies—e.g., EEG—are significantly impacted by the choice of medication. For example, methohexital is useful for increasing the frequency and amplitude of spikes.[7,8] Mild hyperventilation can also lower the seizure threshold and improve EEG signaling during intraoperative mapping.

In the specific case of MEG, benzodiazepines drastically increase the failure rate. Propofol decreases the frequency of spikes, particularly for nonlesional epilepsy; conversely, dexmedetomidine does not produce signal artifacts, which may make it preferable to propofol for MEG.[9]

Surgical Resection of Seizure Foci

The goal is resection of a lesion or area of cortex that has been shown to be related to seizure generation and propagation. The most common location of seizure foci is the temporal lobe, which is involved with complex partial seizures (50% of new epilepsy cases each year) that are often related to mesial temporal sclerosis or a structural lesion of the temporal lobe. Although many epileptogenic foci are located in the region of the temporal lobe, they may be located in any area of the cerebral cortex.

A major concern for resection of seizure foci is to avoid harming brain tissue that controls vital functions such as motion, sensation, speech, and memory, referred to as eloquent cortex. Removal of this area and loss of that specific function would have a deleterious effect on neurologic outcome.

Advances in neurophysiologic monitoring (EEG and electrocorticography [ECoG]) have increased the ability to safely perform resections in functional areas of the brain. Typically low levels of anesthetic are necessary for these types of monitoring in order to map seizure foci and propagation. Sometimes, cortical stimulation of the motor cortex is performed to observe motor movement of the area of the homunculus. Here, muscle relaxants must be avoided to enable visualization of the stimulated area. Asleep craniotomy is appropriate for lesions that are not located in or deep to eloquent areas of the brain. Awake neurosurgical procedures are most important for those patients requiring interventions close to or partially overlapping eloquent brain. There are no randomized controlled trials comparing the safety or efficacy of these various techniques. Further, in the pediatric population, not all patients will tolerate awake craniotomy, and individualized patient selection is paramount. Typically, older children are better candidates, but the key is a real assessment of level of maturity and thorough preoperative discussions to ensure appropriateness.[10]

Awake Craniotomy

Potentially cooperative older children can assist in determination of the limits of safe cortical resection if speech and motor functions can be continually assessed intraoperatively during an awake craniotomy.

There are two basic approaches for an awake craniotomy. All procedures (line placement, local anesthesia for pinning and surgical exposure) can be done with the patient awake or with minimal sedation and the patient kept at a similar state during surgery. Alternatively, short-acting sedatives and analgesics such as propofol or fentanyl can be titrated to unconsciousness with the maintenance of spontaneous ventilation for the aforementioned procedures, after which the patient lightened to an awake or slightly sedated state for surgical resection of the seizure focus. Following surgical resection, sedatives and analgesics can be restarted or increased for patient comfort during surgical closure.

In children, with the advancement of neuromonitoring, awake craniotomy is performed less often these days.

Asleep–Awake–Asleep Technique

This technique allows the painful portions of the procedure to be performed under general anesthesia. The patient does not have to tolerate a potentially uncomfortable and claustrophobic position for a long duration as with an awake craniotomy.

Anesthesia is induced and airway control is maintained with a supraglottic device. General anesthesia is maintained for line placement, placement of head pins, and dural opening. The patient is then awakened, the supraglottic airway carefully removed, and resection of the seizure foci performed. When surgical resection has been completed, general anesthesia is again induced and the supraglottic airway reinserted for closure of the dura, skull, and skin. Following closure, the patient is awakened from general anesthesia.

There are several disadvantages to the asleep–awake–asleep approach. Airway management while the patient is in head pins can be quite difficult. Cervical spine injuries or scalp lacerations can occur during intraoperative emergence and propofol should be administered when the patient coughs or bucks while the head is immobilized in head pins. Brain swelling is a major concern as it may worsen during spontaneous ventilation from the combined vasodilatory effects of hypercapnia and volatile agents. Mannitol and furosemide can be given, but the patient then becomes very uncomfortable with sensations of thirst and urinary urgency. Hyperventilation or doxapram have been used, but the patients quickly tire of this effort. Slight elevation of the head of the bed, ensuring the neck veins are not compromised by clothing and monitors or extreme rotation, often quickly relieves the problem. If none of these maneuvers work, the patient may have to undergo general anesthesia and controlled ventilation.

With either the awake craniotomy or the asleep–awake–asleep approach, it is crucial for the anesthesiologist to have a discussion with the patient and family with respect to intraoperative needs and expectations, particularly the possibility of awareness during the surgery. It is important to communicate that not all patients are candidates for "awake" craniotomy.

In general, children who are younger than 10 years old or uncooperative patients of any age will likely not tolerate the awake craniotomy approach and will require general anesthesia throughout the whole procedure. In these scenarios, a variety of intraoperative electrophysiological techniques such as somatosensory evoked potentials, EEG, ECoG, and motor stimulation may be used to help localize and determine the function of the site of the planned resection.

Electrocorticography (ECoG)

ECoG is an invasive electrophysiological technique.[11] It is commonly employed at 60–70% of North American centers. ECoG is obtained via an array of electrodes, which were historically rigid but are now typically flexible. Arrays of strips and grids of electrodes are useful for analysis of superficial structures, but depth electrodes can be used for analysis of deeper tissues.

The signals obtained via ECoG are large amplitude (0–50 microvolts/mm) and fall within a typical frequency range (0.5–70 Hz). The waveform varies based on electrode location, preexisting lesions, preoperative medications, and anesthetic drugs. Whereas preexisting lesions are of lower amplitude and frequency, seizures caused by anesthetic drugs are typically of higher frequency and have sharper contour. Thus, in order to localize seizure foci, it can be necessary to utilize medications to activate pathological spiking activity.

The best marker of seizure foci is interictal epileptiform activity (IEA), which can manifest as spikes, polyspikes, sharp-and-slow wave complexes, or any combination thereof. IEA usually represents the irritative zone and carries a high positive predictive value for epilepsy in otherwise neurologically normal patients. In general, a high amplitude corresponds to closer proximity to the epileptogenic focus.

Increasing depth of anesthesia changes ECoG readings in a stepwise fashion. In sequence, the obtained waves progress through alpha (8–12 Hz), beta (13–30 Hz), theta (5–7 Hz), and delta (1–4 Hz) phases, and finally burst suppression. Different medications have variable effects on waveform activity. Sedative doses of propofol and dexmedetomidine have little effect on IEAs. Although small boluses of opioids likewise have little effect, large boluses can increase interictal spikes. The halogenated volatile anesthetics tend to shift occipitally dominant alpha waves to the frontal lobe and resemble sleep spindles; nitrous oxide causes fast, frontally dominant, high-frequency activity but may suppress spikes at concentrations >50%.

If ECoG observes no spontaneous discharges, it may be necessary to activate the epileptogenic foci. The end goal is to increase frequency and distribution of spiking while being mindful of where and how different medications have an effect. All intravenous (IV) opioids activate epileptiform activity, with alfentanil being the best studied; their efficacy in this regard is attenuated by prior benzodiazepine. Although the exact mechanism is unknown, the leading hypotheses are disinhibition of gamma-aminobutyric acid-ergic

(GABAergic) interneurons and inhibition of hyperpolarization-activated potassium currents.

Of the sedative hypnotic drugs, methohexital is the most commonly employed, though it may ultimately be too nonspecific. Etomidate has a high activation rate, but can also cause myoclonus and pain. Ketamine is globally active, but poorly studied. All of the inhaled agents cause activation and deterioration of spikes, and engender poorer specificity with increasing concentration. The effects of inhaled agents are exaggerated with hypocapnia.

Subdural Grids and Strips Electrodes

In some patients, the seizures are so generalized that detecting the site of origin can be very difficult. When this occurs, further evaluation with perioperative intracranial EEG monitoring ("grids and strips") may be accomplished by direct ECoG placement and observation of the patient over a period of time (typically several days) in the hospital to attempt to find a seizure focus (Figure 13.2).

Patients undergo a craniotomy under general anesthesia where leads are placed on the surface of the cerebral cortex. Intraoperative EEG monitoring

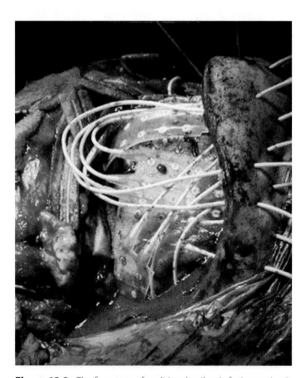

Figure 13.2. The first stage of traditional epileptic foci mapping is to directly place the grids and strips electrodes on the surface of the brain through a large craniotomy.

during the initial placement ensures that all leads are functional. The actual monitoring for seizures and mapping of seizure foci takes place over the next several days to see if a focus can be identified and eventually surgically resected.

The patient must be observed carefully during this period because several complications can develop with the electrodes on the brain. Infections can develop from a foreign body in the brain. Pneumocephalus can occur as air persists in the skull for up to 3 weeks after a craniotomy. These patients should not have nitrous oxide administered to them for subsequent procedures (i.e., seizure focus resection and/or removal of the ECoG leads) until their dura has been opened to avoid the development of tension pneumocephalus.

A peripheral intravenous central catheter (PICC) can be placed during the initial craniotomy as patients will receive IV antibiotic therapy during the period of time the electrodes are in place and avoids the discomfort of multiple IV insertions.

These patients typically return in 1 week for repeat craniotomy for the removal of the grids and strips and resection of the seizure foci.

Nonfocal Surgical Resection

When a focal resection is not possible, a lobectomy or corpus callosotomy may be attempted.

Patients undergoing the corpus callosotomy are often somnolent for the first few postoperative days, particularly if a "complete" callosotomy is performed. It is more common for surgeons nowadays to initially perform a partial callosotomy, and to then perform a complete callosotomy if necessary. Since the surgical approach is near the sagittal sinus, this procedure can be associated with hemorrhage and venous air embolism (VAE).

Occasionally, small children will undergo a hemispherectomy because their seizures are attributed to an abnormal hemisphere that is already severely dysfunctional, such as when a hemiparesis is already present.[12]

Anatomic hemispherectomy consists of the resection of an entire hemisphere, whereas functional hemispherectomy consists of a partial temporal lobectomy and disconnection of interhemispheric neural networks. The functional hemispherectomy generally involves less blood loss and fewer postoperative long-term complications such as hydrocephalus. These procedures are usually performed when patients are very young, with the intent of allowing the contralateral hemisphere to assume function of both hemispheres and hopefully improve developmental and functional outcome later in life.

Hemispherectomies are very challenging cases for the anesthesiologist, as patients can lose multiples of estimated blood volume; therefore adequate IV access is necessary, which can be difficult in very young children. In order to decrease blood loss, it is reasonable to consider a prothrombotic agent such as tranexamic acid. Some practitioners utilize central venous lines to facilitate central venous pressure monitoring, rapid volume resuscitation, and administration of vasopressors and inotropes. Invasive arterial pressure monitoring is routine for these cases

Less Invasive Surgical Techniques and Implications

Recently, a variety of less invasive techniques for mapping and eliminating discrete seizure foci have become more common. Among these techniques are the use of stereo-electroencephalography (SEEG) and laser interstitial thermal therapy (LITT). These techniques involve the use of stereotactically placed devices through one or a series of burr holes in the skull. The purported advantages of SEEG are improved seizure mapping and localization and avoidance of a craniotomy for placement of the electrodes. LITT is a less invasive technique that avoids a craniotomy and is suitable for seizure foci in deep structures of the brain (see Chapter 15).

LITT grew out of a combination of the ideas of radiofrequency thermal ablation and stereotactic radiosurgery. Basically, a laser catheter is inserted stereotactically into a lesion of interest. The lesion is then ablated using heat, which is then monitored in real time within an MRI. The procedure consists of placement of a head frame that is then used to guide placement of the anchoring bolt and subsequently, the laser catheter. The head frame is then removed and the patient is imaged to confirm proper placement of the catheter. Once proper placement is confirmed, the ablation component of the procedure is performed in the MRI scanner with real-time imaging to assess the ablation. Upon completion of the placement, the patient is removed from the scanner, the catheter is removed, the burr hole closed, and the patient can be awoken. Although functionally this procedure

involves a head frame placement and burr hole, there are numerous anesthetic implications that providers must be aware of.[13,14]

First, this process requires a general anesthetic with a secured airway. The patient will have a head frame on for at least part of the process and access to the airway may be limited, even with more modern stereotactic frames. The anesthesiologist should *always* have immediate access to the tools to remove the frame in case of an emergency. For maintenance of anesthesia, basic neuroanesthesia principles apply. The patient may need to be transported to a variety of locations (depending on the institution) for the entire procedure—e.g., computed tomography (CT), MRI, OR, iMRI, etc. So, care must be taken to prepare and plan for such necessities. Prior to moving into zone IV of an MRI environment, extreme care must be taken to ensure that the patient has had all non-MRI safe devices and monitors removed from their person. This is most often coordinated with an MR technologist. Thus, intimate knowledge of MRI safety principles is absolutely necessary. Different centers approach such things in different manners, although many are still advocating invasive monitoring (as if for a standard craniotomy) and intensive care unit (ICU) stay postoperatively.

SEEG involves the placement of depth electrodes via a series of burr holes. SEEG can be thought of as an extension of the classic subdural grids/strips electrodes, although somewhat less invasive. SEEG allows for a four-dimensional picture of both the epileptogenic region and its patterns of spread across other structures. This is not available with subdural strip/grid electrodes. Advantages of SEEG include the ability to record from deep-seated structures that subdural electrodes cannot precisely interrogate. Also, arrays can be tailored to the individual to attempt to characterize network structures both up- and downstream from the lesion of interest. Finally, there are the advantages of patient comfort and safety in terms of avoidance of a craniotomy for placement and monitoring. SEEG procedures are done using stereotactic frames. Because of the multiple electrodes needed and consequent multiple trajectories required, a growing number of centers utilizing this approach are employing a robot to assist with defining the trajectories (Figure 13.3).[15,16]

Many of the anesthetic implications enumerated above also apply to SEEG placement. Some differences are that an SEEG procedure generally does not involve use of MRI. However, CT guidance is used for

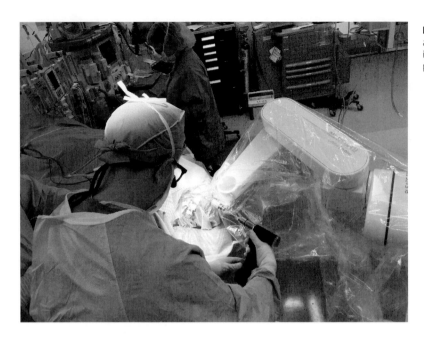

Figure 13.3. The robotic arm can be seen at the right. The robot assists the surgeon in obtaining the optimum trajectory for placement of each SEEG electrode.

navigation once the head frame is placed. Also, another head CT is performed after placement of the electrodes to confirm proper position and evaluate for any complications. These patients are generally taken to the ICU postoperatively for close neuromonitoring. Following mapping and characterization of the lesion in question, a variety of approaches can be utilized to surgically treat the seizures. Depending on the lesion, a traditional craniotomy and focus resection may be the best approach. Alternatively, some lesions may lend themselves to treatment via LITT as described above.

Vagal Nerve Stimulator

The vagal nerve stimulator (VNS) is another advance in the surgical treatment of epilepsy. Although its exact mechanism of action is not understood, it appears to inhibit seizure activity at the brainstem or cortical levels.[17] Its placement has shown benefit with minimal side effects in many patients who are disabled by intractable seizures. It is estimated that there is a 60% to 70% improvement in seizure control in children receiving VNS, with the best results in those who suffer from drop attacks.

The VNS is a programmable device similar to a cardiac pacemaker, and is placed subcutaneously under the left anterior chest wall. Bipolar platinum stimulating electrode coils, which are implanted around the left vagus nerve, are connected to the generator by subcutaneously tunneled wires. The device automatically activates for up to 30 seconds every 5 minutes.

Stimulation of the vagal nerve in this manner may affect vocal cord function, and sudden bradycardia or transient asystole has been reported but without resultant morbidity. When patients with VNS return for subsequent surgeries, it may be appropriate to deactivate the stimulator while the patient is under general anesthesia to prevent vocal cord motion. A magnet placed over the generator will deactivate the stimulator.[18]

General Anesthesia Issues

Positioning

The positioning of the patient will depend mostly on the location of the seizure focus, which is typically over one of the temporal or parietal lobes. Therefore, the most common position for this type of surgery is supine with the head turned over one shoulder, often supported by a shoulder roll. In most of these cases, the elevation of the operative field (i.e., the head) relative to the heart leads to an increased risk of VAE.

The head of the patient is usually placed in a pinning system for the duration of the procedure. Care should be taken to ensure that the endotracheal tube is properly positioned, mindful the head may be turned laterally for the procedure. The supine position is also utilized for many other types of seizure surgery such as corpus callosotomy, hemispherectomy, and VNS placement.

For the awake craniotomy, the face must always be accessible to the anesthesiologist in case airway manipulation is necessary due to oversedation or the generation of a seizure. This also facilitates communication and facial observation during the neuropsychological assessment. The patient must also be in a comfortable position.

Induction and Maintenance

Induction and maintenance of general anesthesia in patients who are undergoing seizure surgery is similar to that of other patients undergoing intracranial procedures. Care should be taken not to exacerbate any existing intracranial hypertension. Also, if intraoperative seizure mapping is planned, one may have to tailor the anesthetic technique.

As mentioned earlier, anticonvulsant drugs affect the metabolism of other drugs, specifically muscle relaxants and narcotics.[18] It seems that first-generation antiepileptic drugs (AEDs) (i.e., phenytoin, phenobarbital, valproate) tend to have a higher potential for interactions and adverse effects due to hepatic enzyme induction or inhibition, whereas the newer AEDs have a greater safety profile and fewer drug interactions. In terms of affecting anesthetic drug dosing, the requirements for muscle relaxants and narcotics are increased to maintain the same depth of anesthesia and muscle relaxation. Phenytoin, which is commonly given intraoperatively, can lead to hypotension and arrhythmias when given rapidly; fatalities have been reported.

Induction can be performed via either an inhalational agent or an IV agent, depending on the clinical circumstances. There is some concern that sevoflurane has epileptogenic potential; however, it has a much faster uptake than isoflurane and is less of an airway irritant, making it more suitable to an inhaled induction. If there is concern for aspiration from vomiting due to increased intracranial pressure, a rapid sequence induction should be performed.

Maintenance of anesthesia can be performed with several techniques as long as one is aware of the effects of the anesthetic agents chosen. Inhaled agents can depress the metabolic demand of the brain tissue, but also can lead to cerebrovascular dilation. They can ultimately decrease cerebral perfusion pressure

mostly by decreasing the patient's mean arterial pressure. Conversely, IV agents decrease the cerebral metabolic demand but do not lead to cerebrovascular dilation. Both inhaled and IV agents can depress EEG and ECoG. Opioids produce quality analgesia with minimal EEG depression, but can lead to side effects of respiratory depression and sedation postoperatively.

There is much controversy as to whether anesthetic agents can increase or lower the seizure threshold. In fact, some anesthetics can produce both proconvulsant and anticonvulsant properties at different doses or in different physiologic situations. It seems that lower anesthetic doses have a proconvulsant tendency while higher doses have anticonvulsant tendencies. Sevoflurane may lead to epileptiform activity, but usually does not convert to convulsions. Low doses of propofol have definite anticonvulsant effects.

Given the propensity for significant blood loss and consequent volume administration, it is important to choose IV fluids wisely. Normal saline is typically used for neurosurgical procedures, as it is mildly hyperosmolar and should minimize cerebral edema; however, large quantities of normal saline are associated with hyperchloremic acidosis. Significant blood loss should be replaced with colloid such as 5% albumin or packed red blood cells. If patients become hypovolemic to the point of hemodynamic instability, vasopressor support may be necessary.

Approximately 16% of patients experience a seizure during craniotomy for seizure focus excision. Most often this occurs as the neurosurgeon stimulates the area of interest. It may be typical of the patient's seizures before surgery or different, depending on the relationship of the surgical stimulation to the patient's intrinsic seizure focus. It is important to quickly communicate to the surgeon that you are observing a seizure. Often the seizure is localized to the face or an extremity initially but rapidly becomes generalized if not immediately interrupted.

The neurosurgeon can irrigate the area with iced Ringer's lactate to rapidly and reliably interrupt the seizure. A small bolus of propofol intravenously will stop a seizure. Both of these interventions also interrupt the electrocorticography briefly, but are quickly reversible. Administration of IV barbiturates or benzodiazepines as anticonvulsants will interrupt the ability to stimulate and monitor for seizures for a longer time. These longer acting medications also take longer to control the seizure and may cause significant delays until effective monitoring can resume. If the patient goes into a persistent seizure, you must protect him or her from personal injury and protect the airway while continuing to administer medications appropriately.

Monitoring

Monitoring for these patients is similar to that for other patients undergoing intracranial procedures: invasive BP monitoring is almost always used for intracranial procedures to ensure adequate mean arterial pressure and therefore cerebral perfusion pressure throughout the case. An arterial line also allows for serial blood gas sampling and lab draws. VNS placement typically does not require invasive BP monitoring.

Given the elevation of head above the heart, these procedures carry a high risk of VAE. A precordial Doppler, in conjunction with end-tidal CO_2 monitoring, should enable the practitioner to detect minute VAE early enough before any significant hemodynamic instability can develop. The probe is best placed on the anterior chest, typically over the right of the sternum at the fourth intercostal space.

Blood glucose levels should be monitored intraoperatively as well. Neonates with underdeveloped gluconeogenesis may require glucose to maintain IV fluids; however, this should be done cautiously, as hyperglycemia should always be avoided in neurosurgical procedures as it may exacerbate neurologic injury if ischemia develops.

Continuous monitoring of neuromuscular blockade (NMB) is imperative as the response to NMBs is quite unpredictable in the context of antiepileptic medications.

Neuromonitoring

During seizure surgery, various modes of intraoperative neuromonitoring are often used to aid in delineation of seizure foci.[19] Such techniques may involve ECoG, cortical stimulation, or electromyography. It is important to discuss the requirements of intraoperative mapping and neuromonitoring with the neurosurgeon, neurologist, and neurophysiologist in order to tailor the anesthetic technique. For example, if it will be necessary to induce seizure activity, long-acting agents that elevate the seizure threshold may be avoided. In the case of concurrent ECoG monitoring, one may minimize the dosage of a benzodiazepine given preoperatively for the anxious child. Occasionally, it may be necessary to induce seizure activity (i.e., administration of methohexital) to help locate seizure foci.

Postoperative Considerations

For patients who have undergone primary resection of a seizure focus, or temporal lobectomy, the postoperative considerations are similar to those of other patients who have undergone craniotomy. Intracranial procedures can be associated with the syndrome of inappropriate antidiuretic hormone secretion (SIADH) leading to hyponatremia, or diabetes insipidus or cerebral salt wasting syndrome leading to hypernatremia. These patients must go to ward locations where serial neurologic examinations can be performed.

Monitoring for seizure activity should continue and a plan for treatment should be agreed upon. When patients have subdural electrodes (grids/strips) placed, the goal is to have the patient seize postoperatively in a controlled and monitored setting in order to generate a map of the seizure focus. There should be a plan in place to address longer, uncontrolled seizure activity that does not cease on its own.

These patients may be somewhat somnolent depending on the number of electrodes left in place with higher numbers seeming to increase somnolence. Conversely, pain may be more significant in these patients and the analgesic technique should be adjusted accordingly. Typically, IV opioids are titrated to treat pain. However, opioid-induced respiratory depression can lead to hypoxemia and hypercarbia. If the patient requires large amounts of opioids and is old enough to do so, patient-controlled analgesia (PCA) can be utilized.

Furthermore, these patients will need continued IV antibiotic coverage while the electrodes are in place (which may be up to 2 weeks). Therefore, a PICC line placed during the initial craniotomy is beneficial.

Patients who undergo hemispherectomy or corpus callosotomy are often extremely somnolent for the first several days postoperatively. Therefore, the patient may be kept intubated at the conclusion of the surgical procedure, taken to the ICU, and extubated when appropriate.

Of note, patients undergoing VNS can be sent home the day of surgery as long as there are no anesthetic or surgical concerns after the procedure has been completed.

Takeaway Concepts

1. These surgeries are associated with significant blood loss. One should always be prepared with adequate IV access and blood products for resuscitation of the patient.

2. Given the numerous AEDs and the differing effects on metabolism of other drugs, the anesthesiologist must be attentive to the effects they can have on anesthetic agents, particularly muscle relaxants and narcotics.

3. Different modalities of neuromonitoring require certain anesthetic techniques. It is important to know ahead of time if the surgeons plan on using EEG, ECoG, cortical stimulation, or the neurological examination from an awake patient.

References

1. Depositario-Cabacar DT, Riviello JJ, Takeoka M. Present status of surgical intervention for children with intractable seizures. *Curr Neurol Neurosci Rep.* 2008;**8**(2):123–9.

2. Chui J, Venkatraghavan L, Manninen P. Presurgical evaluation of patients with epilepsy: the role of the anesthesiologist. *Anesth Analg.* 2013;**116**(4):881–8.

3. Abdallah C. Considerations in perioperative assessment of valproic acid coagulopathy. *J Anaesthesiol Clin Pharmacol.* 2014;**30**(1):7–9.

4. Soriano SG, Martyn JA. Antiepileptic-induced resistance to neuromuscular blockers: mechanisms and clinical significance. *Clin Pharmacokinet.* 2004;**43**(2):71–81.

5. Rabito MJ, Kaye AD. Tuberous sclerosis complex: perioperative considerations. *Ochsner J.* 2014;**14**(2):229–39.

6. Soysal E, Gries H, Wray C. Pediatric patients on ketogenic diet undergoing general anesthesia—a medical record review. *J Clin Anesth.* 2016;**35**:170–5.

7. Ford EW, Morrell F, Whisler WW. Methohexital anesthesia in the surgical treatment of uncontrollable epilepsy. *Anesth Analg.* 1982;**61**(12):997–1001.

8. Modica PA, Tempelhoff R, White PF. Pro- and anticonvulsant effects of anesthetics (Part II). *Anesth Analg.* 1990;**70**(4):433–44.

9. Konig MW, Mahmoud MA, Fujiwara H, Hemasilpin N, Lee KH, Rose DF. Influence of anesthetic management on quality of magnetoencephalography scan data in pediatric patients: a case series. *Paediatr Anaesth.* 2009;**19**(5):507–12.

10. McClain CD, Landrigan-Ossar M. Challenges in pediatric neuroanesthesia: awake craniotomy, intraoperative magnetic resonance imaging, and interventional neuroradiology. *Anesthesiol Clin.* 2014;**32**(1):83–100.

11. Chui J, Manninen P, Valiante T, Venkatraghavan L. The anesthetic considerations of intraoperative electrocorticography during epilepsy surgery. *Anesth Analg.* 2013;**117**(2):479–86.

12. Flack S, Ojemann J, Haberkern C. Cerebral hemispherectomy in infants and young children. *Paediatr Anaesth.* 2008;**18**(10):967–73.

13. Curry DJ, Gowda A, McNichols RJ, Wilfong AA. MR-guided stereotactic laser ablation of epileptogenic foci in children. *Epilepsy Behav.* 2012;**24**(4):408–14.

14. Starr PA, Markun LC, Larson PS, Volz MM, Martin AJ, Ostrem JL. Interventional MRI-guided deep brain stimulation in pediatric dystonia: first experience with the ClearPoint system. *J Neurosurg Pediatr.* 2014;**14**(4):400–8.

15. Fomenko A, Serletis D. Robotic stereotaxy in cranial neurosurgery: a qualitative systematic review. *Neurosurgery.* December 14, 2017. doi:10.1093/neuros/nyx576. Epub ahead of print.

16. Gonzalez-Martinez J, Bulacio J, Thompson S, Gale J, Smithason S, Najm I, Bingaman W. Technique, results, and complications related to robot-assisted stereoelectroencephalography. *Neurosurgery.* 2016;**78**(2):169–80.

17. McLachlan RS. Vagus nerve stimulation for intractable epilepsy: a review. *J Clin Neurophysiol.* 1997;**14**(5):358–68.

18. Kofke WA. Anesthetic management of the patient with epilepsy or prior seizures. *Curr Opin Anaesthesiol.* 2010;**23**(3):391–9.

19. Soriano SG, Bozza P. Anesthesia for epilepsy surgery in children. *Childs Nerv Syst.* 2006;**22**(8):834–43.

Traumatic Brain Injury

David Levin, Monica S. Vavilala, and Sulpicio G. Soriano

Introduction

Traumatic brain injury (TBI) is a leading killer of children over 1 year of age, most often due to falls, and second most often due to motor vehicle crashes. However, the incidence of nonaccidental abusive head trauma (AHT) and sports-related head injury continues to rise in children. The sequelae of TBI affect the patient and the entire family unit for years after the initial injury. Mortality is highest after severe TBI, but the public health burden is from the large number of patients with mild TBI. In the acute phase TBI can present along a continuum from a brief change in mental status or consciousness (concussion or mild TBI classified by Glasgow Coma Scale score [GCS] > 8; Table 14.1) to an extended period of unconsciousness or amnesia after the injury (severe TBI classified by GCS < 9). After TBI, patients may have seizures, motor or sensory deficits, inability to protect the airway, respiratory insufficiency, and hemodynamic instability. In the healthy brain, homeostasis is maintained through a complex and well-coordinated system that includes, but is not limited to, an intact blood-brain barrier, cerebrovascular autoregulation with good matching of local cerebral blood flow with cerebral metabolic rate for oxygen ($CMRO_2$), and

Table 14.1 Glasgow Coma Scale and Modification for Young Children

Glasgow Coma Scale	Pediatric Coma Scale	Infant Coma Scale	Score
Eyes	*Eyes*	*Eyes*	
Open spontaneously	Open spontaneously	Open spontaneously	4
Verbal command	React to speech	React to speech	3
Pain	React to pain	React to pain	2
No response	No response	No response	1
Best verbal response	*Best verbal response*	*Best verbal response*	
Oriented and converses	Smiles, oriented, interacts	Coos, babbles, interacts	5
Disoriented and converses	Interacts inappropriately	Irritable	4
Inappropriate words	Moaning	Cries to pain	3
Incomprehensible sounds	Irritable, inconsolable	Moans to pain	2
No response	No response	No response	1
Best motor response	*Best motor response*	*Best motor response*	
Obeys verbal command	Spontaneous or obeys verbal command	Normal spontaneous movements	6
Localizes pain	Localizes pain	Withdraws to touch	5
Withdraws to pain	Withdraws to pain	Withdraws to pain	4
Abnormal flexion	Abnormal flexion	Abnormal flexion	3
Extension posturing	Extension posturing	Extension posturing	2
No response	No response	No response	1

neurohormonal output that can modulate blood osmolarity, cardiac output, and ventilation. TBI can result in derangements in any of these homeostatic mechanisms. The sequela of TBI are the result of both the "primary injury," caused by direct mechanical insult to the brain parenchyma or vascular supply, and the "secondary injury," marked by diffuse cerebral swelling due to second insults caused by edema, hypoxia, hypotension, intracranial hypertension, and inflammation. The goals of anesthetic and perioperative management are focused around providing adequate surgical conditions while best preserving normal physiologic function, thereby limiting secondary injury. Achieving these goals requires an understanding of the various manifestations of TBI, and the interventions available to limit their progression and to compensate for their dysfunction.[1] Given that many children with TBI will have polytrauma, a multisystem assessment is imperative. Basic life support algorithms including Advanced Trauma Life Support (ATLS) and Pediatric Advanced Life Support (PALS) provide a framework for the initial resuscitation and should be immediately applied to ensure optimal oxygenation and circulation.[2] The 2012 Pediatric Guidelines for managing children with severe TBI have been published by a multidisciplinary group and provide evidence-based guidance on the treatment of pediatric patients.[3]

Approach to the Pediatric Trauma Patient

Acute Resuscitation

Definitions of hypotension have varied across the published TBI literature, but most agree that systemic hypotension is associated with poor outcomes. Systolic blood pressure (SBP) < 5th percentile for age, and SBP < 70 + 2 (age) are the most commonly used definitions of systolic hypotension. This roughly corresponds to a SBP < 90 mmHg for children over 11 years of age. With polytrauma, hypotension and hypovolemic shock are often due to blood loss from solid organs, large vessels, and long bone injuries. Infants can present with hypovolemic shock even with an isolated TBI due to the relatively large head-to-body ratio and the vascularity of the scalp. Additionally, both TBI and spinal cord injury can lead to neurogenic shock and hypotension refractory to volume resuscitation, requiring the use of vasoactive agents. Hypoxia during the preoperative period

can compound the adverse effect of hypotension.[4] In the context of polytrauma, a multidisciplinary team including the relevant surgical specialists, anesthesiologists, radiologists, and intensivists should triage which surgical interventions are required following a "damage control" approach. Appropriate hemodynamic resuscitation has resulted in a reduction in hospital mortality and low GCS at discharge.[5] Acute traumatic coagulopathy is also associated with high mortality,[6] and blood loss should be treated with timely and specific blood component therapy.

Cerebral Perfusion Pressure

An important reason to correct systemic hypotension is to optimize cerebral perfusion pressure (CPP),[2,3] which is defined as mean arterial pressure (MAP) minus the greater of the intracranial pressure (ICP) or the central venous pressure (CVP). CPP represents the driving pressure for flow through the brain. Since arterial pressure and ICP are objective data points often available in TBI patients, CPP has become a target of interest as a clinical endpoint, with clinicians targeting a range of CPP that avoids cerebral hypoperfusion and hyperemia. Both under- and overperfusion to the injured brain can worsen secondary injury following TBI, the former by worsening ischemia and the latter by worsening edema or hemorrhage. There is paucity of data to suggest the best target CPP in pediatric TBI based on age, but there is some evidence an age-related continuum does exist. On the other hand, studies aiming to determine the lower limit of autoregulation (LLA) show that even young children may have an LLA of 60 mmHg, close to the resting MAP and that the LLA varies within age (see Chapter 2).[7,8] Cerebral autoregulation is often compromised in TBI and is associated with a poor prognosis.[9] Perioperative assessments of cerebral autoregulation have been attempted in acute TBI, but these experimental modalities are not widely available.[10–12] Therefore, in general, hypotension secondary to trauma should be aggressively treated. This can be achieved by ensuring large bore intravenous access and restoration of fluid deficits with crystalloid and blood products, as well as with vasopressors. Level III evidence from the multidisciplinary Pediatric Guidelines for TBI recommend that CPP < 40 mmHg be avoided after severe TBI.[13,14] Additional Level III evidence supports keeping CPP between 40 and 50 mmHg.[3] Given the variability of the LLA, especially in TBI, empiric CPP management may not have an expected effect on CBF.[7,10] In the absence of ICP monitoring, supranormal SBP may be targeted to ensure an adequate CPP. Maintenance of CPP > 40 mmHg during craniotomy for TBI is associated with improved discharge survival, and TBI guideline adherence overall is associated with survival benefits.[15]

Airway Management

Children with a GCS score < 9 are considered unable to protect their airway and are at high risk for upper airway obstruction and/or pulmonary aspiration. These patients require tracheal intubation followed by emergent neuroimaging to delineate the extent of the injuries.[16] Immobilization of the cervical spine is essential to avoid secondary spinal cord injury, especially during manipulation of the airway, until clinical and/or radiological clearance is confirmed. It should be noted that infants and young children are predisposed to C1–2 cervical disruptions, which may be difficult to diagnose in cervical spine x-rays. There should be minimal cervical spine manipulation during tracheal intubation of infants with TBI. Spinal cord injury without radiological abnormalities (SCIWORA) manifests as neurological deficit without fracture due to ligamentous and paraspinous muscle laxity. Nasotracheal intubations are relatively contraindicated in these patients because of the possibility of basilar skull fractures.

Abusive Head Trauma (AHT)

Infants with AHT often present with a myriad of chronic and acute subdural hematomas.[17,18] When compared to nonintentional TBI, patients with AHT tend to be younger and present with apnea and seizures.[18] As with all TBI, the presence of other coexisting injuries, fractures, and thoracic and abdominal trauma should be identified and stabilized.[19] Patients with injuries out of proportion to the history of TBI should be considered at risk of AHT.

Concussion

A concussion may lead to secondary injury due to worsening functional and biochemical changes in the brain and can lead to diffuse axonal injury. The impact of general anesthesia in pediatric patients with a recent concussion or mild TBI is unknown and is a major knowledge gap in perioperative medicine.[20,21] Although neuroimaging studies (computed tomography (CT) and magnetic resonance imaging (MRI)) are normal in 78% of pediatric patients with concussions, intracranial and intraparenchymal hemorrhages, nonhemorrhagic contusion, and nonspecific white matter changes are noted in the rest.[22] General anesthesia is frequently associated with alterations of blood pressure and arterial partial pressure of carbon dioxide, and large volumes of intravenous fluids may be administered in response to surgical blood loss and hypotension due to anesthesia-induced vasodilation. Significant systemic hypotension, hypo- or hypercarbia, intracranial hypertension, and hyperglycemia have been observed in a cohort of pediatric patients with TBI undergoing extracranial surgery.[23] A recent study of hospitalized children with sports-related concussion demonstrated impaired cerebral autoregulation.[24] Therefore, close intraoperative monitoring of these hemodynamic variables is essential in preventing secondary injury to a vulnerable brain.[23,24] Many clinicians consider it best practice to delay elective surgery in patients with known concussion until the patient is free of symptoms.

Indications for Surgery

Refractory Intracranial Hypertension

The goal of neurosurgery in TBI is to terminate the vicious cycle of brain swelling and intracranial hypertension. Brain edema worsens intracranial hypertension, which reduces CPP, cerebral blood flow (CBF), and brain oxygenation. Physical examination and neuroimaging will dictate the need for emergent surgery and placement of ICP monitors. Indications for expediting neurosurgical interventions include the following:

1. Cranial

    a. Epidural hematoma
    b. Subdural hematoma
    c. Penetrating injury
    d. Medically refractory intracranial hypertension with or without herniation

2. Extracranial

    a. Long bone fractures
    b. Abdominal visceral injury
    c. Thoracic injuries
    d. Spine injuries

Patients with severe brain swelling with sulci effacement and midline shift on CT or refractory intracranial hypertension are candidates for decompressive craniectomy. A randomized trial comparing decompressive craniectomy versus advanced medical management in patients with severe and refractory intracranial hypertension resulted in decreased mortality and ICP, but increased adverse events and disability in the surgical cohort.[25] The increased frequency of diffuse swelling in the pediatric population makes children more frequently candidates for such treatment.[26] Decompressive craniectomy with duraplasty may be considered when intracranial hypertension reaches or approaches medical refractoriness in salvageable patients where the ICP elevation and its effects are felt to be the major threat to recovery.[3] Unilateral craniectomy is appropriate for lateralized swelling. Bifrontal decompression is selected for diffuse edema, which in a mixed population of head injured patients resulted in favorable outcome in patients with (1) preoperative ICP < 40 mmHg, (2) treatment within 48 hours of presentation, and (3) age < 18 years.[27] Early decompressive craniectomy within 24 hours after the time of injury is associated with a significant decrease in ICP and improved 6-month outcome in children.[28] Bifrontal or frontotemporal craniectomy for management of refractory intracranial hypertension from AHT resulted in a significant decrease in mortality in the craniectomy group when compared to the medically managed children.[29] Early decompressive craniotomy resulted in 16 out of 23 children surviving, with 81% of the survivors returning to school with a reasonable quality of life.[30] Other studies in children demonstrate the utility of decompressive craniectomy in reducing refractory intracranial hypertension.[31] Therefore, decompressive craniectomy may have a dual role as an early and late attempt at managing moribund head injured infants and children.[32]

Skull Fractures

Skull fractures are the most common head injuries in pediatric patients and are frequently caused by falls. Most asymptomatic linear skull fractures do not require treatment and are observed. Compound, open, or depressed skull fractures may cause dural and/or parenchymal injury and need to be surgically explored, debrided, and repaired.

Mass Lesions

Surgical evacuation of mass lesions in comatose patients should be performed expeditiously. Epidural hematomas can expand rapidly and should be evacuated in comatose patients. Subdural hematomas that are greater than 10 mm thick or produce a midline shift of > 5 mm are associated with herniation. Enlarging intraparenchymal mass lesions manifest as progressive neurological deterioration and can lead to refractory intracranial hypertension. If there is minimal or no intracranial mass effect, penetrating injury may be managed with local debridement and watertight closure. Reduction of severe, refractory intracranial hypertension may warrant surgical resection of hemorrhagic and edematous brain tissue.

Surgical Decision Making and Perioperative Communication

Neurosurgical intervention for TBI often occurs early in the acute phase when active resuscitation is ongoing. Clear and ongoing communication between the entire perioperative team should address whether there is a need to stage the procedure, the extent of ongoing blood loss, systemic stability, and any other unanticipated events that might alter the procedure, including the decision to abort if necessary. Intraoperative blood transfusion greater than 40 mL/kg is associated with an increased incidence of 30-day mortality, clearly demonstrating a correlation between the volume of red blood cells transfused and incidence of adverse outcomes.[33] This finding provides a metric for terminating the surgery and stabilizing the patient if prudent. Once the neurosurgical procedure is completed, tracheal intubation and mechanical ventilation should be maintained, and the patient must be managed in an intensive care unit with full hemodynamic monitoring.

Cerebral Resuscitation

Intracranial Pressure Monitoring

The use of ICP monitoring in infants and children with severe TBI with a GCS ≤ 8 may be considered (Level III evidence).[3,34] However, a recent report related that routine ICP monitoring in pediatric TBI did not improve functional outcome.[35] Symptoms of increased ICP are nonspecific in children. Intermittent apnea may be the first sign of raised ICP in infants. Generally, low thresholds are maintained for monitoring unconscious patients since physiologic parameters are less sensitive than mental status changes. In infants, widening sutures and protuberant fontanels are evidence of increasing ICP. With TBI, the $CMRO_2$ and oxygen extraction can be low, and if intracranial hypertension develops, there is a corresponding decrease in CBF.[36] These findings reveal that cerebral hemodynamics and $CMRO_2$ are in flux after TBI. Level III evidence recommends that the treatment may be considered for an ICP threshold of 20 mmHg. ICP measurements from ventricular catheters and fiberoptic intraparenchymal transducer have a good correlation.[37] Ventricular catheters have the advantage of acting as a conduit to withdraw cerebrospinal fluid, which can be a therapeutic option to reduce ICP.

Medical Management of Raised ICP

Intracranial hypertension can be medically managed initially. Therapeutic interventions to lower ICP include measures to improve venous drainage, encourage fluid shifts out of the brain parenchyma, and reduce the cerebral metabolic rate. Improvements in venous drainage can be achieved by elevating the head of the bed, ensuring appropriately fitted neck immobilization collars or endotracheal tube ties, and minimizing intrathoracic pressures (by minimizing ventilation pressures and the use of positive end expiratory pressure [PEEP] or with neuromuscular blockade). Hyperosmolar therapy can encourage free water shifts out of the brain parenchyma. Mannitol can be given at a dose of 0.25 to 1.0 g/kg intravenously. However, repeated dosing may theoretically worsen cerebral edema.[38] The administration of hypertonic saline has been shown to improve various clinical parameters but not survival rate.[39] Hypertonic saline (3% NaCl) decreases ICP and increases CPP, with a loading dose of 3–5 mL/kg followed by an infusion of 0.1–1.0 mL/kg/hr.[40] Its utility to maintain serum osmolarity below 360 mOsm/L is supported by Level III evidence.[3] A reduction in the $CMRO_2$ may be accomplished with a variety of sedative-hypnotic drugs. High-dose barbiturate therapy can be titrated to produce a burst suppression pattern on the electroencephalogram, which results in a reduction in $CMRO_2$. Refractory intracranial hypertension can be treated with thiopental infusions, but volume loading and inotropic support may be needed to counter myocardial depression and hypotension. The empiric administration of steroids in not supported by Level II evidence.

Hyperventilation has traditionally been utilized to acutely treat intracranial hypertension.[41] Current guidelines recommend maintaining normocapnia except in the presence of impending herniation when brief hyperventilation can be used as a tool to temporize the situation.[3] Hyperventilation, and the resultant cerebral vasoconstriction, and increased $CMRO_2$ may worsen the supply demand perfusion ratio to tissue already compromised by injury.[42,43] Aggressive hyperventilation in the absence of cerebral herniation is associated with poor discharge survival.[15] Thus, it is particularly important to recognize that small children are subject to inadvertent overventilation and that hyperventilation-associated cerebral ischemia can occur. Careful monitoring of blood gases, minute ventilation, and use of end-tidal carbon dioxide tensions are recommended. If these maneuvers fail to control elevated ICP, decompressive craniectomy should be considered (see above). Neurogenic pulmonary edema and acute respiratory distress syndrome can compromise oxygenation and should be treated expectantly.

Induced Hypothermia

Head cooling and mild hypothermia have been demonstrated to be protective in asphyxiated neonates.[44] However, induced hypothermia in adult TBI has shown mixed results. An international multicenter trial of induced hypothermia in pediatric patients reported that hypothermia did not improve the neurologic outcome and may increase mortality.[45] A National Institutes of Health (NIH) sponsored phase III trial (CoolKids) revealed that hypothermia for 48 hours with slow rewarming did not reduce mortality or global functional outcome.[46] Interestingly, the International Hypothermia in Aneurysm Surgery Trial (IHAST) in adults also failed to demonstrate any advantage of hypothermia over normothermia intraoperatively during surgical clipping of intracranial aneurysms.[47]

Summary

TBI continues to be the most common yet poorly studied cause of morbidity and mortality in pediatric patients. There are a number of predictors of poor outcome, these include:[48]

1. Age < 4 years
2. The need for cardiopulmonary resuscitation
3. Polytrauma
4. PaO_2 < 60 mmHg

5. $PaCO_2$ < 35 mmHg
6. Glucose > 250 mg/dl
7. Temperature > 38°C
8. SBP < 5th percentile for age
9. ICP > 20 mmHg
10. Poor rehabilitation

Despite the wealth of laboratory and clinical investigations published in the trauma literature, there are only a few studies that have directly addressed the pathophysiology of TBI in infants and children. Clinician investigations continue to evolve and modify the management of these vulnerable patients. Fortunately, published best practice recommendations provide a basic understanding of age-dependent variables and the interaction of management issues that are essential in minimizing perioperative morbidity and mortality. TBI management that can be supported with evidence includes:[3]

1. Level II evidence (should be considered)

   a. Steroids: not indicated
   b. Hypothermia: 32–33°C for only 24 hours should be avoided; 32–33°C 8 hours after injury for 48 hours should be considered
   c. Nutrition: not indicated
   d. Hypertonic saline: indicated

2. Level III evidence (may be considered)

   a. ICP: treatment for ICP > 20 mmHg
   b. CPP: maintain CPP > 40 mmHg and 40–50 mmHg
   c. Neuroimaging: routine imaging not recommended
   d. Brain oxygenation: maintenance of PbO_2 ≥10 mm Hg
   e. Hyperventilation: avoidance of $PaCO_2$ <30 mmHg

References

1. Hardcastle N, Benzon HA, Vavilala MS. Update on the 2012 guidelines for the management of pediatric traumatic brain injury—information for the anesthesiologist. *Paediatr Anaesth*. 2014;**24**:703–10.

2. American Heart Association. *Pediatric Advanced Life Support Provider Manual*. Dallas: American Heart Association; 2012.

3. Kochanek PM, Carney N, Adelson PD, Ashwal S, Bell MJ, Bratton S, et al. Guidelines for the acute medical management of severe traumatic brain injury in infants, children, and adolescents—second edition. *Pediatr Crit Care Med*. 2012;**13**(suppl 1):S1–82.

4. Vavilala MS, Bowen A, Lam AM, Uffman JC, Powell J, Winn HR, Rivara FP. Blood pressure and outcome after severe pediatric traumatic brain injury. *J Trauma*. 2003;**55**:1039–44.

5. Kannan N, Wang J, Mink RB, Wainwright MS, Groner JI, Bell MJ, et al. Timely hemodynamic resuscitation and outcomes in severe pediatric traumatic brain injury: preliminary findings. *Pediatr Emerg Care*. 2018;**34**(5):325–9.

6. Liras IN, Caplan HW, Stensballe J, Wade CE, Cox CS, Cotton BA. Prevalence and impact of admission acute traumatic coagulopathy on treatment intensity, resource use, and mortality: an evaluation of 956 severely injured children and adolescents. *J Am Coll Surg*. 2017;**224**:625–32.

7. Brady KM, Mytar JO, Lee JK, Cameron DE, Vricella LA, Thompson WR, et al. Monitoring cerebral blood flow pressure autoregulation in pediatric patients during cardiac surgery. *Stroke*. 2010;**41**:1957–62.

8. Lee JK. Cerebral perfusion pressure: how low can we go? *Paediatr Anaesth*. 2014;**24**:647–8.

9. Udomphorn Y, Armstead WM, Vavilala MS. Cerebral blood flow and autoregulation after pediatric traumatic brain injury. *Pediatr Neurol*. 2008;**38**:225–34.

10. Donnelly JE, Young AMH, Brady K. Autoregulation in paediatric TBI—current evidence and implications for treatment. *Childs Nerv Syst*. 2017;**33**:1735–44.

11. Young AMH, Guilfoyle MR, Donnelly J, Smielewski P, Agarwal S, Czosnyka M, Hutchinson PJ. Multimodality neuromonitoring in severe pediatric traumatic brain injury. *Pediatr Res*. 2018;**83**:41–9.

12. Brady KM, Lee JK, Kibler KK, Easley RB, Koehler RC, Czosnyka M, et al. The lower limit of cerebral blood flow autoregulation is increased with elevated intracranial pressure. *Anesth Analg*. 2009;**108**:1278–83.

13. Chambers IR, Jones PA, Lo TY, Forsyth RJ, Fulton B, Andrews PJ, et al. Critical thresholds of intracranial pressure and cerebral perfusion pressure related to age in paediatric head injury. *J Neurol Neurosurg Psychiatry*. 2006;**77**:234–40.

14. Downard C, Hulka F, Mullins RJ, Piatt J, Chesnut R, Quint P, Mann NC. Relationship of cerebral perfusion pressure and survival in pediatric brain-injured patients. *J Trauma*. 2000;**49**:654–8; discussion 658–9.

15. Vavilala MS, Kernic MA, Wang J, Kannan N, Mink RB, Wainwright MS, et al. Acute care clinical indicators brain injury. *Crit Care Med*. 2014;**42**:2258–66.

16. Wright JN. CNS injuries in abusive head trauma. *AJR Am J Roentgenol.* 2017; **208**:991–1001.

17. Duhaime AC, Christian CW, Rorke LB, Zimmerman RA. Nonaccidental head injury in infants—the "shaken-baby syndrome." *N Engl J Med.* 1998;**338**:1822–9.

18. Miller Ferguson N, Sarnaik A, Miles D, Shafi N, Peters MJ, Truemper E, et al. Abusive head trauma and mortality—an analysis from an international comparative effectiveness study of children with severe traumatic brain injury. *Crit Care Med.* 2017;**45**:1398–407.

19. Lee JK, Brady KM, Deutsch N. The anesthesiologist's role in treating abusive head trauma. *Anesth Analg.* 2016;**122**:1971–82.

20. Abcejo AS, Savica R, Lanier WL, Pasternak JJ. Exposure to surgery and anesthesia after concussion due to mild traumatic brain injury. *Mayo Clin Proc.* 2017;**92**:1042–52.

21. Vavilala MS, Ferrari LR, Herring SA. Perioperative care of the concussed patient: making the case for defining best anesthesia care. *Anesth Analg.* 2017;**125**:1053–5.

22. Ellis MJ, Leiter J, Hall T, McDonald PJ, Sawyer S, Silver N, et al. Neuroimaging findings in pediatric sports-related concussion. *J Neurosurg Pediatr.* 2015;**16**:241–7.

23. Fujita Y, Algarra NN, Vavilala MS, Prathep S, Prapruettham S, Sharma D. Intraoperative secondary insults during extracranial surgery in children with traumatic brain injury. *Childs Nerv Syst.* 2014;**30**:1201–8.

24. Vavilala MS, Farr CK, Watanitanon A, Clark-Bell BC, Chandee T, Moore A, Armstead W. Early changes in cerebral autoregulation among youth hospitalized after sports-related traumatic brain injury. *Brain Inj.* 2018;**32**:269–75.

25. Hutchinson PJ, Kolias AG, Timofeev IS, Corteen EA, Czosnyka M, Timothy J, et al. Trial of decompressive craniectomy for traumatic intracranial hypertension. *N Engl J Med.* 2016;**375**:1119–30.

26. Bruce DA, Alavi A, Bilaniuk L, Dolinskas C, Obrist W, Uzzell B. Diffuse cerebral swelling following head injuries in children: the syndrome of "malignant brain edema." *J Neurosurg.* 1981;**54**:170–8.

27. Polin RS, Shaffrey ME, Bogaev CA, Tisdale N, Germanson T, Bocchicchio B, Jane JA. Decompressive bifrontal craniectomy in the treatment of severe refractory posttraumatic cerebral edema. *Neurosurgery.* 1997;**41**:84–92; discussion 92–4.

28. Taylor A, Butt W, Rosenfeld J, Shann F, Ditchfield M, Lewis E, et al. A randomized trial of very early decompressive craniectomy in children with traumatic brain injury and sustained intracranial hypertension. *Childs Nerv Syst.* 2001;**17**:154–62.

29. Cho DY, Wang YC, Chi CS. Decompressive craniotomy for acute shaken/impact baby syndrome. *Pediatr Neurosurg.* 1995;**23**:192–8.

30. Jagannathan J, Okonkwo DO, Dumont AS, Ahmed H, Bahari A, Prevedello DM, et al. Outcome following decompressive craniectomy in children with severe traumatic brain injury: a 10-year single-center experience with long-term follow up. *J Neurosurg.* 2007;**106**:268–75.

31. Jacob AT, Heuer GG, Grant R, Georgoff P, Danish SF, Storm PB, Stein SC. Decompressive hemicraniectomy for pediatric traumatic brain injury: long-term outcome based on quality of life. *Pediatr Neurosurg.* 2011;**47**:81–6.

32. Young AMH, Kolias AG, Hutchinson PJ. Decompressive craniectomy for traumatic intracranial hypertension: application in children. *Childs Nerv Syst.* 2017;**33**:1745–50.

33. Goobie SM, DiNardo JA, Faraoni D. Relationship between transfusion volume and outcomes in children undergoing noncardiac surgery. *Transfusion.* 2016;**56**:2487–94.

34. Alali AS, Gomez D, Sathya C, Burd RS, Mainprize TG, Moulton R, et al. Intracranial pressure monitoring among children with severe traumatic brain injury. *J Neurosurg Pediatr.* 2015;**16**(5):1–10.

35. Bennett TD, DeWitt PE, Greene TH, Srivastava R, Riva-Cambrin J, Nance ML, et al. Functional outcome after intracranial pressure monitoring for children with severe traumatic brain injury. *JAMA Pediatr.* 2017;**171**:965–71.

36. Sharples PM, Stuart AG, Matthews DS, Aynsley-Green A, Eyre JA. Cerebral blood flow and metabolism in children with severe head injury. Part 1: Relation to age, Glasgow coma score, outcome, intracranial pressure, and time after injury. *J Neurol Neurosurg Psychiatry.* 1995;**58**:145–52.

37. Gambardella G, Zaccone C, Cardia E, Tomasello F. Intracranial pressure monitoring in children: comparison of external ventricular device with the fiberoptic system. *Childs Nerv Syst.* 1993;**9**:470–3.

38. McManus ML, Soriano SG. Rebound swelling of astroglial cells exposed to hypertonic mannitol. *Anesthesiology.* 1998;**88**:1586–91.

39. Shackford SR, Bourguignon PR, Wald SL, Rogers FB, Osler TM, Clark DE. Hypertonic saline resuscitation of patients with head injury: a prospective, randomized clinical trial. *J Trauma.* 1998;**44**:50–8.

40. Khanna S, Davis D, Peterson B, Fisher B, Tung H, O'Quigley J, Deutsch R. Use of hypertonic saline in the treatment of severe refractory posttraumatic

intracranial hypertension in pediatric traumatic brain injury. *Crit Care Med*. 2000;**28**:1144–51.

41. Meng L, Gelb AW. Regulation of cerebral autoregulation by carbon dioxide. *Anesthesiology*. 2015;**122**:196–205.

42. Coles JP, Minhas PS, Fryer TD, Smielewski P, Aigbirihio F, Donovan T, et al. Effect of hyperventilation on cerebral blood flow in traumatic head injury: clinical relevance and monitoring correlates. *Crit Care Med*. 2002;**30**: 1950–9.

43. Coles JP, Fryer TD, Coleman MR, Smielewski P, Gupta AK, Minhas PS, et al. Hyperventilation following head injury: effect on ischemic burden and cerebral oxidative metabolism. *Crit Care Med*. 2007;**35**:568–78.

44. Shankaran S, Pappas A, McDonald SA, Vohr BR, Hintz SR, Yolton K, et al. Childhood outcomes after hypothermia for neonatal encephalopathy. *N Engl J Med*. 2012;**366**:2085–92.

45. Hutchison JS, Ward RE, Lacroix J, Hebert PC, Barnes MA, Bohn DJ, et al. Hypothermia therapy after traumatic brain injury in children. *N Engl J Med*. 2008;**358**:2447–56.

46. Adelson PD, Wisniewski SR, Beca J, Brown SD, Bell M, Muizelaar JP, et al. Comparison of hypothermia and normothermia after severe traumatic brain injury in children (Cool Kids): a phase 3, randomised controlled trial. *Lancet Neurol*. 2013;**12**:546–53.

47. Todd MM, Hindman BJ, Clarke WR, Torner JC. Intraoperative Hypothermia for Aneurysm Surgery Trial Investigators. Mild intraoperative hypothermia during surgery for intracranial aneurysm. *N Engl J Med*. 2005;**352**:135–45.

48. Vavilala MS, Soriano SG, Krane EJ. Anesthesia for neurosurgery. In: Davis PJ, Cladis FP, eds. *Smith's Anesthesia for Infants and Children*, 9th ed. Philadelphia: Elsevier; 2017:744–73.

Chapter 15

Anesthesia for Minimally Invasive Neurosurgery

Petra M. Meier and Thomas O. Erb

Introduction and Anesthetic Goals

Minimally invasive neurosurgery has greatly impacted pediatric neurosurgery during the past few decades. Technological advances in optics, imaging, and computing and the availability of three-dimensional image-guided navigational systems (frameless stereotaxy, stealth technology) and micro-surgical tools allow access to areas of the brain for-merly reachable only through large surgical incisions. Currently the most common indications for infants and children undergoing neuroendoscopic proce-dures are conditions ranging from hydrocephalus, brain tumors, and congenital intracranial cysts to craniosynostosis and stereotactic procedures (Table 15.1). The potential benefits of minimally invasive neurosurgery result from reduced invasive-ness, smaller incisions, limited need for brain retrac-tion, decreased intraoperative blood loss, shorter operating times, and shorter hospital stay compared with corresponding open procedures. With these new surgical techniques come requirements for expertise, simulation training, and specific modifications of intraoperative anesthesia care (Table 15.1). The neuroanesthetic goals remain unchanged also under special interventional conditions: (1) preserva-tion of cerebral blood flow, (2) control of intracranial pressure (ICP), (3) immobility of the patient, (4) facilitation of intraoperative neurophysiologic mon-itoring techniques, and (5) rapid emergence from anesthesia and return of neurological/cognitive func-tion for prompt neurologic assessment.

Ventricular Neuroendoscopy

The cerebrospinal fluid (CSF) channels provide the working environment for ventricular neuroendo-scopy. The CSF space is transparent and therefore allows excellent visualization of deep brain struc-tures. Ventricular neuroendoscopy permits inspec-tion of the ventricular system, treatment of hydrocephalus by procedures such as endoscopic

third ventriculostomy (ETV), choroid plexus abla-tion, intraventricular cyst fenestration, tumor biopsy and resection, irrigation and removal of hemorrhage, and endoscopic placement of cathe-ters.[1] The surgical technique employs burr hole placement in the skull through which a flexible or rigid endoscope is inserted into the ventricle. Endoscopes provide the advantage of excellent visualization and illumination at angles not neces-sarily available when using a surgical microscope. While flexible endoscopes allow greater degrees of freedom, this goes at the expense of comparatively impaired optic quality. They are available with working channels allowing the use of single or multiple instruments and an irrigation port. Adequate visualization requires continuous irriga-tion of the ventricles with warmed normal saline or lactated Ringer's solution and simultaneous drainage of CSF and irrigating fluid through the scope.

ETV is a mainstay treatment for *occlusive hydro-cephalus* (Figures 15.1, 15.2, 15.3) and in selected cases with choroid plexus cauterization.[2] The setting of isolated lateral ventricular hydrocephalus secondary to unilateral obstructions at the foramen of Monro (trapped lateral ventricle) is another form of hydro-cephalus, in which endoscopic-aided procedures have proven to be useful. *Endoscopic septostomy for trapped lateral ventricle* may be performed to create a communication between the lateral ventricles; here endoscopic-guided intervention has been demon-strated to eliminate the need for CSF shunting or ventricular catheters.

Regarding *endoscopic cyst fenestration, decompres-sion, and resection,* intracranial cysts are often seen in children located in the intraventricular, paraventricu-lar, cisternal, or subarachnoid spaces. Advances in neuroendoscopic-guided techniques have resulted in most cysts being treated with endoscopic fenestration, decompression, and resection (Figure 15.4). The fenestration is completed either into a nearby

Table 15.1 Common Indications for Minimally Invasive Surgery and Perioperative Anesthesia Considerations/Implications

Diagnosis	Intervention	Perioperative Anesthesia Implications
Obstructive hydrocephalus	Third ventriculostomy ± CPC for – Aqueductal stenosis – 4th ventricular outlet obstruction	Increased ICP, altered mental status: primary disease, intraventricular clots, obstructed egress of irrigation fluid
Isolated lateral ventricular hydrocephalus due to unilateral obstruction at Foramen of Monro	Septostomy to form a communication between the lateral ventricles	Vomiting and hypovolemia Aspiration Arrhythmias
Multiloculated hydrocephalus or complex ventricular anatomy	Endoscopic external ventricular drainage	Hemorrhage, basilar artery aneurysmal formation
		Damage to midbrain structures Hypothermia (use warm irrigation fluid) Ventriculitis and postoperative fever
Intracranial arachnoid cysts	Fenestration, removal	Increased ICP (obstructive hydrocephalus) Vomiting and hypovolemia Aspiration
		Hemorrhage
Intra-, paraventricular tumor	Biopsy	Hemorrhage
Cranial synostosis	Endoscopic-assisted strip craniectomy	Difficult airway with craniofacial syndromes Endotracheal tube displacement with neck flexion/extension Positioning: supine or modified prone Potential for blood loss Potential for venous air embolism
Deep seated, difficult to access, inoperable lesions, brain metastases, gliomas, radiation necrosis, epilepsy foci	Stereotactic procedures	Frame can interfere with airway management Damage to midbrain structures Increased ICP Hemorrhage from biopsy site: – Direct surgical manipulation – Abrupt alterations in blood pressure (cave during emergence)

CPC = choroid plexus cauterization

cistern or into the closest abutting ventricle in an attempt to create a connected CSF space.

Endoscopic biopsy and resection of tumors within the ventricles of the brain include intra- and paraventricular tumors including pineal region tumors, optic hypothalamic tumors, and craniopharyngeomas. Biopsy is often the initial intervention of choice to accurately diagnose the pathology before a definitive treatment plan can be established. Some tumors may be hemorrhagic, and thus bleeding may be encountered at the time of biopsy,

which requires irrigation at the site of the biopsy, electrocautery, and/or insertion of a ventricular drain.

Endoscopic Third Ventriculostomy (ETV)

By far the most commonly performed intraventricular neuroendoscopic procedure is ETV for hydrocephalus.[3,4] Indications include primary congenital anomalies such as aqueductal stenosis (narrowing of the duct connecting the third ventricle to the fourth

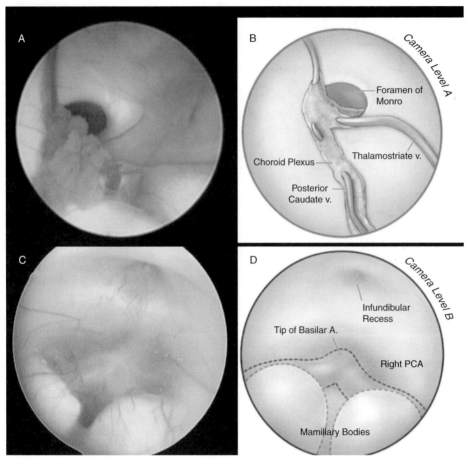

Figure 15.1. Endoscopic view of the foramen of Monro (A, B) obtained with a rigid endoscope positioned in the frontal horn of the right lateral ventricle. After advancing the endoscope through the foramen of Monro, the floor of the third ventricle is identified (C, D). Note the tip of the basilar artery and the two posterior cerebral arteries are visible through the floor of the third ventricle. Reprinted with permission from Meier et al., *Paediatr Anaesth* 2014[3] and from Guzman et al., *J Neurosurg Pediatr* 2013.[4]

ventricle), meningomyelocele/Chiari malformation and idiopathic causes, obstruction secondary to pineal tumors, aqueductal stenosis secondary to tectal gliomas, and cisternal arachnoid cysts. ETV is also used as a viable and efficacious alternative to treat cases of obstructive hydrocephalus, previously treated by ventriculoperitoneal shunting, that present with a shunt failure. The burr hole in the skull is typically placed at the same location where the ventriculoperitoneal (VP) shunt would be inserted (lateral to the right sagittal suture and anterior to the coronal suture in the mid-pupillary line). An endoscope is placed through the burr hole into the frontal horn of the lateral ventricle, through the foramen of Monro into the third ventricle, and then directed toward the anterior floor of the third ventricle. An opening is created in the floor of the third ventricle posterior to the infundibular recess, which creates a bypass within the brain allowing the CSF to drain, avoiding the placement of a ventricular peritoneal shunt. Figure 15.1 demonstrates the endoscopic and schematic view of the anatomy of the foramen of Monro and the anterior translucent floor of the third ventricle. Figure 15.2 illustrates the different surgical steps in performing ETV and Figure 15.3 the fenestration of the third ventricular floor using Fogarty occlusion balloon (Edwards, Irvine, CA) or NeuroBalloon (Integra, Saint-Priest, France) catheters with view into the prepontine cistern.[3,4]

Preoperative Issues

Much of the preoperative considerations and anesthetic care is dictated not by the specific endoscopic procedure but by the patients' conditions including

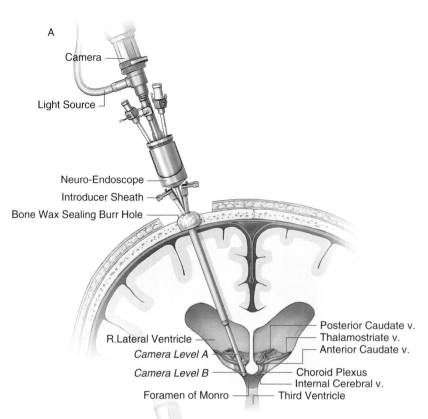

A

Camera

Light Source

Neuro-Endoscope

Introducer Sheath

Bone Wax Sealing Burr Hole

R.Lateral Ventricle

Camera Level A

Camera Level B

Foramen of Monro

Posterior Caudate v.

Thalamostriate v.

Anterior Caudate v.

Choroid Plexus

Internal Cerebral v.

Third Ventricle

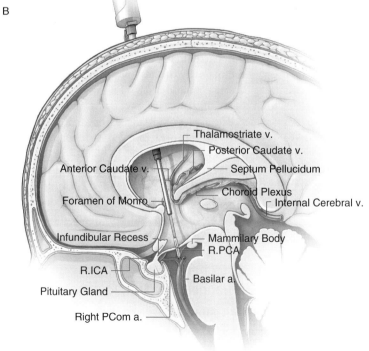

B

Thalamostriate v.

Posterior Caudate v.

Anterior Caudate v.

Septum Pellucidum

Foramen of Monro

Choroid Plexus

Internal Cerebral v.

Infundibular Recess

Mammilary Body

R.PCA

R.ICA

Basilar a.

Pituitary Gland

Right PCom a.

Figure 15.2. Endoscopic third ventriculostomy. (A) Illustration demonstrates the advancement of the endoscope from a right frontal burr hole through the frontal horn of the right lateral ventricle, through the foramen of Monro into the third ventricle. (B) The balloon catheter is positioned across the floor of the third ventricle to perform the fenestration. Reprinted with permission from Meier et al., *Paediatr Anaesth* 2014.[3]

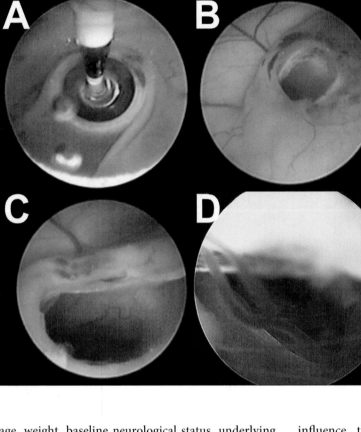

Figure 15.3. Surgical steps of endoscopic third ventriculostomy using a rigid endoscope. (A) After the puncture with a 4-F Fogarty balloon catheter through the thin, translucent third ventricular floor along the anterior aspect of the tuber cinereum, the balloon is slowly inflated. Be aware of possible bradycardia during this maneuver. In cases where bleeding is encountered from the floor of the third ventricle, the balloon may remain inflated for an extended period and used for tamponade. (B) Completion of the balloon dilation after removal of the Fogarty balloon from the field. (C) Through the fenestration, the clivus is visible. The surgeon ascertains that there is no flow obstruction in the prepontine cisterns such as the Lilequist membrane. (D) The basilar artery, the left posterior cerebral artery, and perforator branches can be appreciated. Reprinted with permission from Meier et al., *Paediatr Anaesth* 2014[3] and from Guzman et al., *J Neurosurg Pediatr* 2013.[4]

age, weight, baseline neurological status, underlying disease process, associated medical illnesses, and current state of health.[5] Patients may range in age from preterm newborns to adolescents. Some patients presenting for ETV may have had prior shunt placements with shunt systems extending from the ventricles to the peritoneal/pleural cavity or the right atrium or central vascular locations. The need for repeated surgical procedures secondary to malfunction or infections can result in added morbidity to the patient. A standard preoperative workup should address the patient's systematic illnesses as well as the current underlying primary disease process (e.g., intraventricular hemorrhage). Preoperative evaluation must be focused on the neurological status; for example, patients with hydrocephalus or a primary lesion resulting in obstruction of CSF pathways may present with symptoms of increased ICP. Patients with prolonged vomiting may have significant dehydration and/or electrolyte abnormalities, requiring correction prior to the surgical procedure. Associated medical illnesses especially cervical spine abnormalities, syndromes, and current medication regimen might

influence the perioperative anesthesia planning. As these procedures have a potential for blood loss, our current practice includes laboratory testing for the majority of these patients (including coagulation and a type and cross). Preoperative medication (e.g., benzodiazepines) may not be required or desired because of potentially associated problems such as presence of intracranial hypertension and/or altered mental status and the need for postoperative rapid awakening to expedite a neurological examination. Treatment with anticonvulsants or other therapeutic agents should usually be continued during the perioperative period, and pharmacological interactions with neuromuscular blocking agents have to be taken into account and appropriately monitored.[6]

Intraoperative Management

The intraoperative anesthesia care should be guided by the fact that endoscopic intraventricular neurosurgical interventions are short, noninvasive procedures performed in supine position without neurosurgical head pins. For the majority of these semielective

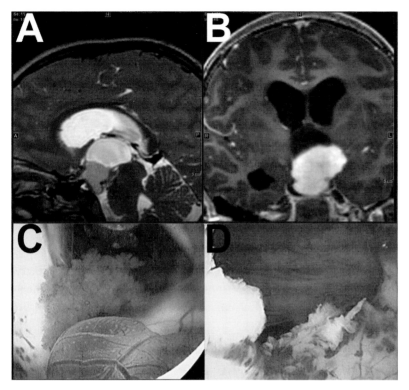

Figure 15.4. Four-year-old child with a cystic tumor obstructing the third ventricle as seen in a sagittal T2-weighted (A) and a coronal T1-weighted (B) MR image. An endoscopic transventricular approach through the right lateral ventricle was chosen for cyst fenestration (C). Note the incidental choroid plexus cyst (C). View into the tumor cavity after cyst fenestration and the biopsy (D). Cerebrospinal fluid pathways were restored after this procedure. Reprinted with permission from Meier et al., *Paediatr Anaesth* 2014.[3]

procedures, intravenous induction or inhalational induction represent equally good options. However, for urgent indications, such as the presence of increased ICP, nausea, and vomiting, a modified rapid sequence induction should be taken into account. Endotracheal intubation is required secondary to the muscle relaxation needed to prevent patient movement during the delicate intraventricular surgical maneuvers. Ventilation must be carefully controlled, especially in small infants when the proportionate increase in dead space along with small tidal volumes may cause end-tidal CO_2 to underestimate $PaCO_2$, resulting in hypercapnia and associated alterations in ICP. Anesthesia monitoring includes the standard monitors (electrocardiogram, pulsoxymetry, capnography, noninvasive blood pressure). An arterial line and central line are usually not required except in the presence of serious comorbidities. Often a second access of a peripheral vein is advisable. In case of central line placement, VP/ventriculoatrial shunt locations need to be explored to avoid unintended puncture of the peripheral shunt tubing. For maintenance anesthesia, in our practice, the combination of an inhalation anesthesia (without nitrous oxide) and wound infiltration with local anesthetics (at the site of the burr hole at the beginning of the procedure) aiming to minimize the administration of opioids is sufficient. The burr hole approach creates minimal postoperative pain, so small doses of short-acting narcotics and acetaminophen are satisfactory. The anesthetic goals should focus on intraoperative immobilization, cardiovascular stability, control of ICP and preservation of cerebral blood flow, and rapid emergence for early neurologic examination. After emergence from anesthesia, the surgical team will perform the first neurological examination in the operating room (OR). Thereafter, the patient is moved to the postanesthesia care unit (PACU) and thereafter to the ward with frequent follow-up neurological examinations.

A standard OR layout, including adequate positioning of the equipment and view of the monitors, must be carefully considered. To facilitate surgical exposure and surgical access to the patient, the patient and bed are often turned 90° to 180°. The anesthesia team and equipment are usually situated on the left side of the patient. The surgical team is positioned directly around the head of the patient, observing the video monitors, which are located at the foot of the patient while navigating the endoscope. Importantly, the OR table must be absolutely immobile when the endoscope is maneuvered inside the ventricular system.

Avoidance of Complications and Postoperative Concerns

Prevention of intraoperative complications requires control of ICP and irrigation pressures, and mastery of the intraventricular anatomy to minimize tissue trauma. Despite the minimally invasive nature of these procedures, acute bradycardia and other cardiovascular complications may occur. During the procedure, there is a constant flow of irrigation solution (normal saline or lactated Ringer's solution) through the endoscope to irrigate the ventricular space. These irrigation fluids should be warmed to body temperature, as cold fluid can cause bradycardia and hypothermia. The difference in chemistry between CSF and irrigation fluid may cause toxic reactions such as meningitis, fever, headache, and an increased cell count.[7,8] Normal saline irrigation may cause CSF acidosis, and use of lactated Ringer's has been reported to result in postoperative increased potassium serum levels.[9] Acute increases in ICP will occur if egress of the irrigating fluid is not maintained, mandating a constant evaluation of the amount of fluid infused and the amount retrieved. Otherwise, a Cushing-type response may result with refractory hypertension and tachycardia/bradycardia as an indicator of impaired brain perfusion and/or stimulation of the preoptic area,[10,11] which require vigilant recognition and correction to prevent serious and potentially irreversible injury. The development of neurogenic pulmonary edema after vigorous intraventricular irrigation may be another acute intraoperative complication requiring postoperative ventilation and treatment in the intensive care unit (ICU).[12] Intraoperative acute bradycardia might occur during the process of fenestration through a thickened third ventricular floor (reported up to 41%), which is mostly self-resolving with cessation of the surgical stimuli.[13]

Occasionally bleeding may occur during intraventricular endoscopic procedures.[14] The scope must then be maintained within the field and continuous irrigation with warm irrigation fluid generally stops the bleeding. Cauterization may be attempted if a bleeding site can be identified and a ventricular drain may be left in place along the endoscopic tract to allow for drainage of the intraventricular hemorrhage in rare cases if mild bleeding persists. If the bleeding is catastrophic, rapid conversion to open craniotomy has to be considered.

The importance of mastering the intraventricular anatomy and landmarks is paramount to limiting complications.[15] The endoscope is navigated along the desired trajectory through the foramen of Monro; care should be taken to avoid injury to the fornix, which might result in transient memory loss, personality changes, and injury to cranial nerves III and VI. Lateral entry can result in injury to the hypothalamus entailing endocrine problems such as syndrome of inappropriate antidiuretic hormone, diabetes insipidus, secondary amenorrhea, loss of thirst, seizures, or trancelike states. Fenestration along the anterior floor risks injury to the pituitary, and fenestration posteriorly risks injury to the mammillary bodies and brainstem. Injury to the basilar artery, the most feared surgical complication, might cause hemorrhage, formation of a pseudoaneurysm, or stroke, and may even result in intraoperative death.

A report of 368 patients with an average age of 6.5 years over a 15-year period (1989–2004) from multiple Canadian centers cited a complication rate of 14%, with the most common complications being CSF leak 3.6%, meningitis 2.8%, hemorrhage 1.4%, hypothalamic injury 1.4%, cranial nerve injury 1.4%, seizure 1.4%, and other 1.4%.[14]

After an uneventful surgical procedure, the majority of patients can be discharged with apnea monitoring from the PACU to the ward when the patient is fully awake, the neurological exam is at baseline, and the PACU course is uneventful. Patients should be monitored for signs of central nervous infections, and if clinically indicated, monitoring of serum electrolytes might be warranted.

Endoscopic-Assisted Strip Craniectomy for Craniosynostosis Repair

Craniosynostosis is a congenital anomaly characterized by the premature fusion of one or more cranial sutures, with an incidence of about 1:2,000 live births. Surgical intervention is indicated to improve appearance and prevent complications of increased ICP such as cognitive impairment and auditory and visual loss.

Correction of craniosynostosis includes various surgical techniques, some of which are associated with substantial blood loss. In the last two decades, less invasive alternatives have evolved to treat infants with craniosynostosis.[16] One such technique, endoscopic-assisted strip craniectomy (ESC), has been typically offered to young infants 3–6 months of age. The fused suture is accessed through small incisions and, with the use of an endoscope for visualization, the affected suture(s) is removed. Subsequently, the skull shape is modified by helmet therapy redirecting the growth after the surgical procedure. Conceptually this turns the treatment of synostosis into a deformational problem. With this technique, the surgical intervention needs to be performed early in infancy to maximize successful reshaping of the skull with the helmet during the time period of maximum rapid brain growth. In contrast, the open surgical techniques involve wide scalp dissections with multiple osteotomies followed by reshaping and stabilization of these cranial bones. Consequently, these procedures are lengthy (4–6 hours), and almost universally require blood transfusion; estimated percentage of blood volume loss ranges from 25% (open linear strip craniectomies, pi procedure) to as high as 500% (total calvarial vault remodeling), and is associated with increased perioperative morbidity, and a typical 4- to 5-day hospital course with ICU admission.[17,18] ESCs have comparable cosmetic and volumetric outcomes to open cranial vault remodeling techniques, but with less operative time (<1 hour), blood loss (blood transfusion required in 5–10% of infants), and length of hospitalization (discharge first postop day) and lower costs.[19–21]

Surgical Procedure ESC

ESC can be used to treat craniosynostosis of any cranial suture. While the majority of ESC procedures are single suturectomies, ESC can be also considered for multiple suture craniosynostoses.

Sagittal ESC and lambdoid ESC are usually performed in prone position, often using special headrests and metopic and coronal ESC in supine position, commonly using the cerebellar headrest. Small skin incisions are performed perpendicular to the stenosed sutures (Figure 15.5) and deepened to the level of the periosteum. Cranial burr holes are drilled through the midline of each scalp incision. An endoscope is inserted parallel to a suction tip to improve the visibility of emissary veins, dural attachments, and ensure hemostasis. The epidural suturectomy (usually < 1 cm in width) is typically performed with bone-cutting scissors or an ultrasonic bone-cutting device (e.g.,

metopic ESC). The closed suture is resected and removed through the burr hole. Bone bleeding is controlled using bone wax and thrombin-soaked absorbable gelatin (Gelfoam; Pharmacia and Upjohn, Kalamazoo, MI).[22] Within 1 week of surgery, cranial molding helmets are individually fitted with frequent progress evaluations and adjustments. The average duration of helmet therapy is 22 hours per day for 7.5 months (Figure 15.6).

Patient positioning remains one of the paramount concerns during neuroendoscopic procedures in providing surgical access and optimal exposure of the suture.[3,5] Infants undergoing sagittal or lambdoid ESC are placed in different modifications of prone positions, including "sphinx" or "sea lion" positioning on the bean bag or a modified prone head holder (Figure 15.5A). The neck is extended and the endotracheal tube has to be carefully placed in midtracheal position to prevent inadvertent extubation.

Preoperative Assessment

The surgical procedure is optimally performed by 3 months of age and up to 6 months of life. At this time, the infant is at the physiologic nadir of hematocrit value.

Preoperative laboratory tests should include complete blood count (CBC), electrolyte, and coagulation study. Although blood loss and blood transfusion are significantly decreased with ESC, there is a risk of significant blood loss secondary to bleeding of an emissary vein of the sagittal sinus. Blood products should be immediately available in the OR during the procedure.

Craniofacial anomalies can be associated with syndromes (Apert, Crouzon, Muenke, Saethre Chotzen, Pfeiffer), a compromised airway, and cardiac and other congenital anomalies. Although the incidence of sleep disorder and obstructive sleep apnea syndrome is high in syndromic infants, it is often unrecognized and adds to the perioperative morbidity in these infants. Obstructive sleep apnea symptoms occur in almost half of the children during episodes of upper respiratory tract infections.

Ophthalmologic examinations may show papilledema and optic atrophy with chronically raised ICP. Syndromic craniosynostoses with shallow, deformed orbits and exorbitism increase the risk of corneal abrasion and ocular trauma and require appropriate protection during the surgical procedure.

Congenital heart disease, both repaired and unrepaired, has been shown to increase the risk for

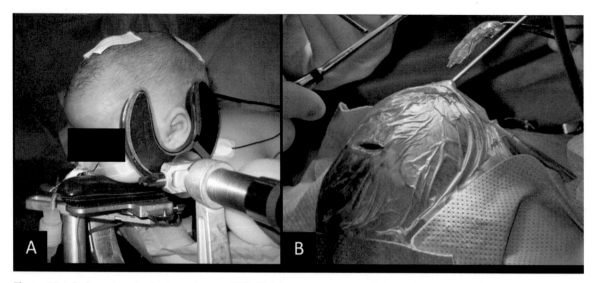

Figure 15.5. Endoscopic-assisted strip craniectomy (ESC). (A) Infant in prone position for sagittal ESC on a modified prone head holder in sphinx position. It illustrates the extended head position and the significant distance between the highest point of the surgical field to the right atrium, a risk factor for venous air embolism (VAE) or paradoxical air embolism. (B) Intraoperative picture of sagittal ESC with two skin incisions perpendicular to the stenosed sagittal suture: one posterior to the coronal sutures and the other at the junction of the lambdoids. After endoscopic suturectomy, the 1- to 2-cm-wide bone strip of the fused sagittal suture is removed. Reprinted with permission from Meier et al., *Paediatr Anaesth* 2014.[3]

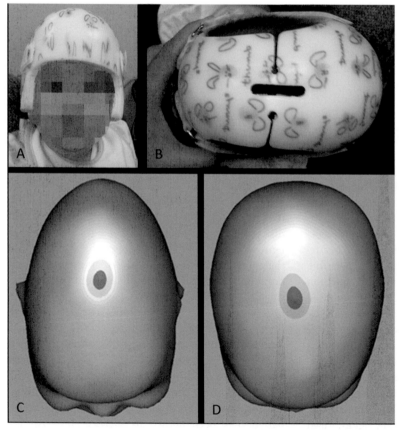

Figure 15.6. Postoperative orthosis after endoscopic-assisted strip craniectomy (ESC) (A and B) Infant with sagittal craniosynostosis after ESC wearing the helmet with openings at the side that allows the growing brain to push the skull out, which finally results in the desired round head form. (C and D) Preorthotic (left) and postorthotic (right) laser scan documenting the change in head shape and improvement in cranial index in an infant with sagittal synostosis. Reprinted with permission from Meier et al., *Paediatr Anaesth* 2014.[3]

anesthesia and any surgery. Infants with patent foramen ovale or ductus arteriosus are at risk for paradoxical air emboli.

Cervical vertebra anomalies, particularly in Apert, Pfeiffer, and Crouzon syndromes, limit neck motion (flexion and extension) and can increase the difficulty of intubation, and positioning for ESC needs to be carefully assessed.

Infants receiving anticonvulsants should have their dosing optimized preoperatively and continue their treatment during the perioperative period.

Intraoperative Management

The intraoperative anesthesia care of ESCs should be based on their short duration of approximately 30–45 minutes, relatively low blood loss, and low incidence of blood transfusion (8%; associated predictors: body weight < 5 kg, syndromic craniosynostosis, suture type) and venous air embolism (VAE; 2–8%).[16,19,23] The sagittal ESC can have a higher risk of bleeding secondary to emissary veins from the sagittal sinus and the metopic ESC due to the thickness of the bone. The low risk of VAE is most likely related to the low average of blood loss. Therefore, the rate of ICU admission is low (8%; mostly for respiratory and hemodynamic monitoring after blood transfusion and respiratory complications), and the majority of patients are discharged on postoperative day 1.

Most infants undergo an inhalational induction and tracheal intubation under neuromuscular blockade. Correct midtracheal placement of the endotracheal tube is essential and should be clinically tested with flexion and extension of the head simulating surgical positioning to prevent inadvertent extubation or bronchial mainstem intubation. Invasive arterial blood pressure monitoring is rarely needed. However, two large bore peripheral intravenous (IV) catheters suitable for intraoperative venous blood sampling and fluid administration are especially important for infants with higher risk of bleeding. For all infants, typed and crossed blood products must be readily available in the OR. Careful positioning and appropriate padding are essential. Although the risk of VAE is low, all infants undergoing ESC procedures should be monitored with precordial Doppler probe for early detection of VAE. The limited anesthesiologist's access to the patient throughout the procedure mandates careful securing of the endotracheal tube, lines, and

monitoring devices. Because of concern for rapid systemic absorption from the scalp, a reduction of the maximum dose of bupivacaine should be considered (e.g., from 2.5 to 1.25 mg/kg and epinephrine 1:200000). Analgesia can be usually provided with short-acting opioids and acetaminophen, followed by small doses of longer acting opioids after extubation to facilitate an early neurological examination and feeding. Usually these infants can be extubated in the OR and transferred to the PACU.

Postoperative Concerns

The infants should be monitored for infection, CSF leak, and neurologic injury. Given an uneventful perioperative anesthesia course, postoperative early feeding is important to facilitate discharge on postoperative day 1.

Stereotactic Techniques and MRI-Guided Laser Ablation

Magnetic resonance imaging (MRI)-guided laser interstitial thermal therapy (LITT) is a stereotactically guided percutaneous minimally invasive procedure that delivers light energy to target tissue via a fiberoptic catheter, resulting in selective thermal ablation of targeted tissue. Recent technological advances in LITT have improved safety and efficiency by providing the ability to monitor tissue ablation in real time and reduced ablation times.[24] LITT is used for treatment of deep-seated, difficult-to-access, inoperable lesions, brain metastases, gliomas, radiation necrosis, and epilepsy foci (beneficial when dealing with deep, focal lesions, such as hypothalamic hamartomas or hippocampal sclerosis).[25] Although MRI-guided LITT is an invasive intracranial procedure that requires a burr hole and general anesthesia in children, it provides a potential benefit over the noninvasive stereotactic radiosurgery by delivering photogenic energy for thermocoagulation instead of ionizing radiation. However, the long-term effects of thermal necrosis have not yet been clearly elucidated. Successful management of patients undergoing MRI-guided LITT requires interdisciplinary collaboration. As the use of MRI-guided LITT is still in its infancy, indications and contraindications are still being worked out. Potential benefits of stereotactic laser ablations might include decreased length of hospital stay, reduced procedure-related discomfort, and improved access to surgical treatment for patients less likely to be considered for an open resective procedure.

Surgical Procedure

In our institution, the experience with MRI-guided LITT is limited to the Visualase System (Medronic, Minneapolis, MN), which includes a diode laser, a cooled laser applicator probe with an outer cooling catheter, and an image-processing computer workstation that communicates with MRI. The workstation is used during therapy to generate real-time magnetic resonance color-coded "thermal" images (MRTI) and an estimation of the ablation zone. During ablation, temperatures surrounding the laser tip are continuously updated and depicted in various colors, which are then used to generate "damage" images, depicting the area of tissue that has been successfully ablated on the basis of the Arrhenius model of thermal ablation. Treatment concludes when the "damage zone" in a damage image covers the entire target area. If temperatures exceed the programmed thresholds, the laser shuts down automatically to prevent damage to adjacent normal brain tissue. An important difference of MRI thermometry versus radiofrequency ablation is the ability to measure not only temperature at the device tip (the only temperature monitored in radiofrequency ablation) but also the temperature of tissue any distance from the tip during heating, thus providing near real-time confirmation of the ablation zone relative to off-target structures.

In the neurosurgical MRI-OR, the preoperative MRI examination identifies the target lesion and entry site. Using intraoperative neuronavigation, a small burr hole is made through which a bone anchor is placed into the skull in the exact target trajectory identified by neuronavigation. The cooling catheter is advanced through the anchor to the desired target and fixed to the bone anchor. Then the laser probe is inserted into the cooling catheter and locked into place. Once the location of the laser probe and the laser fiber insertion is confirmed, the skull frame is removed and the patient is transported under anesthesia to the MRI suite. In the MRI scanner the fast-spoiled gradient recalled phase images are obtained at the patient's body temperature to serve as a baseline for all intraprocedural thermal measurements. Once the cooling system begins to circulate, a test pulse of 3–4 W for 30–60 seconds is administered to determine the exact location of the distal 1-cm segment of the laser probe. This is important because thermal energy is emitted from the distal-most 1-cm segment of the laser fiber, and knowing its exact location within the target lesion is crucial to ensuring the accuracy of ablation. Ablation is performed by applying treatment doses of 10–15 W for 30–180 seconds until the damage zone covers the entire area of the target lesion. As described above, intraprocedural MRTI allows the neurosurgeon to visualize ablation in real time. After completion of the procedure, the probe, catheter, and anchor are removed and the small skin puncture site will be closed in the radiology anesthesia area.[24]

Preoperative Issues

Initial evaluation includes assessment of the underlying disease. Near real-time MR LITT requires clearance for MRI, excluding patients with implantable devices. Children with focal, medically intractable seizures who are considered for MR LITT should undergo a comprehensive preoperative anesthetic evaluation prior to surgery. For details, see Chapter 13 on epilepsy. The nature and manifestation of the patient's seizure patterns and associated psychomotor behavior should be inquired preoperatively. Many patients are relatively young and fit from a cardiovascular and respiratory standpoint. Several rare medical conditions, such as neurofibromatosis (intracranial tumors, airway compromise from tumors involving the respiratory tract, cranial nerve involvement) and tuberous sclerosis (cardiac dysrhythmias, intracardiac tumors, renal dysfunction, aneurysms), are associated with epilepsy. Pulmonary status might be compromised from chronic aspiration syndrome, pulmonary hypertension, and cor pulmonale. Medication history is important for preoperative laboratory test selection and prediction of intraoperative drug interactions. Anticonvulsants (e.g., phenytoin, carbamazepine) can significantly increase dose requirements for non-depolarizing muscle relaxants and opioids and elevate liver function parameters. Sedation and lethargy are common side effects of many antiepileptic agents. Chronic topiramate intake can be associated with metabolic acidosis, likewise a ketogenic diet. Valproic acid intake results in dose-related thrombocytopenia and platelet dysfunction.

Epilepsy has a pervasive effect on patients and is associated with a higher incidence of cognitive dysfunction and severe behavioral and developmental decline, which can be a challenge in the preoperative holding area requiring planning for oral or I/M premedication. Neuropsychological testing is often performed to assist in identification of dysfunction that is relevant for localization and proximity to key structures involved in cognition, language, and memory. The most common indications for laser ablation in children are mesial temporal sclerosis, hypothalamic hamartomas (non-neoplastic developmental malformations centered around the tuber cinereum), other focal lesions and low-grade glioneural tumors such as ganglioglioma, and dysembryoplastic and neuroepithelial tumors (DNET).

Intraoperative Management

A general anesthesia with endotracheal intubation is performed with inhalational agents for maintenance during the surgical part of the procedure and total intravenous anesthesia (TIVA) (propofol infusion) during the transport periods, opioid infusion (e.g., fentanyl, sufentanil) for adequate analgesia, and muscle relaxation for immobility of the patient throughout the whole procedure. As the surgical procedure is a burr hole/placement of the laser probe with little associated blood loss, placement of 1–2 peripheral IV catheters is sufficient; A-line insertion is necessary only in the presence of significant comorbidities or anticipated protracted length of the procedure. The common goals for neurosurgical anesthesia include preservation of cerebral blood flow, control of systemic blood pressure and ICP, and rapid emergence from anesthesia and return of neurological/

cognitive function for prompt neurologic assessment. Administration of preoperative antibiotics within 1 hour of incision and steroids per surgical request before performing the ablation to decrease treatment-associated edema need to be timed accordingly. Active warming is used when the patient is not on transport or in the scanner.

The procedure is divided into two portions: (1) placement of the laser probe using a stereotactic frame system (e.g., the Cosman-Roberts-Wells [CRW], Brown-Roberts-Wells) and MRI-based confirmation of the probe location; and (2) transport to the MRI suite with subsequent laser ablation.[25]

After anesthesia induction the stereotactic skull frame, for example the CRW, is placed while the patient is in a semisitting position. Care must be taken to measure the systemic blood pressure on heart level and maintain sufficient brain perfusion. It is a ring structure applied to the skull with screws, on which the localizer and the plastic phantom cage are placed (Figures 15.7A, 15.7B). The required position of the CRW ring frame makes the access to the airway difficult and the breathing tube needs to be placed in midtracheal position and secured safely. The patient is imaged with the frame in place to provide an external relationship to the internal structures of the brain. This planning study is uploaded to the planning software of the workstation and the neurosurgical team selects the surgical target, trajectory, and entry point best suited for the patient. The resulting CRW coordinates are entered into the

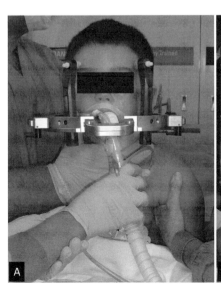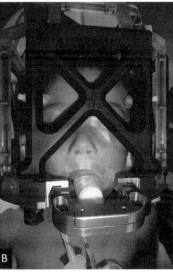

Figure 15.7. The stereotactic frame is placed under anesthesia for a localizing study. (A) A 2-year-old child is positioned in a semiupright position with the 4 pin MRI-safe Cosman-Roberts-Wells (CRW) skull frame and (B) with the plastic phantom cage.

CRW precision arc and accuracy confirmed with the CRW phantom base. After the phantom cage is removed, the patient is positioned on the Mayfield adaptor, prepped, and draped, the sterile precision arc is placed on the frame, and the C-Arm is aligned with the arc rings for later confirmation of the target. The CRW trajectory determines the entry point at which the incision is made, and the burr hole is drilled. The precision arc is used to introduce the stylet through the selected entry point, and its arrival is confirmed at the target. The stylet is removed and the bolt is placed in the skull for laser sheath placement to target location, and catheter and laser fixation (Figures 15.8A–C). Another MRI scan is obtained to verify correct laser location (Figure 15.9). If no further laser adjustments are needed, the stereotactic equipment is removed and the patient is moved to a transport stretcher for transport to the 3T MRI suite for laser treatment. The patient's anesthesia is switched to TIVA, and is transported fully monitored and ventilated by the anesthesia team and the laser probe/laser fiber system is handled by the neurosurgical team. The 3T MRI suite must be equipped with an anesthesia induction/emergence work space as well as an anesthesia work space within the scanner room with ferromagnetic-free equipment. On arrival the patient is transferred and positioned on the MRI bed and the catheter and laser are connected to the Visualase System. The radiology and neurosurgical team will proceed with the laser calculations and applications with intermittent scanning. Immediately after completion of the laser treatment, a contrast-enhancing brain MRI is performed for confirmation of target lesion ablation. Thereafter the patient is moved to the emergence anesthesia work space of the MRI suite for sterile removal of the laser, catheter, and bolt, with subsequent wound closure. The patient is extubated and a first neurological exam is performed before the patient is transported to the ICU.

Complications and Postoperative Concerns

Pediatric patients usually spend one night in the ICU for frequent neurological evaluations. The hospital stay varies, but for cases without complications it usually is 24–48 hours. The most common complications include neurologic deficits (dysphagia, weakness, hemianopsia, minor seizures), 13% of which either resolve spontaneously or respond to steroid administration within days and weeks.[24] The next most common complications include new progressive or permanent neurologic symptoms (3%), intracranial hemorrhage (2.5%), and deep venous thrombosis (2.5%). Life-threatening complications include intracranial hemorrhage, ventriculitis, meningitis, and refractory intracranial hypertension (cerebral edema) after simultaneous use of multiple probes to treat a large irregular lesion.

References

1. Choudhri O, Feroze AH, Nathan J, Cheshier S, Guzman R. Ventricular endoscopy in the pediatric population: review of indications. *Childs Nerv Syst.* 2014;**30**(10):1625–43.

2. Stone SS, Warf BC. Combined endoscopic third ventriculostomy and choroid plexus cauterization as primary treatment for infant hydrocephalus: a prospective North American series. *J Neurosurg Pediatr.* 2014;**14**(5):439–46.

3. Meier PM, Guzman R, Erb TO. Endoscopic pediatric neurosurgery: implications for anesthesia. *Paediatr Anaesth.* 2014;**24**(7):668–77.

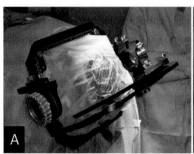
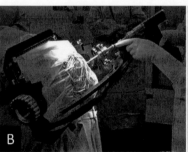
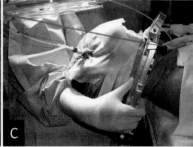

Figure 15.8. (A) The child's head is in the stereotactic frame, covered with a clear drape and the CRW localizer arc is applied to the three holes of the frame. (B) The burr hole is drilled and the precision arc is used to introduce the stylet through the selected entry point. (C) The catheter and the laser fiber are fixed with the bolt and the precision arc is removed.

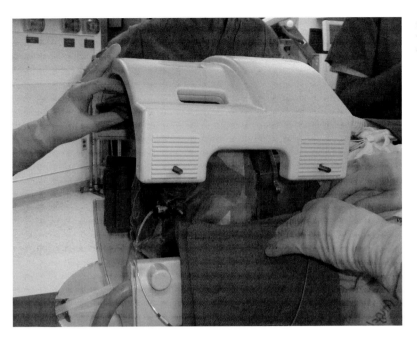

Figure 15.9. The child's head is placed on the coil so an MRI scan can verify the correct laser position.

4. Guzman R, Pendharkar AV, Zerah M, Sainte-Rose C. Use of the NeuroBalloon catheter for endoscopic third ventriculostomy. *J Neurosurg Pediatr.* 2013;**11**(3): 302–6.

5. Johnson JO, Jimenez DF, Tobias JD. Anaesthetic care during minimally invasive neurosurgical procedures in infants and children. *Paediatr Anaesth.* 2002;**12**(6): 478–88.

6. Ornstein E, Matteo RS, Schwartz AE, Silverberg PA, Young WL, Diaz J. The effect of phenytoin on the magnitude and duration of neuromuscular block following atracurium or vecuronium. *Anesthesiology.* 1987;**67**(2):191–6.

7. El-Dawlatly AA. Endoscopic third ventriculostomy: anesthetic implications. *Minim Invasive Neurosurg.* 2004;**47**(3):151–3.

8. El-Dawlatly AA. Blood biochemistry following endoscopic third ventriculostomy. *Minim Invasive Neurosurg.* 2004;**47**(1):47–8.

9. Anandh B, Madhusudan Reddy KR, Mohanty A, Umamaheswara Rao GS, Chandramouli BA. Intraoperative bradycardia and postoperative hyperkalemia in patients undergoing endoscopic third ventriculostomy. *Minim Invasive Neurosurg.* 2002;**45**(3):154–7.

10. van Aken J, Struys M, Verplancke T, de Baerdemaeker L, Caemaert J, Mortier E. Cardiovascular changes during endoscopic third ventriculostomy. *Minim Invasive Neurosurg.* 2003;**46**(4):198–201.

11. Kalmar AF, Van Aken J, Caemaert J, Mortier EP, Struys MM. Value of Cushing reflex as warning sign for brain ischaemia during neuroendoscopy. *Br J Anaesth.* 2005;**94**(6):791–9.

12. Davidyuk G, Soriano SG, Goumnerova L, Mizrahi-Arnaud A. Acute intraoperative neurogenic pulmonary edema during endoscopic ventriculoperitoneal shunt revision. *Anesth Analg.* 2010;**110**(2):594–5.

13. El-Dawlatly AA, Murshid WR, Elshimy A, Magboul MA, Samarkandi A, Takrouri MS. The incidence of bradycardia during endoscopic third ventriculostomy. *Anesth Analg.* 2000;**91**(5):1142–4.

14. Drake JM, Canadian Pediatric Neurosurgery Study Group. Endoscopic third ventriculostomy in pediatric patients: the Canadian experience. *Neurosurgery.* 2007;**60**(5):881–6.

15. Chowdhry SA, Cohen AR. Intraventricular neuroendoscopy: complication avoidance and management. *World Neurosurg.* 2013;**79**(2 suppl): S15e1–0.

16. Jimenez DF, Barone CM, Cartwright CC, Baker L. Early management of craniosynostosis using endoscopic-assisted strip craniectomies and cranial orthotic molding therapy. *Pediatrics.* 2002;**110**(1 pt 1):97–104.

17. Faberowski LW, Black S, Mickle JP. Blood loss and transfusion practice in the perioperative management of craniosynostosis repair. *J Neurosurg Anesthesiol.* 1999;**11**(3):167–72.

18. Stricker PA, Shaw TL, Desouza DG, Hernandez SV, Bartlett SP, Friedman DF, et al. Blood loss, replacement, and associated morbidity in infants and children undergoing craniofacial surgery. *Paediatr Anaesth.* 2010;**20**(2):150–9.

19. Meier PM, Goobie SM, DiNardo JA, Proctor MR, Zurakowski D, Soriano SG. Endoscopic strip craniectomy in early infancy: the initial five years of anesthesia experience. *Anesth Analg.* 2011;**112**(2): 407–14.

20. Erb TO, Meier PM. Surgical treatment of craniosynostosis in infants: open vs closed repair. *Curr Opin Anaesthesiol.* 2016;**29**(3):345–51.

21. Meier PM, Zurakowski D, Goobie SM, Proctor MR, Meara JG, Young VJ, et al. Multivariable predictors of substantial blood loss in children undergoing craniosynostosis repair: implications for risk stratification. *Paediatr Anaesth.* 2016;**26**(10):960–9.

22. Berry-Candelario J, Ridgway EB, Grondin RT, Rogers GF, Proctor MR. Endoscope-assisted strip craniectomy and postoperative helmet therapy for treatment of craniosynostosis. *Neurosurg Focus.* 2011;**31**(2):E5.

23. Tobias JD, Johnson JO, Jimenez DF, Barone CM, McBride DS Jr. Venous air embolism during endoscopic strip craniectomy for repair of craniosynostosis in infants. *Anesthesiology.* 2001;**95**(2): 340–2.

24. Medvid R, Ruiz A, Komotar RJ, Jagid JR, Ivan ME, Quencer RM, et al. Current applications of MRI-guided laser interstitial thermal therapy in the treatment of brain neoplasms and epilepsy: a radiologic and neurosurgical overview. *Am J Neuroradiol.* 2015;**36**(11):1998–2006.

25. Buckley R, Estronza-Ojeda S, Ojemann JG. Laser ablation in pediatric epilepsy. *Neurosurg Clin N Am.* 2016;**27**(1):69–78.

Chapter 16

Intraoperative Neuromonitoring in Pediatric Neurosurgery

John McAuliffe

Introduction

Pediatric neurosurgical procedures, for which intraoperative neuromonitoring (IONM) is utilized, can be divided into three broad categories: intracranial, extracranial decompression/stabilization, and extracranial mass lesion excisions. In adults IONM is frequently used for neurovascular procedures such as aneurysm clipping, arterial bypass procedures, and carotid endarterectomies. These procedures are uncommon in children; however, tumor resections, especially posterior fossa lesion resections, are far more frequently monitored in the pediatric population. These cases pose a number of challenges to the IONM team that increase with the size of the tumor and inversely with the age of the patient. Supratentorial lesions may pose risk to motor and sensory pathways directly, by virtue of their location, or indirectly by disturbing the vascular supply to motor/sensory pathways.

When IONM is used, it is important to understand the pathways that can be monitored and the limitations of the IONM data.[1] For example, transcranial motor evoked potentials (TcMEPs) may be normal in a patient incapable of volitional movement due to injury to the supplemental motor area or the basal ganglia. A normal auditory brainstem response (ABR) is compatible with a preserved auditory pathway to the level of the inferior colliculus, but gives no information about the status of the primary auditory cortex. A full discussion of the limitation of IONM in the pediatric neurosurgical settings is beyond the scope of this chapter, but the major pathways monitored by each modality and the surgical procedures for which the modalities can provide useful information to the surgeon will be discussed. Prior to discussing the application of IONM to pediatric neurosurgical procedure, it is important to understand the combined impact of anesthesia and development on each of the IONM modalities that might be used during a given procedure.

The Impact of Anesthesia and Development of Specific Modalities

Signals that are recorded during IONM can be divided into two broad categories: (1) spontaneous activity such as cerebral electrical activity recorded as electroencephalography (EEG) and muscle activity that can be recorded as electromyography (EMG), and (2) evoked potentials. Evoked potentials are electrical responses to a specific stimulus. The response is typically recorded for a finite period of time after the stimulus; the relationship between stimulus and recording interval is known as time locking. Time locking can be used to advantage to reduce the admission of noise or to signal average multiple repetitions of a stimulus/recording trial, as is typically done for somatosensory evoked potentials and ABRs. In other cases such as TcMEPs the signals are sufficiently robust and have very high signal-to-noise ratios (SNR) that only a single trial is needed to obtain the desired data. Additionally, certain reflexes, such as the bulbocavernosus reflex, may be obtained on a single trial, if conditions are permissive.

Somatosensory Evoked Potentials

Somatosensory evoked potentials (SSEPs) are generated by repetitive stimulation of large peripheral nerves such as the ulnar, median, or posterior tibial nerve (PTN). The stimulus causes depolarization of 1A and B fibers that carry proprioceptive, vibration, and light touch information.[2] The nerve impulses ascend ipsilaterally in the dorsal columns to either the cuneate (upper extremities) or gracile (lower extremities and trunk) nuclei in the medulla. A cervical response can be recorded at the level of the fifth cervical vertebra as the impulses in the dorsal columns pass beneath the recording electrode.

The presence of this potential provides an indication that the spinal cord pathways are intact to the C5 level. SSEP latencies to the C5 level will be less affected by marginal perfusion than motor evoked potentials because white matter is less metabolically active than gray matter. However, once the impulses that generate the component potentials of the SSEPs reach the intracranial level, both white and gray matter are involved and the effects of marginal perfusion are more easily detected by changes in latency and amplitude (Table 16.1).

The next named potential is generated as the impulses reach the cuneate, or gracile, nucleus. If the impulses arrive at the brainstem nuclei in synchrony, the impulses are transmitted to the ventral-posterior lateral tiers of the thalamus via the arcuate fibers and medial lemniscus. As the impulses arrive at the thalamus, yet another potential is generated (P18). The impulses are relayed from the thalamus to the primary cortex. A potential known as the N20 marks the arrival of the impulses at the primary somatosensory cortex.[3] The commonly named potentials for both a median nerve and PTN SSEPs are shown in Figures 16.1A and 16.1B, respectively. The peripheral potentials (usually recorded at Erb's point), the cervical potential, and the median (ulnar) nerve cortical potentials are referred to as "near-field" potentials as the recording electrode is proximate to the site of generation. On the other hand the subcortical potential (N14–18) is a far-field potential, as the medial lemniscus is not near the recording sites. Far-field potentials are less sensitive to inexact placement of the recording electrodes than are near-field potentials.

The latencies of the various waves are affected by both anesthesia and postnatal development. Peripheral nerve conduction velocities increase with postnatal age and are not typically affected by anesthetic agents at clinical concentrations. Distances between stimulus site and recording site are much smaller than in an adult; consequently, peripheral (N9) and cervical potential (N13) latencies are much shorter in infants and toddlers than in adults. However, central conduction times are longer due to lack of myelination of central pathways. Myelination of the central pathways is generally complete by 2 years of age; the medial lemniscus is usually fully myelinated by 12 months and the thalamocortical projections by 12–18 months of age.[4] Once the signals reach the medullary nuclei (gracile and cuneate), the effects of incomplete myelination manifest as a prolonged peripheral to cortical interpeak latency. Even in the absence of anesthesia, the amplitude of the

Table 16.1 CNS Structures and Their Vascular Supplies Assessed by Median Nerve SSEPs

Structure	Vascular Supply	Potential Affected
Dorsal columns	Posterior spinal artery	N11 (P11) dorsal root entry zone
	Anterior serratus anterior (variant)	
Gracile/cuneate nucleus	Anterior spinal artery	N13
	Derived from ventriculoatrial (VA)	
Medial lemniscus	Anterior spinal artery; vertebral arteries; paramedian branches of basilar artery; quadrageminal and medial posterior choroidal	P14
Thalamus–ventral posterolateral tier	Posterior choroidal artery	N18
Thalamocrtical projections	Lenticulostriates	
Primary somatosensory cortex	M3 and M4 branches of MCA and A4 of ACA	N20, P25, P37 (PTN SSEPs)

Notes:

(1) The vascular supplies listed derived from diagrams in *Neuroanatomy: An Atlas of Structures, Sections, and Systems*, D.E. Haines, 2008, Lippincott, Williams, and Wilkins.

(2) The listed vascular supplies are typical, but individual variation exists; for example, 30%, or more, of the total area of the dorsal columns has been shown to be supplied by branches of the anterior spinal artery in some individuals.

(3) The names assigned to the potentials are those assigned for adult patients. For patients younger than 8 years, N11 is N8, N14 is N9, and N20 is N16.

A

SEP Upper Left: 15.0

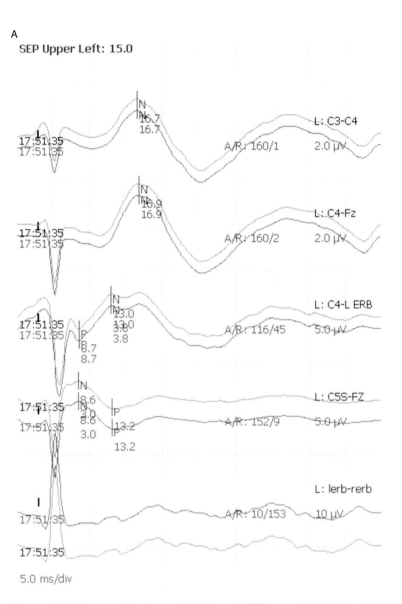

5.0 ms/div

Figures 16.1. Ulnar nerve (A) and posterior tibial nerve (B) SSEPs, respectively. (A) From the bottom to top, the montages represent the peripheral potentials recorded at Erb's point, a cervical level response, the subcortical response, and the cortical response (top two). The short latencies of the Erb's, cervical, and subcortical responses are due to the age of the patient. The Erb's point to cortical interpeak latency is comparable to an adult indicating relative maturation of the central conduction pathways (see text). (B) The recording was obtained from a preteen undergoing a posterior spinal fusion. The bottom trace was recorded from electrodes in the popliteal fossa, the next trace up from the mastoid with a frontal reference, and the top three cortical montages provide data to determine the orientation of the dipole in 3-space.

cortical signals is attenuated compared to the adult due to dispersion of conduction velocities. The addition of anesthetic effects results in the near absence of recognizable cortical potentials in infants less than 1 month of age as SSEP latencies increase and amplitudes decrease in a dose-dependent manner with anesthetics. The only exception is etomidate, which increases the amplitude of evoked potentials compared to other agents.[5] Median nerve SSEPs are typically recorded using a 100-μsec stimulus, applied at a rate of near 4 Hz in adults. When recording from infants, longer pulse lengths and lower stimulus frequencies must be used to record cortical signals on a consistent basis. This phenomenon can be partially overcome by using a lower stimulus frequency and longer pulse times.[6,7]

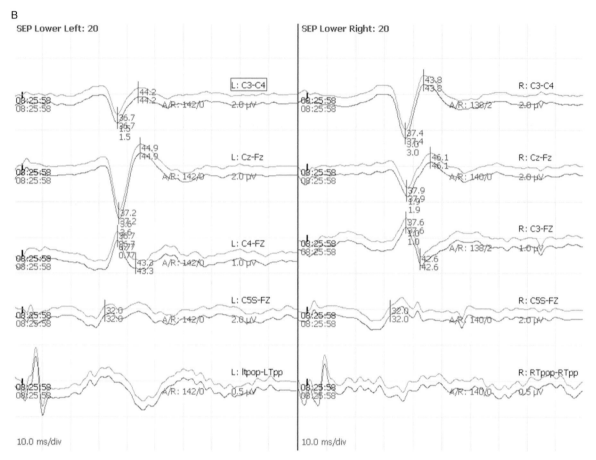

Figures 16.1. (cont).

Incomplete myelination in the spinal cord has a greater effect on the PTN SSEPs than on median nerve or ulnar nerve SSEPs because of the distance the impulses must travel within the spinal cord before reaching the medullary nuclei. Myelination of the dorsal columns proceeds in a cranial-caudal fashion and is complete at around 8 years of age. As a consequence of the delayed myelination of the dorsal columns, there tends to be greater dispersion of signals traveling on the dorsal columns of a 2-year-old than an adult resulting in a lower likelihood of generating a useable PTN cortical SSEP in the 2-year-old. Failure to obtain cortical PTN SSEPs in children less than 2 years of age is not uncommon;[8] the rate of failure increases in the face of pathology within the spinal cord and with anesthesia/sedation. As in the case of the median nerve SSEPs, alteration of stimulus parameters is necessary when attempting to record PTN SSEPs from very young children.

SSEPs can also be used to locate the central sulcus when it is necessary to directly stimulate the primary motor cortex. A 1 × 4 grid can be placed on the brain while the median nerve on the contralateral wrist is stimulated. An upright N20 from a grid location indicates that the point is over the sensory cortex, while an inverted N20 indicates the grid point is over the motor cortex. Care must be taken to ensure that a transition from an upright to inverted N20 is clearly present in order to properly identify the central sulcus.

Transcranial Motor Evoked Potentials (TcMEPs)

Intraoperative and postoperative motor deficits can occur in the absence of changes in the SSEPs. Therefore, it is necessary to monitor the functional integrity of the entire motor pathway independently of the sensory tracts. Transcranial (Tc) and direct cortical (dc) motor evoked potentials (MEPs) serve this function (Table 16.2). TcMEPs are elicited by applying a high-voltage, short-duration stimulus to the scalp overlying the primary motor cortex.[9] This electrical stimulus directly depolarizes the axons on the pyramidal neurons generating (D-waves) and activates cortical interneuronal networks in the motor cortex generating I-waves. The D-waves may initiate one of three or four locations within the intracranial portion of the corticospinal tract (CST), while the I-waves always originate from the cortex.[10] Even in adults, lower extremity TcMEPs are more sensitive to anesthetic effects than upper extremity TcMEPs.[11] Both D- and I-waves are conducted along the CST to depolarize a population of spinal alpha motor neurons (αMNs). The common teaching has been that D-waves are relatively resistant to the effects of anesthesia, but D-wave latency has been demonstrated to increase in a dose-dependent fashion when isoflurane is used for anesthesia.

Table 16.2 CNS Structures and Their Vascular Supplies Assessed by MEPs

Structure	Vascular Supply
Primary motor cortex	M3 and M4 branches of MCA and A4 of ACA
Corona radiata internal capsule	Lenticulostriate arteries
	Anterior choroidal artery
Intracranial CST	Quadrageminal and posterior choroidal
	Basilar artery
	Vertebral artery
Pyramidal decussation	Anterior spinal artery
	Derived from VA
Intraspinal CST	Anterior spinal artery (SC level)
Alpha motor neurons	Anterior spinal artery (SC level)

Notes:

(1) Cortical ischemia will result in reduction of, or loss of, I-wave recruitment with consequent significant attenuation or loss of MEPs on the contralateral side.

(2) Partial or complete occlusion of the leticulostriates or the anterior choroidal artery can result in rapid attenuation or loss of MEPs on the contralateral side.

The generation of I-waves is inhibited by anesthetics, volatile agents having a greater effect than propofol; thus multipulse techniques are used to elicit TcMEPs under anesthesia.

The MEP is a compound muscle action potential (CMAP) recorded from the motor unit depolarized by the descending D- and I-waves (Figure 16.2). All anesthetics decrease the resting membrane potential of the αMNs; the increase in membrane potential from the combined effects of the D- and I-waves must exceed firing threshold for the αMN to depolarize. The neuromodulatory influences of serotonin and noradrenaline have a significant effect on αMN excitability by regulating channel open-state time and resting membrane potential.[12] Volatile agents reduce seratoninergic output, while ketamine may potentiate it. Dexmedetomidine reduces central noradrenaline and can inhibit TcMEPs in a dose-dependent fashion.[13] All of the adverse effects of anesthetic agents on MEP generation are more prominent in young children due to immaturity of the motor system. Although direct CST to αMN connections are present in the αMNs innervating muscles of the hand at birth,[14] the same is not true for connections between the CST and the αMNs innervating lower extremity muscles. As a consequence of these factors, special techniques such as temporal or spatial facilitation may be required to elicit MEPs in very young children. The temporal facilitation technique, also called double-train stimulation, can be very effective for obtaining TcMEPs from young children.[15,16] Spatial facilitation is technically more difficult and is limited to the homonymous muscle in a single (or two, upper or lower) limb(s), whereas temporal facilitation has no such limits.

During complex intracranial procedures there may be selective loss of the I-waves for various reasons. Loss of the I-waves due to cortical ischemia or ischemia within the internal capsule may result in complete loss of the TcMEPs or significant attenuation of TcMEP amplitude. Compromise of blood flow to the anterior choroidal artery or the lenticulostriates can produce ischemia in the internal capsule resulting in loss or severe attenuation of the TcMEPs. Thus the TcMEPs are highly informative during procedures during which retraction near these vessels is likely to be performed. In addition to somatic muscle TcMEPs, it is possible to record TcMEPs from muscles innervated by cranial nerves, especially from CN VII,[17] X,[18] and XII. Special techniques are required to generate

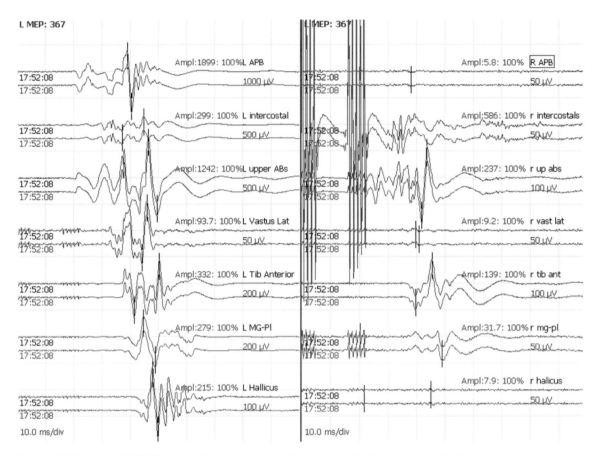

Figure 16.2. Transcranial MEPS. These recordings were obtained from a 2-year-old with congenital scoliosis using a double-train technique.

these TcMEPs, but they can be very useful during posterior fossa tumor resection involving the floor of the fourth ventricle when used in conjunction with direct motor mapping.

In some cases, the motor cortex may be directly exposed making the use of TcMEPs on the operative side impossible. In this case, either a ball probe or a grid electrode may be used to directly stimulate the motor cortex. The central sulcus can be positively identified using a phase reversal of the N20 of a cortically recorded median nerve SSEP (see above). Unlike TcMEPs, dcMEPs can be performed frequently during a procedure because there is no movement associated with the application of the stimulus.[19]

If tumor resections involve dissection in subcortical regions near the internal capsule, or any part of the intracranial CST, the distance between the resection margin and the CST may be accurately estimated using subcortical mapping. A ball probe or other device, such as a modified suction, can be used to deliver pulse trains of increasing current until an MEP is elicited. The current, in mA, required to produce an MEP closely approximates the distance, in millimeters, between the stimulus and the CST.[20] When used in combination with dcMEPs, this technique can provide meaningful real-time feedback to the surgeon concerning the functional state of the CST and the distance between the CST and the resection margin.

Electromyography (EMG)

Direct mechanical or thermal injury to motor nerve roots or cortical spinal tracts can result in electrical activity in skeletal muscle. The electrical activity of the muscle, or the electromyogram, can be recorded using either subdermal or intramuscular needles. Activity triggered by direct trauma to motor nerves is called neurotonic activity; the magnitude and frequency of the activity are related to the rate at which energy is absorbed by the nerves. Other types of EMG activity can result from pathology within the nervous system such as denervation, chronic nerve irritation, or intrinsic muscle disease. During certain neurosurgical procedures, such as tethered cord release, structures are directly stimulated by the surgeon, in an attempt to distinguish nerve tissue from non-nerve tissue. EMG responses to the stimulus serve to make the distinction as stimulation of nerve tissue result in activation of skeletal muscle either directly or reflexively. The EMG of an infant differs from that of an adolescent because the muscle mass of infants and young children is reduced compared to adults; the diameter of individual fibers is about one-fourth that of an adult at birth. Fiber diameter increases in size through puberty. Additionally, the mean duration of motor unit action potentials is significantly shorter in infancy and early childhood than at 20 years of age.

Direct mechanical or thermal trauma to the CST within the spinal cord may cause EMG firing in muscle groups innervated many levels below the point of injury.[21] This phenomenon is known as suprasegmental discharges. EMG bursts from the muscles of the lower extremities may indicate CST injury during a cervical or thoracic procedure.

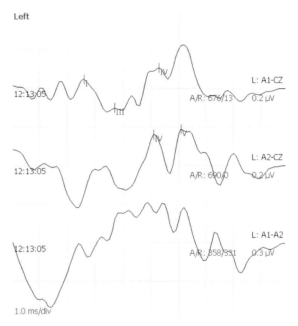

Figure 16.3. Brainstem auditory evoked response. This recording was obtained from the patient whose MRI is shown in Figure 16.5 at the end of the tumor resection. The latency of the wave V was reduced compared to preresection. Wave V is typically the largest peak in the montage recorded on the side contralateral to the ear being stimulated.

Brainstem Auditory Evoked Responses (BAERs)

Auditory evoked responses are used to monitor the integrity of CN VIII. The classes of BAERs are typically divided into short, middle, and long latency responses. During surgery, only the short latency responses are resistant to the effects of anesthetic agents and are useful for assessing the integrity of the eighth cranial nerve and the ascending auditory pathways to the level of the inferior colliculus. The short latency responses all have latencies less than 10 milliseconds and have labels that include Roman numerals I through V. Waves III, IV, and V have generators within the brainstem, while waves I and II originate from the cochlear nerve itself. Wave III originates from the cochlear nucleus and wave V from the termination of the lateral lemniscus in the inferior colliculus[22–24] (Figure 16.3). Neurosurgical procedures that involve retraction of the brainstem or cerebello-pontine angle have the potentials to adversely affect CN VIII function; BAERs are useful for detecting injury to the eighth nerve before the damage results in permanent hearing loss. Developmental influences

impact the BAERs less than SSEPs or TcMEPs. Term infants will have wave I latencies similar to those of adults; wave III and V latencies reach adult values by 18–36 months of age.[25] The value of BAERs is limited by the fact that the potentials are very low amplitude (< 0.5 μV) in a background in the tens of microvolts; therefore, signal averaging of many trials (500–2,000) is sometimes required. This process can take 2–3 minutes. Early notification of the surgeon concerning replicating changes in the BAERs is important, given the time required to acquire the signals.

Bulbocavernosus Reflex (BCR)

Monitoring the bulbocavernosus reflex has been proposed by Skinner as a means of preserving lower sacral nerve function during intradural and extradural surgeries at the level of conus medullaris, cauda equina, sacral plexus, and the pudendal nerve.[26] Acquisition of the reflex requires use of a multipulse technique applied as a double train with a long intertrain interval (Figure 16.4). Alternatively, a double-tap technique can be used. In either case the acquisition time must be sufficiently

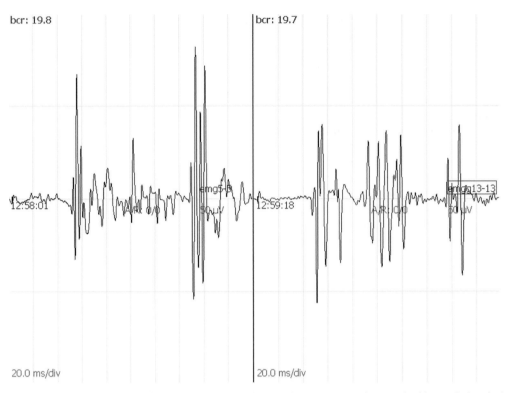

bcr: 19.8   bcr: 19.7

12:58:01   20.0 ms/div

12:59:18   20.0 ms/div

Figure 16.4. Bulbocavernosus reflex. The recording was obtained during resection of an intradural lipoma below the level of the conus. The response to stimulating the pudendal nerve is recorded from the anal sphincters bilaterally. Here a brisk response from the sphincters is obtained in response to stimulation of the pudendal nerve on the right. This reflex is sensitive to thermal injury to afferent fibers from bipolar or laser use during lipoma resection.

long to capture the response. The reflex is also sensitive to anesthetic technique in young children and infants; total intravenous anesthesia (TIVA) is the preferred anesthetic technique for acquisition of this reflex. Recording electrodes are placed in the anal sphincters bilaterally; these same electrodes can be used to record TcMEPs from the anal sphincter. Loss of the BCR but not the anal sphincter TcMEP suggests damage to the efferent pathways in the reflex arc. We record BCRs during complex tethered cord releases, lipoma resections, and similar procedures. The presence of a preexisting major urodynamic abnormality may make recording the BCR difficult to impossible, while mild abnormalities are not incompatible with recording the BCR.

Common Pediatric Neurosurgical Procedures Utilizing IONM

A summary of common pediatric surgical procedures and the IONM modalities utilized during these procedures is shown in Table 16.3. A detailed discussion of some of the listed procedures follows.

Dorsal Rhizotomy

Selective dorsal rhizotomies are done to decrease spasticity in children with cerebral palsy. In children who are ambulatory, the reduction in spasticity may be permanent, while in nonambulatory children spasticity may recur after a period of years. The best results are obtained when there is no injury to structures such as the basal ganglia and vestibular apparatus. The spasticity results from abnormal regulation of the gamma motor neurons and abnormal connections between 1A afferents and αMNs. The combination results in the classic cog-wheel behavior seen with passive movement of a joint. Excitatory influences dominate at the αMNs, leading to spasticity and contractures.

Surgically, afferent (sensory) dorsal nerve roots from L1 to S1 are divided into rootlets and the rootlets are selectively cut to reduce the spasticity. Each rootlet is sequentially tested, initially with a 1 to 2 Hz constant current pulse to determine the threshold current needed to elicit a stable EMG response. The threshold current is then applied for 1 second at 50 Hz and the response noted. The response is graded by the number of muscles exhibiting EMG activity, and the intensity and duration of the activity. Responses involving muscles contralateral to the stimulated root are always pathological. Muscle relaxants must be avoided and excessive depth is undesirable as the technique relies on αMNs responding to input form homonymous 1A afferents. Preservation of the clonus response helps ensure that EMG responses can be elicited using reasonable stimulating currents. Therefore, the goal of IONM is to help the surgeon to restore the balance between the inhibitory and excitatory motor influences, while preserving as much sensory innervation as possible. Postoperatively this procedure results in improved muscle tone, elimination of clonus, and increased passive range of motion (if fixed contractures were not present).

Table 16.3 CNS Structures and Their Vascular Supplies Assessed by BAERs (ABRs)

Structure	Vascular Supply	Potential Affected
Cochlea	Labyrinthine artery	Waves I & II
Cochlear nerve	Labyrinthine artery	
Cochlear nucleus	Anterior inferior cerebellar artery (AICA)	Wave III
Olivary complex	Paramedian branches of basilar artery	Wave IV ?
Lateral lemniscus	Paramedian and long circumferential branches of basilar artery	Wave IV ?
Inferior colliculus	Lateral branches of quadrageminal artery	Wave V

Note:
(1) Brainstem compression caused by mass lesions in the posterior fossa can prolong BAER (ABR) latencies and distort waveforms.

Tethered Cord Release

Tethered cords occur because the conus medullaris is prevented from migrating cephalad as the child grows. Tethered cord can be diagnosed clinically or radiographically. The most common signs and symptoms are leg muscle weakness and sensory loss, bowel or bladder dysfunction, back or leg pain, and disturbed gait. Magnetic resonance imaging (MRI) may reveal a displaced cord, scar, lipoma, or tight filium. Pathophysiologically there is a mechanical process that distorts the cord and neuronal components. A growth spurt can cause increased tension on the distal portion of the cord, causing stretch injury, or in severe cases, impaired blood flow and cord ischemia. Complex tethering results when the tissue restricting cord movement infiltrates or encases nerve tissue. EMG evoked by direct stimulation of putative neural tissue allows the surgeon to differentiate the nerve tissue from non-neural tissue prior to resection or transection of the structure. Frequent or extended bipolar use can result in thermal injury to the delicate afferent fibers that are essential for sacral reflexes. Frequent trials of the BCR are especially useful in signaling potentially reversible change in the function of both the afferent and efferent loops of the reflex, as the BCR is very sensitive to injury to afferent circuits. The utility of the BCR is enhanced by monitoring bowel and bladder function via anal sphincter and detrusor muscle TcMEPs. The anal sphincter TcMEP may be preserved and the BCR lost if the afferent pathways are injured and the efferent pathways spared.

Craniotomy for Resection of Tumor/Mass Lesion

Central nervous system (CNS) lesions, requiring resection, may reside in the brain or spinal cord. The intracranial lesions pose special challenges because so many areas are silent to our current monitoring techniques when patients are under general anesthesia. The specific IONM modalities used will be a function of the location of the lesion and the proposed surgical procedure and approach. During resection of supratentorial tumors the CST or its vascular supply may be close to the resection margins. The location of the incision may prevent optimal placement of electrode for eliciting TcMEPs. In some cases, sterile electrodes may be placed in the field or the motor strip must be identified using phase reversal of the median nerve SSEP N20 and direct cortical stimulation. Subcortical mapping, using cathode stimulation, is useful to determine this distance between the resection margin and the CST and to estimate the likelihood of residual deficits associated with the subcortical resection.

Monitoring cranial nerve function is frequently done during resection of infratentorial lesions (Figure 16.5). Individual cranial nerves may be monitored by use of cranial nerve EMG. EMG from specific cranial nerves is very sensitive to the effects of neuromuscular blockade (NMB), consequently these drugs should be avoided if CN EMG is employed. Special techniques have been described to elicit MEP from CN VII, X, and XII. Cranial nerve EMG displays specific patterns predictive of later dysfunction, especially so for the facial nerve. EMG responses to direct stimulation of the floor of the fourth ventricle (rhomboid fossa) may be used to map the location of cranial nerves and their nuclei in order to find a safe entry point for tumor resection. The location of critical structures in the rhomboid fossa may be significantly distorted depending on the location of a brainstem lesion. While much attention is paid to the location of the facial colliculus, it is important to remember that the hypoglossal nucleus and the motor nucleus of CN X are in close proximity to the floor of the fourth ventricle in the caudal segment of the rhomboid fossa and the nucleus of CN VI lies near the facial colliculus. These mapping techniques cannot guarantee the integrity of the corticobulbar tracts however; these must be monitored by either direct cortical stimulation or by transcranial techniques.[18] Hemispheric stimulation is the technique of choice for eliciting cranial nerve TcMEPs in children in order to minimize the probability of direct stimulation of the facial nerve on the side of interest.[17] Correct placement of the anode over the face motor area is key to successful acquisition of CN VII and XII TcMEPs. High frequency pulses (1 msec ISI) appear to work well with 75 μsec pulses. The actual latency of the facial nerve TcMEP may be normal or significantly prolonged at baseline depending on the size, location, and secondary effects of the mass lesion (see Figure 16.5).

The only afferent pathway that can be monitored is BAER, which provides information concerning the integrity of the auditory nerve, cochlear nucleus, and lateral lemniscus. Sudden significant changes in heart rate and/or blood pressure may be the only indications

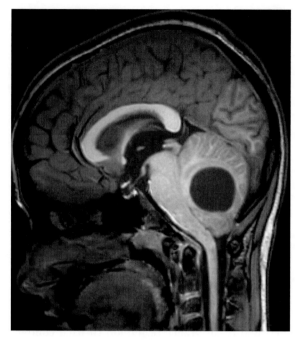

Figure 16.5. Sagittal T1 MRI of posterior fossa tumor. A large cystic component and solid components can be seen compressing the brainstem. Multiple cranial nerves, including VIII, as well as SSEPs and TcMEPs, were monitored during the resection of this tumor.

of irritation of CN IX/X afferent pathways and should prompt immediate notification of the surgeon by the anesthesia team.

Monitoring of tumor resections in the posterior fossa requires a highly skilled IONM team and careful attention to the anesthetic management. The techniques used to elicit TcMEPs for intracranial surgery are different from those used during spine surgery. The region of the CST depolarized on the anode side must be as close to the axon hillock as possible to avoid depolarization of the CST beyond the region at risk. In most cases, acquisition of TcMEPs from the intrinsic muscles of the hand and digital flexors is sufficient to provide information regarding the integrity of the motor pathways. Exceptions to this generalization include lesions near the lateral part of the crus cerebri, as the CST fibers projecting the αMN innervating lower extremity muscles are in close proximity. Excessive depth, producing burst suppression, or use of volatile agents in young children may prevent eliciting lower extremity TcMEPs when appropriate stimulating conditions for intracranial surgery are utilized. Further, smaller changes in the amplitude of the MEPs are needed to achieve alarm criteria during intracranial surgery than for spine surgery and the time window for corrective action is shorter during intracranial surgery than for spine surgery. Despite extensive and careful monitoring postoperative deficits, particularly problems with gag and swallowing, may occur due to injury to afferent pathways that are unable to be monitored under anesthesia.

A close working relationship between the anesthesiologist, the surgeon, and the neuromonitoring team increases the likelihood of a successful outcome during complex neurosurgical procedures. Ideally, the anesthesiologist has an in-depth understanding of the surgical procedure, and an understanding of the impact of anesthetic techniques on the acquisition and interpretation of IONM data.

References

1. Sala F, Krzan MJ, Deletis V. Intraoperative neurophysiological monitoring in pediatric neurosurgery: why, when, how? *Childs Nerv Syst*. 2002;**18**:264–87.

2. Fagan ER, Taylor MJ, Logan WJ. Somatosensory evoked potentials: part I. A review of neural generators and special considerations in pediatrics.*Pediatr Neurol*. 1987;**3**:189–96.

3. Leeman SA. SSEPs: from limb to cortex. *Am J Electroneurodiagnostic Technol*. 2007;**47**:165–77.

4. Eyre JA, Miller S, Ramesh V. Constancy of central conduction delays during development in man: investigation of motor and somatosensory pathways. *J Physiol*. 1991;**434**:441–52.

5. Koht A, Schutz W, Schmidt G, Schramm J, Watanabe E. Effects of etomidate, midazolam, and thiopental on median nerve somatosensory evoked potentials and the additive effects of fentanyl and nitrous oxide. *Anesth Analg*. 1988;**67**:435–41.

6. Gilmore R. The use of somatosensory evoked potentials in infants and children. *J Child Neurol*. 1989;**4**:3–19.

7. Gilmore R. Somatosensory evoked potential testing in infants and children. *J Clin Neurophysiol*. 1992;**9**:324–41.

8. McIntyre IW, Francis L, McAuliffe JJ. Transcranial motor-evoked potentials are more readily acquired than somatosensory-evoked potentials in children younger than 6 years. *Anesth Analg*. 2016;**122**:212–18.

9. Macdonald DB, Skinner S, Shils J, Yingling C, American Society of Neurophysiological Monitoring. Intraoperative motor evoked potential monitoring—a position statement by the American Society of Neurophysiological Monitoring. *Clin Neurophysiol*. 2013;**124**:2291–316.

10. Amassian VE, Stewart M. Motor cortical and other cortical interneuronal networks that generate very high frequency waves. *Suppl Clin Neurophysiol*. 2003;**56**: 119–42.

11. Chong CT, Manninen P, Sivanaser V, Subramanyam R, Lu N, Venkatraghavan L. Direct comparison of the effect of desflurane and sevoflurane on intraoperative motor-evoked potentials monitoring. *J Neurosurg Anesthesiol*. 2014;**26**:306–12.

12. Heckman CJ, Mottram C, Quinlan K, Theiss R, Schuster J. Motoneuron excitability: the importance of neuromodulatory inputs. *Clin Neurophysiol*. 2009;**120**:2040–54.

13. Mahmoud M, Sadhasivam S, Salisbury S, Nick TG, Schnell B, Sestokas AK, et al. Susceptibility of transcranial electric motor-evoked potentials to varying targeted blood levels of dexmedetomidine during spine surgery. *Anesthesiology*. 2010;**112**: 1364–73.

14. Eyre JA, Miller S, Clowry GJ, Conway EA, Watts C. Functional corticospinal projections are established prenatally in the human foetus permitting involvement in the development of spinal motor centres. *Brain*. 2000;**123**(pt 1):51–64.

15. Journee HL, Polak HE, De Kleuver M. Conditioning stimulation techniques for enhancement of transcranially elicited evoked motor responses. *Neurophysiol Clin*. 2007;**37**:423–30.

16. Journee HL, Polak HE, de Kleuver M, Langeloo DD, Postma AA. Improved neuromonitoring during spinal surgery using double-train transcranial electrical stimulation. *Med Biol Eng Comput*. 2004;**42**:110–13.

17. Dong CC, Macdonald DB, Akagami R, Westerberg B, Alkhani A, Kanaan I, Hassounah M. Intraoperative facial motor evoked potential monitoring with transcranial electrical stimulation during skull base surgery. *Clin Neurophysiol*. 2005;**116**:588–96.

18. Deletis V, Fernandez-Conejero I, Ulkatan S, Rogic M, Carbo EL, Hiltzik D. Methodology for intra-operative recording of the corticobulbar motor evoked potentials from cricothyroid muscles. *Clin Neurophysiol*. 2011;**122**:1883–9.

19. Szelenyi A, Langer D, Beck J, Raabe A, Flamm ES, Seifert V, Deletis V. Transcranial and direct cortical stimulation for motor evoked potential monitoring in intracerebral aneurysm surgery. *Neurophysiol Clin*. 2007;**37**:391–8.

20. Seidel K, Beck J, Stieglitz L, Schucht P, Raabe A. The warning-sign hierarchy between quantitative subcortical motor mapping and continuous motor evoked potential monitoring during resection of supratentorial brain tumors. *J Neurosurg*. 2013;**118**: 287–96.

21. Skinner SA, Transfeldt EE, Mehbod AA, Mullan JC, Perra JH. Electromyography detects mechanically-induced suprasegmental spinal motor tract injury: review of decompression at spinal cord level. *Clin Neurophysiol.* 2009;**120**: 754–64.

22. Moller AR, Jannetta P, Moller MB. Intracranially recorded auditory nerve response in man. New interpretations of BSER. *Arch Otolaryngol.* 1982;**108**:77–82.

23. Moller AR, Jannetta PJ. Comparison between intracranially recorded potentials from the human auditory nerve and scalp recorded auditory brainstem responses (ABR). *Scand Audiol.* 1982;**11**:33–40.

24. Moller AR, Jho HD, Yokota M, Jannetta PJ. Contribution from crossed and uncrossed brainstem structures to the brainstem auditory evoked potentials: a study in humans. *Laryngoscope.* 1995;**105**:596–605.

25. Salamy A. Maturation of the auditory brainstem response from birth through early childhood. *J Clin Neurophysiol.* 1984;**1**:293–329.

26. Skinner SA, Vodusek DB. Intraoperative recording of the bulbocavernosus reflex. *J Clin Neurophysiol.* 2014;**31**:313–22.

Chapter 17

Anesthesia for Neurointerventional Radiology

Mary Landrigan-Ossar

Introduction

Anesthesiologists caring for pediatric patients in the neurointerventional suite have many tasks. As experts in the physiology of anesthesia and its expected alterations during a proposed procedure, they are the final arbiters of whether a patient is medically prepared to undergo a procedure in an offsite location with limited access to backup. They coordinate the team in the procedure room, ensuring that every person regardless of their role is focused on patient safety and procedural success (in that order). They act as a psychological support to fearful patients and parents prior to the procedure. Only by successfully integrating all of these tasks can a consistently safe and successful pediatric neurointerventional service be facilitated.

For many anesthesiologists, the interventional radiology (IR) suite is a supremely undesirable anesthetizing location. With the currently rare exception of hybrid angiography operating rooms, IR is remote from the main operating rooms and is perceived as terra incognita for many reasons: unfamiliar staff and equipment, unfamiliar procedures, and greater patient acuity. This prejudice against the supposed terrors of IR must fall before the fact that it is increasingly utilized for the treatment of patients with neurosurgical pathology, particularly neurovascular issues.

This chapter deals with several common procedures that are encountered in a pediatric neurointerventional suite, with suggestions for their safe and effective management.

Case 1

An 8-year-old female with suspected moyamoya syndrome presents for diagnostic cerebral angiography in preparation for an upcoming craniotomy and pial synangiosis. She had experienced several seizures; magnetic resonance imaging (MRI) showed carotid narrowing concerning for moyamoya.

Diagnostic Angiography

Diagnostic cerebral angiography is the most common pediatric neurointerventional procedure. It is fortunately the procedure resulting in the least physiologic derangement. While noninvasive imaging such as computed tomography (CT) and MRI continually gains in sophistication, catheter-based angiography remains the gold standard for characterizing neurovascular pathology. Cerebral angiography may be used to investigate vasculature in the setting of hemorrhage, stroke, and vasculopathies such as moyamoya disease and after operative cerebrovascular interventions.

Preoperative Issues

Preoperative preparation for procedures in the neurointerventional suite is most safely accomplished when it mirrors preanesthesia workup for the main operating room. Consistent standards for chart review and the need for communication with consulting services will ensure that patients receive appropriate assessment and optimization before they arrive in radiology for their procedure. For uniformity throughout an institution, this is ideally accomplished by, or in close consultation with, the anesthesiology department. In a similar vein, anesthesia equipment should be as similar as practicable to that used in the operating rooms. Unfamiliar machines and monitors in a remote anesthetizing location increase user discomfort and the risk of error in an already challenging physical location (Figure 17.1).[1]

While simple cerebral angiography itself does not warrant anything more than a day surgical visit, careful consideration must be given to patient comorbidities that would increase patient risk with anesthesia and perhaps warrant pre- or postprocedure admission. For example, moyamoya disease risk is increased in patients with conditions including sickle cell disease, trisomy 21, and neurofibromatosis. Consultation with

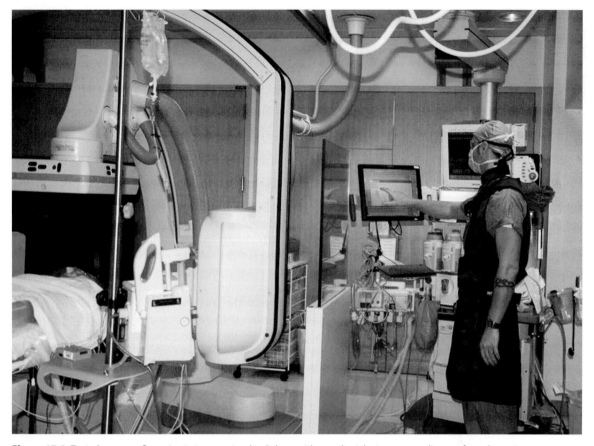

Figure 17.1. Typical room configuration in interventional radiology, with anesthesiologist at some distance from the patient.

a patient's specialty services to ensure preoperative medical optimization and consideration of the issues that go along with those conditions are necessary when planning for anesthesia.[2]

Intraoperative Management

Cerebral angiography is a relatively short procedure, usually taking less than 1 hour. Intermittent periods of apnea are ideal for suitable images. An emotionally mature teenager may be able to tolerate the procedure without sedation or with anxiolysis; deeper levels of sedation run the risk of a disinhibited patient, or a patient too sleepy to cooperate with breath holding. For this reason, it is common to perform the procedure on younger or more anxious patients with general anesthesia and an endotracheal tube. Should anesthesiologists determine that sedation is the safest choice for a patient, it is essential that they discuss this with their neuroradiology colleague to determine if this will result in acceptable image quality.

When anesthetizing any patient with potential cerebrovascular disease, careful consideration must be given to blood pressure and fluid management. Especially on induction of anesthesia, one must avoid hypotension that can put patients with a vasculopathy such as moyamoya at risk for cerebral hypoperfusion. It may be advisable to schedule such patients early in the day to minimize their fasting time. On the other hand, acute hypertension that could precipitate catastrophic bleeding in an unstable aneurysm or arteriovenous malformation (AVM) must also be avoided. An arterial line for this short procedure is generally unnecessary if reliable readings can be obtained from a noninvasive blood pressure cuff. Normocapnia is desirable in the vast majority of cases, and any proposed acute hypocapnia should be discussed with the neuroradiologist. While the risk of significant bleeding is extremely low, intravenous access that is sufficient to allow for adequate hydration is necessary. Normo- to slight hypervolemia will offset the diuretic effect of nonionic contrast medium and reduce the slight chance of any contrast-induced nephropathy.

Postoperative Concerns

Complications after cerebral angiography in pediatric patients are quite rare. Several series from high volume pediatric centers have demonstrated rates less than 0.4% with experienced neuroradiologists.[3] The most common of these rare problems is bleeding or hematoma at the site of femoral puncture. Neurologic or vascular problems as a result of catheterization are very rare, as are nephrologic consequences of contrast administration.

One major challenge for a pediatric patient after a cerebral angiogram is that they must lie flat for several hours to ensure hemostasis of the femoral artery. While behavioral techniques and the presence of parents can help reassure and distract an older or more cooperative child, medications have a role for younger or less cooperative children. Deep extubation when feasible and a period of quiet sleep in the recovery area with narcotics, benzodiazepines, or α-2 agonists as adjuncts can make this experience much less stressful. Pain after the procedure is minimal, and most patients are discharged from the recovery room needing only nonopiate pain medications thereafter.

Case 2

A 3-day-old male is scheduled to come to IR for embolization of a massive vein of Galen AVM (Figure 17.2). He was born in high-output heart failure and is currently intubated and being treated with vasopressor infusions.

Case 3

A 10-year-old girl, as part of an investigation into her history of headaches, had an MRI demonstrating a cerebral AVM. She presents to IR for embolization of the lesion prior to surgical excision (Figure 17.3).

Neuroembolization

Indications for therapeutic neurointerventional procedures include embolization of intracranial

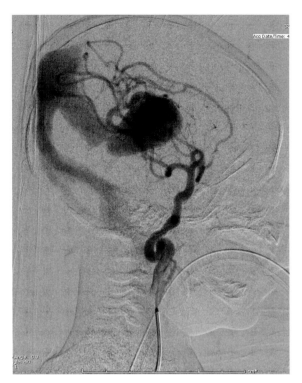

Figure 17.2. Cerebral angiogram demonstrating massive vein of Galen malformation in a neonate.

vascular anomalies, such as AVM, arteriovenous fistulae and aneurysms, targeted injection of intraarterial chemotherapy for tumors (see below), and presurgical embolization of both AVMs and tumors of the head and neck.

Preoperative Issues

As the two case scenarios above make clear, patients needing neuroembolization for arteriovenous anomalies can demonstrate a range of clinical presentations that go from a neurologically intact child to a child in full-blown heart failure or devastated from intracranial hemorrhage.[4] Preprocedure preparation in the former case is no more challenging than preparing any other healthy child for a long anesthetic. Preparation and optimization of the latter cases will likely require coordination with services such as cardiology to ensure that heart failure is well managed, or neurosurgery to determine if emergent surgery will be necessary to decrease intracranial pressure before proceeding for embolization. In these more medically fraught cases, a

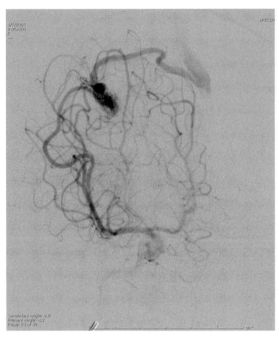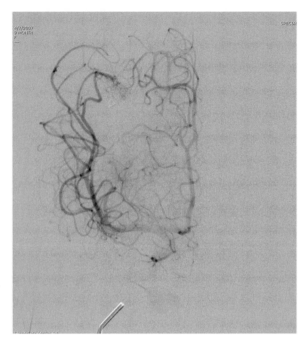

Figure 17.3. Cerebral angiograms demonstrating an arteriovenous malformation pre- and postembolization.

balance must be sought between perfect preanesthetic optimization and starting an embolization that if successful may improve issues such as cardiac overload.

Intraoperative Management

Therapeutic embolizations of cerebrovascular anomalies are some of the longest procedures performed in the neurointerventional suite, not uncommonly lasting 6–8 hours.

With very few exceptions, neurointerventions in children are performed on patients under general endotracheal anesthesia with consistent muscle relaxation. Frequent periods of apnea are generally required, and patient motion while catheters are deployed in the brain could be catastrophic. Careful attention must be paid to patient positioning and padding; it may be impossible to reposition a patient during a procedure.

As is the case with diagnostic angiography, in experienced hands the chance for blood loss is quite low. However, good intravenous access is necessary for fluid administration, with the goal of euvolemia. It is important to recognize that to reduce the risk of microemboli, the neuroradiologist continuously infuses heparinized saline via the femoral sheath through the guide catheter. This can result in a significant amount of fluid, invisible to the anesthesia team and maybe not quantifiable until pressure bags are taken down, being delivered to the patient by the neuroradiologist.

Close control of blood pressure usually mandates an arterial catheter. The neurointerventionalist and anesthesiologist prior to the case should mutually determine blood pressure parameters. A reasonable goal is a blood pressure within the normal range for age. Deliberate hypotension and even induction of asystole have been described in adult patients to facilitate injection of glue into high-flow lesions; these have not been well described for pediatric patients. The technique of balloon-assisted glue embolization may render such radical measures unnecessary. It is uncommon in this population to encounter hypertension resistant to anesthetic gas and pain medications. It is more likely that these young patients will tend to become hypotensive with anesthesia and require adjustment of anesthesia levels to maintain adequate perfusion. As abrupt increases in blood pressure can lead to hemorrhage from abnormal cerebral vessels, vasopressor medications should be used with extreme caution.

Hemodynamic alterations may be observed during embolization. Embolization with ethylene vinyl alcohol copolymer glue (Onyx, Covidien, Plymouth, MN) has been reported to induce bradycardia. Embolization of high-flow AVMs, which have already resulted in some degree of high-output heart failure, may result in immediate improvement in the patient's status.[4]

The risk of damage to nearby normal brain tissue during embolization is ever present, either from migration of embolic agent to a nontarget vessel, or because the target vessel perfuses both normal and abnormal tissue. In adult patients, it is not uncommon when embolizing in "eloquent cortex" to perform the procedure under light or no sedation so that a patient's neurologic status can be continuously monitored.[6] Such provocative testing has not been widely described in children, and in fact some groups describe risk factors for failed provocative testing, such as younger age and developmental delay.

Postoperative Concerns

In general, patients will require intensive care unit (ICU) observation at least overnight after embolization of an intracranial vascular lesion. As described above, a period of immobility is necessary after femoral artery access, which might require sedative assistance in younger or less cooperative patients.

Alterations in flow dynamics within an AVM postembolization may result in a period of increased hemorrhage risk; this is particularly true of partial embolizations such as those before a surgical resection where definitive closure of all vessels is not the goal.[7] Descriptions of postprocedure care of these patients have emphasized close control of blood pressure, avoiding abrupt increases that could result in hemorrhage. While there are few descriptions of techniques for achieving this goal, our group has had success with a continuous infusion of dexmedetomidine following extubation for the first night in the ICU.

Embolization of an AVM or a tumor in preparation for surgical resection can occur either under a single anesthetic or in separate sessions. Separate anesthetics are not uncommon since both the embolization and the resection can be very lengthy. If embolization and resection will occur in one session, patients are likely to require transport under anesthesia from the IR suite to the main operating room. While hybrid operating suites that incorporate high-quality angiography exist, they are not widespread. During transport, in addition to maintaining a secure airway, a patient's level of sedation must be carefully maintained to decrease the risk of abrupt increases in blood pressure.

Case 4

A 14-month-old girl with retinoblastoma is referred to IR for a series of injections of intra-arterial chemotherapy. She is otherwise healthy, and has a family history of retinoblastoma on her father's side.

Intra-arterial Chemotherapy

While retinoblastoma is the most common tumor requiring a neurointerventional radiologist's skills, directed delivery of chemotherapy to tumors via the vascular route is described for many cancers. Patients generally will receive several rounds of chemotherapy, in some cases interspersed with exams under anesthesia or MRI/CT to determine the course of treatment.

Preoperative Issues

These patients may have undergone chemotherapy or radiation previously, with potential cardiotoxic effects. Patients may experience decreased blood counts, and consultation with the referring oncologist should precede the case when in doubt.

Intraoperative Management

Injection of intra-arterial chemotherapy carries some unique challenges for the anesthesiologist. The radiologist may require pharmacologic assistance to direct the dispersion of medication; in treatment of retinoblastoma, the use of oxymetazoline nasal spray to preferentially drive flow in the ophthalmic artery to the optic component is utilized. Accessing the ophthalmic artery and/or injection of the chemotherapeutic drug into the artery has been associated with a not insignificant risk of vagal stimulation with bronchospasm and bradycardia; this can often be terminated by asking the radiologist to pull back the catheter.[8] Albuterol is often given preemptively, and occasionally glycopyrrolate is employed. Nausea and vomiting are increased postoperatively in these patients, and aggressive prophylaxis may be necessary to prevent a child with a fresh femoral puncture from repeatedly retching and vomiting.

References

1. Landrigan-Ossar M, McClain CD. Anesthesia for interventional radiology. *Paediatr Anaesth.* 2014;**24**(7):698–702.

2. Hishikawa T, Sugiu K, Date I. Moyamoya disease: a review of clinical research. *Acta Medica Okayama.* 2016;**70**(4):229–36.

3. Burger I, Murphy KJ, Jordan LC, Tamargo RJ, Gailloud P. Safety of digital subtraction angiography in children: complication rate analysis in 241 consecutive diagnostic angiograms. *Stroke.* 2006;**37**:2535–9.

4. Recinos PF, Rahmathulla G, Pearl M, Recinos VR, Jallo GI, Gailloud P, et al. Vein of Galen malformations: epidemiology, clinical presentations, management. *Neurosurg Clin N Am.* 2012;**23**(1):165–77.

5. Theix R, Williams A, Smith E, Scott R, Orbach D. The use of onyx for embolization of central nervous system arteriovenous lesions in pediatric patients. *Am J Neuroradiol.* 2010;**31**:112–20.

6. Wang Q, Chen G, Gu Y, Song D. Provocative tests and parent artery occlusion in the endovascular treatment of distal middle cerebral artery pseudoaneurysms. *J Clin Neurosci.* 2011;**18**: 1741–3.

7. Gross BA, Storey A, Orbach DB, Scott RM, Smith ER. Microsurgical treatment of arteriovenous malformations in pediatric patients: the Boston Children's Hospital experience. *J Neurosurg Pediatr.* 2015;**15**(1):71–7.

8. Kato MA, Green N, O'Connell K, Till SD, Kramer DJ, Al-Khelaifi M, et al. A retrospective analysis of severe intraoperative respiratory compliance changes during ophthalmic arterial chemosurgery for retinoblastoma. *Paediatr Anaesth.* 2015;**25**(6):595–602.

Radiation Therapy

Thejovathi Edala, Rahul Koka, and Babu V. Koka

Introduction

In 2015, it was estimated that more than 10,000 new cases of cancer were diagnosed in children aged 1–14 years in the United States.[1] Although deaths from cancer have declined in the past couple of decades, cancer remains the second leading cause of death in children. Currently, acute lymphocytic leukemia accounts for about 31% of childhood cancer cases, and central nervous system including spinal cord tumors around 21%.

Central Nervous System Tumors in Children

The most common types of brain tumors in children are astrocytoma, medulloblastoma, and ependymoma.

1. Astrocytomas are tumors that arise from astrocyte, star-shaped cells that make up the supportive tissue of the brain. They can appear in various parts of the brain and nervous system, including the cerebellum, the cerebrum, the diencephalon of the brain, the brainstem, and the spinal cord. The different types of astrocytomas are the following:

   a. Pilocytic astrocytoma: these tumors usually stay in the area where they started and do not spread. Less known astrocytomas are cerebellar and desmoplastic infantile gangiloglioma.

   b. Diffuse astrocytoma: these astrocytomas tend to invade surrounding tissue and grow at a relatively slow pace.

   c. Anaplastic astrocytoma: these rare astrocytoma tumors require more aggressive treatment.

   d. Astrocytoma grade IV: primary tumors in this group are very aggressive and are the most common astrocytoma grade IV. The secondary

tumors originate as a lower-grade tumor and then evolve into a grade IV tumor.

2. Medulloblastomas are fast-growing and high-grade and are the most common of the embryonal tumors. They usually are located in the cerebellum, and it is unusual for them to spread outside the brain and spinal cord. Medulloblastomas are relatively rare, accounting for roughly less than 2% of all primary brain tumors.

3. Ependymomas arise from the ependymal cells that line the ventricles of the brain and the spinal cord. Ependymomas can appear in different locations within the brain and spinal column. They account for about 2–3% of the primary brain tumors. Ependymomas can be of four different types:

   a. Subependymomas: typically slow-growing tumors that appear near a ventricle.

   b. Myxopapillary ependymomas: slow-growing tumors that tend to grow in the lower spinal column.

   c. Ependymomas: the most common of the ependymal tumors, located along or within the ventricular system.

   d. Anaplastic ependymomas: these are faster growing, mostly posterior fossa tumors in children.

Considerable advances in cancer treatment have led to an increase in survival rates. In the last four decades, overall survival rates have increased from just 10% to nearly 90% today. Factors contributing to these increased survival rates include sophisticated early detection, better chemotherapeutic agents, refined surgical techniques, and improvement in radiation therapy.

The anesthesiologist remains a key part of the multidisciplinary team that cares for a child with cancer, starting from diagnosis, surgery, chemotherapy, and radiotherapy with pain management to later surveillance. Radiotherapy has an increasing role in brain tumors. Knowledge of the multiple effects of cancer process, treatment, toxic effects, and complications is important for any anesthesiologist involved in the care of these children who undergo radiation therapy.

Goals of Radiotherapy

Radiotherapy may serve as:

- Primary therapy
- Adjuvant or neoadjuvant therapy
- Curative therapy
- Palliative therapy

Therapeutic radiation can be in the form of:

- Ionizing radiation
- Electromagnetic radiation—characterized by high energy and absence of mass, short wavelength, greatest energy on the electromagnetic spectrum
- X-rays produced when a stream of fast-moving electrons accelerated by high voltage strike the target and give up their energy (betatrons, linear accelerators)

The purpose of radiotherapy is to deliver therapeutic doses of radiation to the tumor while limiting damage to the surrounding healthy tissue. Advancements in three-dimensional imaging have produced modalities such as three-dimensional conformational radiation therapy and intensity-modulated radiation therapy,[2–5] which help concentrate the energy beam on the tumor while reducing radiation to the normal surrounding tissue.

Radiosensitivity of a cell is determined by its phase in cell cycle and by its nutrient and oxygen content. Therefore, healthy tissues have by far a greater capacity to repair damage from ionizing radiation, but they need time to do so. For that reason, the total dose of radiation is divided into a series of treatments. Additionally, by applying radiation at different times, the tumor cells that are in a relatively radio-resistant phase during one treatment are likely to cycle to a sensitive phase for a subsequent treatment.

Effects of Radiotherapy on a Cellular Level

Radiotherapy exerts its cytotoxic effects by generating free radicals, which cause lysis of cell membranes, DNA strand breakage, and RNA damage by ionization. Cellular kinetics determine the speed of cell death.

Airway Problems

Tumors involving the airway are relatively rare in pediatric patients. However, central nervous system (CNS) tumors with superior vena cava syndrome, large cervical, and retropharyngeal lymph nodes from leukemic infiltration may present as stridor. Complications to maintenance of the airway may become evident when the patient is lying down or anesthetized. After radiotherapy, these patients need to be evaluated for fibrosis of tissues, as distortion of airway anatomy leads to limited mouth opening, limited neck extension, supra- and subglottic edema, stenosis, and xerostomia. Furthermore, obliteration of lymphatics can lead to postoperative edema that causes airway problems.

Toxicity from Treatment

In cancer patients, the disease process itself has certain implications for anesthesia, depending on the site, type, and extent of involvement, with additional considerations coming from the effects of chemotherapy and radiotherapy (Table 18.1). Toxicity from chemotherapy and radiotherapy is unavoidable. The developing tissues of children are particularly susceptible to these effects. It is very important to evaluate these patients carefully for anesthesia and to detail the anatomical and physiological effects from the cancer, the treatment, and the potential toxicity.[6]

Factors that determine the susceptibility to radiotherapy toxicity[2] include:

- The total and fractionated dose received
- Sensitivity of the tissue
- Anatomy and extent of the tissue irradiated
- Course of the treatment
- Recent surgery and concurrent chemotherapy

Cardiotoxicity

When chemotherapeutic agents like anthracyclines (doxorubicin, daunorubicin, and alkylating agents) and cyclophosphamide are used in chemotherapy or radiation, cardiotoxicity can manifest early to late as myocarditis, pericardial effusion, myocardial depression, arrhythmias, endomyocardial and valvular fibrosis, conduction defects, and cardiomyopathy. Subclinical cardiomyopathy can become evident during the perioperative period. Cardiac failure is the

Table 18.1 Toxicity of Chemotherapy[6]

Chemotherapy Agent	Complications
Anthracyclines	Myelosuppression
	Cardiomyopathy
	Arrhythmias
Bleomycin	Pneumonitis
	Pulmonary fibrosis
	Hypersensitivity
Cisplatin	Neurotoxicity
	Nephrotoxicity
Cyclophosphamide	Myelosuppression
	Cardiomyopathy
	Arrhythmias
	Hepatotoxicity
	Hemorrhagic cystitis
5-fluorouracil	Myelosuppression
	Alopecia
Methotrexate	Myelosuppression
	Pneumonitis, pleural effusion
	Mucositis
	Renal failure
Procarbazine	Myelosuppression
	Pulmonary toxicity
	Neurotoxicity
	Leukemia
Vincristine	Myelosuppression
	Mucositis
	Peripheral neuropathy
	Syndrome of inappropriate ADH secretion

most common nonmalignant cause of death in survivors of Hodgkin's disease. Therefore, the anesthesiologist should look for physical signs and use surveillance echocardiography during preoperative assessment in this group of patients.

Factors that predispose patients to cardiotoxicity from chemotherapy and radiotherapy include:

- Chemotherapy agent and the combination used—lower the total cumulative dose to reduce risk for cardiomyopathy
- Total dose administered (anthracyclines—more than 300 mg/m^2)
- Route of administration—systemic administration leads to multiorgan injury
- Concurrent radiotherapy (anthracyclines—200 mg/m^2 with mediastinal radiation)
- Preexisting heart disease

Cancer survivors who underwent radiation therapy for conditions such as neurofibromatosis type 1, craniopharyngioma, and optic tumors may present with moyamoya syndrome, in which the carotid arteries narrow and develop collaterals. Moyamoya is seen usually 5 years after radiation, particularly in patients who were young at the time of radiotherapy.[7]

Pulmonary Toxicity

Pulmonary toxicity can be evident as an early or late effect. Cancer patients treated with busulfan, bleomycin, methotrexate, carmustine, or cyclophosphamide can present with dyspnea, dry nonproductive cough, and fever. Acutely they can present with malignant pleural effusions that require symptomatic relief with thoracocentesis before anesthesia. Acute noncardiogenic pulmonary edema, bronchiolitis obliterans, and drug-induced pneumonitis that progresses to pulmonary fibrosis are seen as late complications in patients treated with bleomycin. Anesthesiologists should be particularly cognizant of these possible effects because patients presenting for anesthesia after bleomycin chemotherapy need to be titrated carefully to the minimum oxygen possible to maintain oxygenation but at the same time avoid bleomycin-induced lung injury.

At radiation doses greater than 15–20 GY, radiation-induced pulmonary complications appear similar to chemotherapy-induced lung injury. Pulmonary changes are evident as restrictive defects on pulmonary function tests, increased alveolar-arterial gradient, reduction in forced vital capacity, and decreased carbon monoxide diffusing capacity. Anesthesiologists should keep in mind that they should review these tests to assess the severity and effects on anesthesia.

Hematological Toxicity

Myelosuppression can occur as a result of the disease state or after chemotherapy or radiotherapy. Patients with myelosuppression present with neutropenia, thrombocytopenia, and anemia. Anesthesiologists need to remember that this population is more prone to opportunistic infections from immune suppression. They should maintain utmost adherence to aseptic precaution during invasive procedures like accessing the port, and flush the intravenous tubing after the use of propofol, which is a potent culture medium. The patient should be isolated perioperatively, and a protocol should be in place for platelet and packed red blood cell transfusion.

Gastrointestinal Toxicity

Gastrointestinal toxicity includes stomatitis, mucositis presenting as nausea and vomiting, diarrhea, malnutrition, and anorexia. Anesthesiologists may encounter patients with dehydration, electrolyte imbalance, acute renal failure, and pain issues. Mucositis may cause the mucosa to be prone to bleeding during intubation, turning an easy airway into a difficult intubation.

Neuroendocrine Dysfunction

Neuroendocrine dysfunction from radiation of the hypothalamus or pituitary can present acutely or as a late effect, when the patient might present with neurocognitive defects, leukoencephalopathy, gonadotropin deficiency, hyperprolactinemia, growth hormone deficiency, or precocious puberty.

Coexisting Oncological Processes

Risk of secondary cancers[8] raises concern in survivors of childhood cancers. Three main categories in second malignancies after radiotherapy are leukemia, non-Hodgkin's lymphoma, and solid tumors like bone sarcomas and thyroid.

Anesthesia Management for Radiotherapy

Though radiotherapy is a noninvasive and painless procedure, most infants and toddlers require anesthesia. Children can experience considerable anxiety related to separation and are intimidated by the radiation equipment and immobilization devices used to restrain them, which fit tightly over the face and other body structures. Children will have undergone workup procedures before their radiotherapy and may be very apprehensive and suspicious of medical personnel. Older children are often able to go for

radiotherapy without sedation or anesthesia. They do well with distraction, audiovisual interventions like music or an iPad, and a reward after treatment completion.

A basic understanding of the fundamental elements of radiotherapy will help anesthesiologists to plan for and provide anesthesia with ease in the radiotherapy suite. The goal is to provide a precise target localization with accurate translation of anatomy to treatment and delineation of target extent through computed tomography (CT) imaging. Treatment planning techniques aim to administer a high conformal dose and gradient to the tumor and to use precisely reproducible patient positioning and immobilization.

Anesthesia Challenges

Anesthesiologists may have many concerns when planning to provide anesthesia for patients undergoing radiotherapy. These can include:

- Unfamiliar environment, limited space, bulky equipment, and restricted access to the patient
- Location away from main operating theater—immediate assistance, additional drugs, and backup equipment may not be readily available
- Inconsistent staffing
- Low ambient temperatures required for cooling of equipment can result in patient hypothermia
- In case of an adverse event, monitoring challenges may hinder response time, and physical barriers make immediate intervention difficult

It is well worth spending some time to familiarize oneself with the layout of the radiotherapy room to assess the adequacy, availability, and functional condition of monitoring equipment and medications. Anesthesiologists and staff should be briefed on emergency protocols and should be familiar with the location and use of emergency drugs and equipment.

After receiving approval from the oncologist to go for radiotherapy, the child will first undergo a treatment planning session, which is called a simulation. Simulation includes CT imaging, measurements, and reproducing the exact same conditions during radiotherapy sessions with immobilization casts, radio-opaque shields to protect the sensitive tissues, and precise target treatment. The simulation session may be the patient's first anesthetic session with the team, and the patient's airway issues and response to the anesthesia will be better appreciated after a few sessions with the team. This simulation is followed by the first treatment session.

Parents are advised to follow fasting guidelines as suggested by the practitioner, which may vary by institution.

The large majority of patients will have intravascular access in the form of an implanted central venous access device such as a tunneled central venous catheter or an implantable port, either from recent completion of or concomitant chemotherapy. The port can be accessed on the first day with strict aseptic precautions, left in place throughout the week, and removed over the weekend. The process can be repeated on Monday when the patient presents for the week of radiotherapy. The anesthesiologist uses closed-circuit television to monitor the patient, as he or she is unable to remain in the vault during treatment. The patient's monitor feeds to the screen in the control room.

Many techniques and agents have been used to anesthetize children during radiotherapy.[9] However, no randomized controlled studies have shown superiority of any one anesthesia technique in the pediatric population. The ideal anesthesia for radiotherapy should have fast onset, short duration, and quick recovery. It should prevent movement and maintain airway patency and spontaneous respiration.

General anesthesia can be administered by means of inhalational or intravenous routes, alone or in combination. The safe provision of inhalational anesthesia demands adequate monitoring of inspired and expired gases, ventilation, and oxygenation and often requires repeated airway instrumentation.

Anesthetic drugs used for sedation include propofol, ketamine, midazolam, dexmedetomidine, or a combination. Propofol has gained wide popularity as the drug of choice for deep sedation or anesthesia.[10,11] The appeal of propofol lies in its favorable pharmacokinetic profile, providing rapid onset and awakening, together with a lower incidence of nausea.[12]

Induction takes place with the child either on the bed or on the parent's lap. The goal is to provide adequate sedation while preserving spontaneous ventilation. The studies looking into induction dose of propofol in unpremedicated children found that the dose required was larger in preschool children than in older children. Doses in the range of 2.5–3.5 mg/kg are required in healthy unpremedicated children, with a lower range for older children and increasing requirements for younger children.[13,14]

One such approach is an initial propofol bolus in the range of 2–3 mg/kg. Then a maintenance infusion is usually begun at a rate of 250 mcg/kg/min and titrated to response. The patient is gently moved into position on the vault table, and the immobilization device is placed. A capnography catheter secured nasally can allow continuous assessment of ventilation and deliver supplemental oxygen. Once the patient is in a satisfactory position, respiratory efforts and adequacy of ventilation are carefully observed. There is considerable interindividual variation in the dose of propofol required to ensure adequate immobility. Though, over time, this population is exposed to propofol repeatedly, neither the clinical results nor the values derived from the BIS measurements have indicated tolerance to propofol.[15]

Ketamine, an N-methyl-D-aspartate (NMDA) receptor antagonist, is another drug that has been used in combination with midazolam pretreatment.[16–18] An initial ketamine dose of 0.5–1 mg/kg is all that is required for the short treatment session of radiotherapy. Tachyphylaxis has been described with the repeated use of ketamine for radiotherapy.

Dexmedetomidine, an imidazole, α_2-adrenoceptor agonist, also has been used as a sole anesthetic with a loading dose of 1 μg/kg over 10 minutes followed by an infusion of 0.7–0.8 μg/kg/hr.[19–21]

Recovery

A dedicated recovery area in close proximity is preferable. Similar caveats that govern safe recovery in the operating room apply to extubation and postanesthesia care in a radiotherapy location. If the postanesthesia care unit is distant from the radiotherapy location, one option is to keep the child anesthetized during transfer with appropriate monitoring and medications for transport, and then proceed with emergence and extubation in the main recovery area.

Conclusion

Anesthesia for radiotherapy is frequently fraught with the perils of remote and dark treatment rooms, bulky equipment, and personnel who are less experienced at dealing with emergency situations. It falls on the expertise of the anesthesiologist to ensure that despite these challenges, the conduct of anesthesia for these patients takes place in the safest possible way. Thorough preparation, a reliable team, and a safe anesthetic plan form the key elements in any procedural sedation or anesthesia. An understanding of the procedure, pathophysiology, and comorbidities of the patient population will help the anesthesiologist to meet these goals and provide safe anesthesia in this otherwise intimidating environment.

References

1. Howlader N, Noone AM, Krapcho M, Miller D, Bishop K, Altekruse SF, et al., eds. *SEER Cancer Statistics Review, 1975–2013*. Bethesda, MD: National Cancer Institute; April 2016. Available at http://seer.cancer.gov/csr/1975_2013/.

2. Milano MT, Constine LS, Okunieff P. Normal tissue tolerance dose metrics for radiation therapy of major organs. *Semin Radiat Oncol*. 2007;**17**:131–40.

3. Knab B, Connell PP. Radiotherapy for pediatric brain tumors: when and how. *Expert Rev Anticancer Ther*. 2007;7:S69–77.

4. Gibbs IC, Tuamokumo N, Yock TI. Role of radiation therapy in pediatric cancer. *Hematol Oncol Clin North Am*. 2006;**20**:455–70.

5. Kirsch DG, Tarbell NJ. Conformal radiation therapy for childhood tumors. *Oncologist*. 2004;**9**:442–50.

6. Lowenthal RM, Eaton K. Toxicity of chemotherapy. *Hematol Oncol Clin North Am*. 1996;**10**:967–90.

7. Ullrich NJ, Robertson R, Kinnamon DD, Scott RM, Kieran MW, Turner CD, et al. Moyamoya following cranial irradiation for primary brain tumors in children. *Neurology*. 2007;**68**(12):932–8.

8. Hall EJ, Wuu CS. Radiation-induced second cancers: the impact of 3D-CRT and IMRT. *Int J Radiat Oncol Biol Phys*. 2003;**56**:83–8.

9. Anghelescu DL, Burgoyne LL, Liu W, Hankins GM, Cheng C, Beckham PA, et al. Safe anesthesia for radiotherapy in pediatric oncology: St Jude Children's Research Hospital experience, 2004–2006. *Int J Radiat Oncol Biol Phys*. 2008;**71**:491–7.

10. Gottschling S. Propofol versus midazolam/ketamine for procedural sedation in pediatric oncology. *J Pediatr Hematol Oncol*. 2005;**27**(9):471–6.

11. McDowall RH, Scher CS, Barst SM. Total intravenous anesthesia for children undergoing brief diagnostic procedures. *J Clin Anesth*. 1995;7:273–80.

12. Buehrer S, Immoos S, Frei M, Timmermann B, Weiss M. Evaluation of propofol for repeated prolonged deep sedation in children undergoing proton radiation therapy. *Br J Anaesth*. 2007;**99**(4):556–60.

13. Westrin P. The induction dose of propofol in infants 1–6 months of age and in children 10–16 years of age. *Anesthesiology*. 1991;**74**(3):455–8.

14. Aun CST. Induction dose-response of propofol in unpremedicated children. *Br J Anaesth*. 1992;**68**(1):64–7.

15. Keidan I, Peral A, Shabtai EL, Pfeffer RM. Children undergoing repeated exposures for radiation therapy do not develop tolerance to propofol: clinical and bispectral index data. *Anesthesiology*. 2004;**100**(2):251–4.

16. Pellier I, Monrigal JP, Le Moine P, Rod B, Rialland X, Granry JC. Use of intravenous ketamine–midazolam association for pain procedures in children with cancer. A prospective study. *Paediatr Anaesth*. 1999;**9**:61–8.

17. Haeseler G, Zuzan O, Kohn G, Piepenbrock S, Leuwer M. Anesthesia with midazolam and S-(+)-ketamine in spontaneously breathing patients during magnetic resonance imaging. *Paediatr Anaesth*. 2000;**10**:513–19.

18. Tobias JD, Phipps S, Smith B, Mulhern RK. Oral ketamine premedication to alleviate the distress of invasive procedures in pediatric oncology patients. *Pediatrics*. 1992;**90**:537–41.

19. Virtanen R. Characterization of the selectivity, specificity, and potency of Dexmedetomidine as an α_2-adrenoceptor agonist. *Eur J Pharmacol*. 1988;**150**:9–14.

20. Shukry M, Miller JA. Update on dexmedetomidine: use in nonintubated patients requiring sedation for surgical procedures. *Ther Clin Risk Manag*. 2010;**6**:111–21.

21. Shukry M, Ramadhyani U. Dexmedetomidine as the primary sedative agent for brain radiation therapy in a 21-month old child. *Paediatr Anesth*. 2005;**15**(3):241–2.

Chapter 19

Anesthetic-Induced Neurotoxicity

Mary Ellen McCann

Introduction

The safe conduct of anesthesia during the neonatal period and infancy is associated with more complications than during later periods of childhood. Many neonates require immediate surgery during the period in which their circulation and respiratory systems are transitioning from fetal life to postnatal life. Blood pressure is generally at its lowest nadir at this time, and the depressant effects of general anesthesia may further decrease blood pressure to the point of affecting cerebral perfusion.[1] Major congenital defects occur in approximately 3% of all births, with cardiac defects accounting for almost one-half of all serious congenital defects.[2] These anomalies are the leading cause of infant mortality in the United States, with the vast majority of infants born with a serious congenital anomaly requiring surgery in the first year of life. Mortality and morbidity after anesthesia are approximately tenfold greater in neonates compared to older infants, with the mortality after intraoperative cardiac arrest in neonates being 92%.[3] Several studies across many developed countries reveal that approximately 12% of all children will have a general anesthetic before the age of 3, which translates to millions of very young children receiving general anesthesia every year.[4,5] In addition to being concerned about the immediate neurophysiologic effects of general anesthesia on the well-being of our youngest patients, pediatric anesthesiologists are also concerned about the possible neurotoxic effects of general anesthesia on these fragile patients. Laboratory evidence of anesthetic and sedative drugs causing immediate neurotoxic damage and later neurocognitive deficits is incontrovertible. The evidence for direct neurotoxic damage in young humans is much less certain.

This chapter reviews the expanding literature about neurotoxicity in preclinical in vitro and in vivo studies as well as provides an update on the clinical data available.

Laboratory Findings

Developmental neurotoxicity had been demonstrated in laboratory models after exposure to the majority of anesthetic and sedative drugs that are currently used in pediatric anesthetic practices.[6–11] Other types of medications that cause similar laboratory effects include anticonvulsant medications and ethyl alcohol.[12] The implicated general anesthetics include N-methyl-D-aspartate (NMDA) antagonists such as ketamine and nitrous oxide and gamma-aminobutyric acid (GABA) agonists such as the volatile anesthetics, propofol, barbiturates, and benzodiazepines. Susceptibility to these anesthetics in laboratory animals begins in the late fetal life through early development, which in most species is the time of maximal synaptogenesis or the "brain growth spurt." Three distinct neurodevelopmental histologic abnormalities have been shown in juvenile animals: an abnormal degree of neuroapoptosis, abnormal neurogenesis, and altered dendritic formation. Brain development in mammals involves neurogenesis and synaptogenesis. Neurons that do not make synapses are considered redundant and undergo a programmed cell death known as neuroapoptosis. However, general anesthetics administered to young animals that are undergoing brain growth spurts can lead to a fiftyfold increase in neuroapoptosis with a resultant overall loss of neurons compared with young animals that were not exposed to general anesthesia.[6,7] The time frame for rapid synaptogenesis varies from species to species, with young rats demonstrating maximal vulnerability from postnatal days 1 through 14 with a peak at postnatal day 7. In rhesus monkeys the period appears to be the later third of gestation to the first postnatal week. In humans, the brain growth spurt is believed to be during the last trimester of gestation to the first 3 years of life.[13] Exposure to noxious stimuli and stressors such as maternal deprivation, hypoxia, hypoglycemia, and ischemia during these time frames can also induce similar neurodegenerative changes in young animals.

Characterization of Anesthesia-Induced Developmental Neurotoxicity (AIDN)

Pathological Apoptosis

An increase as well as acceleration in neuroapoptosis is the most significant finding after general anesthesia exposure in young animals. Although apoptosis is a normal process by which the body prunes itself of abnormal or redundant neurons, in young animals the apoptotic pathway can be activated by prolonged or repeated exposure to general anesthetics. Apoptosis differs from other types of cell death in that it is almost always executed by caspase enzymes, which are cysteine-dependent aspartate proteases that either initiate the apoptotic process (caspases 2, 8, 9, and 10) or affect the process (caspases 3 and 7). The first pathway usually activated is the intrinsic pathway, which is mitochondrially activated. When the mitochondria are under stress, they can release proapoptotic proteins such as cytochrome C, procaspases, smac/diablo, bin G, adenylate kinase-2, and apoptosis inducing factor (AIF). Stress causes the outer mitochondrial membrane to become porous, and these proapoptotic proteins are released from the space between the inner and outer mitochondrial layers. AIF is unusual in that it can induce cell death without activating the caspase enzyme system.[14] A family of proteins known as the Bcl-2 family includes proteins that act as anti- or proapoptotic regulators within the cytosol. Cellular stress leads to an increase in the BAX proteins (Bcl-2 proapoptotic), which causes an increase in mitochondrial outer wall permeability and release of cytochrome C and other proapoptotic proteins, which activates caspase 9. Volatile anesthetic exposure can cause impaired mitochondrial function and activation of the intrinsic apoptotic pathway. Mitigators that restore mitochondrial integrity such as reactive oxygen species scavengers can ameliorate this response.

The extrinsic pathway involves the activation of the Fas receptor on the cell wall. Tumor necrosis factor (TNF), when it binds the death receptor protein, forms a ligand known as the TNF-related apoptosis inducing ligand or TRAIL. Both these receptors can activate procaspase 8 and initiate the caspase cascade.

Abnormal Neurogenesis

In very young rats, volatile agents and propofol have been shown to cause a loss of neural stem cells with a resultant decrease in neurogenesis. In contrast, isoflurane exposure causes a brief increase in abnormal neurogenesis in the adult rat followed by a loss of these abnormal cells.[15] Isoflurane exposure is also associated with impaired glial cell neurogenesis.[16] The inflammatory response elicited by general surgical trauma is also implicated in causing a decrease in neurogenesis in young animals. The evidence points to a twofold negative effect of general anesthesia exposure in young animals, a decrease in neural stem cells, and a decrease in the remaining stem cells to proliferate and mature into neurons.[17,18]

Altered Dendritic Development

Maximal anesthetic neurotoxicity generally occurs developmentally around the time of maximal synaptogenesis. Very young rodents from postnatal day 5 to day 14 generally exhibit abnormal neuroapoptosis after anesthetic exposure or a decrease in synapse formation. In slightly older animals, abnormal dendritic spines are formed. A dendritic spine generally receives input from a single neuron and is necessary for synaptogenesis. Rat species are generally susceptible to forming abnormal and increased number of dendritic spines at a postnatal age of 15–20 days.[19,20] Implicated anesthetics include propofol, midazolam, volatile agents, and ketamine. The impact of both a decrease for younger rats and an increase in slightly older rats of dendritic spine formation is unknown. New learning tasks in rats that are not exposed to anesthetics are associated with new dendritic spine formation. The altered dendritic spine formation after anesthetic exposure in the different developmental age groups in rats highlights how anesthetic neurotoxicity differs with age.

Aberrant Glial Development

In addition to neuronal apoptosis, neural glial cells are negatively affected by anesthetic exposure at a young age. Glial cells are crucial developmentally because by creating the scaffolding for neurons, they guide the migration of neurons from progenitor layers of neuronal substrate to necessary locations to make appropriate synapses. Isoflurane has been found to decrease the release of brain-derived neurotrophic factor (BDNF) by astrocytes.[21] This factor encourages developing neurons to develop axons to form synapses. Astrocytes are impaired during neural development by exposure to isoflurane. In rhesus monkeys and fetuses, isoflurane is also associated with an increased level of apoptosis.[10,22]

Anesthetic Effects on Spinal Cord

The effects of general anesthesia exposure have been noted to cause neurotoxicity in the spinal cord of young animals. Exposure to isoflurane and nitrous oxide causes an increase in neuroapoptosis of the spinal cord especially in the ventral horn in very young rat pups.[23] However, when these animals were allowed to mature there were no motor functional abnormalities detected. Intrathecal ketamine injections cause an increase in neuroapoptosis and microglial activation in the spinal cords of postnatal day 3 rats and later motor functional disabilities.[24] In contrast, intrathecal morphine and bupivacaine in very young rats given in analgesic and anesthetic doses did not lead to an increased level of spinal cord neuroapoptosis.[25]

Neuroinflammation

Inflammatory conditions in premature human infants are known to lead to poor long-term neurocognitive outcomes. Premature infants that are born small for gestational age, which can be a proxy for intrauterine inflammation, are at an even higher risk for developmental disabilities than age-matched cohorts who were born at a normal weight for gestational age.[26] In adults, activation of the neuroinflammatory cascades such as seen with surgical trauma has been implicated in postoperative cognitive dysfunction. The effects of general anesthetics on activating or deactivating these cascades are mixed. Sevoflurane had been shown to increase neuroinflammatory markers in young but not adult mice.[27] Other studies in young rats have shown that ketamine can ameliorate the neuroapoptotic effects of painful stimuli.[28]

Neurocognitive Function

Most of the studies examining the long-term decrements in neurocognitive function are based on rodent models. In this species, fetal, neonatal, and infant exposure is associated with both long- and short-term memory loss, as evidenced by poor performance on the Morris water navigation test and radial arm

test. After exposure to ketamine and sevoflurane in utero or in early infancy, rhesus monkeys show increased anxiety to the human intruder test and decreased motivation in their performance on the operant test battery.[29]

Relevant Anesthetic Durations and Concentrations

It is clear that anesthetic duration and concentration matter in terms of neurotoxicity for young mammals. Although both are important metrics, the anesthetic duration appears to have a higher impact than anesthetic concentration. Most studies that have shown an effect of anesthetic exposure involved an exposure of at least 4 hours, and in some studies involving monkeys and ketamine, an exposure of 24 hours was necessary before a neurotoxic effect was noted on psychometric testing.[30] There are some studies that have shown that exposure to 0.25 to 0.5% minimum alveolar concentration (MAC) for 6 hours or greater is associated with an uptick of neuroapoptosis as demonstrated by an increase in caspase 3 histologic staining on brain slides.[31] The data are mixed as to whether the volatile anesthetics are equally neurotoxic.[20,32] Some studies suggest that desflurane may be more neurotoxic than sevoflurane or halothane, but other studies in young mice demonstrate an equivalent level of apoptosis for equivalent MAC levels of the volatile anesthetics. There is a suggestion that an anesthetic mixture of a volatile anesthetic with nitrous oxide is more neurotoxic than a volatile anesthetic alone. It is unclear whether this is due to an additive or synergistic effect.

In general opioids do not increase neuroapoptosis, but under some experimental conditions, repeated morphine administration over 7 days is associated with increased apoptosis in the sensory cortex and amygdala of neonatal rats. However, a single dose of morphine given to postnatal day 7 rat pups did not increase neuroapoptosis.[33] Furthermore, daily administration of morphine for 9 consecutive days did not alter dendritic morphology. These areas of the brain are different from those affected by volatile and intravenous anesthetics, which preferentially affect the learning and memory areas (hippocampus) of developing brains.

Alleviation of AIDN

Apoptosis serves a very important function throughout the life span of mammals. During development it is a method of pruning redundant, abnormal, and useless cells of the organism in order to facilitate differentiation within the organ systems. Later it is chiefly a method of ridding cells that are abnormal in order to prevent tumors and other illnesses from occurring. As such it is logical that there are many different molecular pathways for apoptosis to occur and thus many different potential ways to block these pathways. Medications such as lithium, melatonin, estradiol, carnitine, erythropoietin, and dexmedetomidine have been shown to block pathways that lead to apoptosis. Dexmedetomidine, an adjunctive anesthetic agent, is particularly promising as an agent that may be partially neuroprotective during anesthetic exposure. It has been shown in rat pups to decrease isoflurane-induced neuroapoptosis and behavioral deficits.[34] However, extremely high doses of this drug will induce neuroapoptosis in very young rats. Its protective mechanism is unknown, but it is known to induce cell survival signaling pathways at clinically relevant doses. Although the animal data are concerning, there is some evidence that an enhanced and stimulating environment is more important to normal rat development than volatile anesthetic exposure.[35]

NMDA Receptor Antagonists

Ketamine

Neuroapoptosis induced by ketamine has been demonstrated in mice, rats, and rhesus monkeys, with peak effect occurring during the period of peak synaptogenesis. In monkeys this effect occurs in the last trimester of fetal development and the first 6 days postnatally.[30] By 35 days postnatally in monkeys, there is no neuroapoptotic effect found even in monkeys that were exposed to 24-hour infusions of ketamine. The long-term developmental effects of early exposure to ketamine include decreased motivation, color discrimination, anxiety, and short-term memory when the animals are tested at age 2. The doses used to sedate the monkeys were approximately 10 times the dose that is conventionally used to sedate humans and resulted in serum levels 10 times higher. However, the dose of 25–50 mg/kg/hr was the minimal dose required to sedate the monkeys and prevent them from biting their handlers. These differences in dosing requirements between humans and nonhuman primates highlight the difficulties in extrapolating results between the two closely related species. Similar findings have been demonstrated in rats.

Repetitive doses of ketamine at 20–50 mg/kg given every 90 minutes for 7 or more doses will result in histologic evidence of increased neuroapoptosis.[36,37] Repetitive doses of 4 or less did not increase the level of neuroapoptosis. Mice appear to be more sensitive to the neurotoxic effects of ketamine, with a single dose of 10 mg/kg resulting in increased neuroapoptosis and later learning disabilities in P7 mice.[38]

The neurotoxic effects of ketamine are amplified when the drug is combined with a GABAergic agonist such as thiopental or propofol. Mice pups at postnatal day 10 demonstrated neurotoxicity and later learning deficits when exposed to ketamine at 25 mg/kg and either thiopental 5 mg/kg or propofol 5 mg/kg.[39] There were no deficits in the group of mice exposed to a single dose of ketamine.

Ketamine appears to have salutary neuroprotective effects in some situations. Painful inflammatory stimulation in P7 rats such as injection of Freund's adjuvant into the hind paw will induce an uptick in neuroapoptosis seen in the cortical and subcortical regions of the brain, which is ameliorated by concurrent low-dose ketamine sedation.[28]

Nitrous Oxide

Nitrous oxide exposure has been demonstrated to cause an increase in neuroapoptosis in neonatal mice but not rats.[40] This degree of neuroapoptosis is greatly increased when nitrous oxide is combined with isoflurane in both neonatal rats and mice. However, like ketamine, it does have some neuroprotective properties. Juvenile animals show less neuronal cell death after a hypoxic ischemic injury if the injury occurs while the animal is being exposed to nitrous oxide.[41] Adult humans have less chronic pain after major surgery when nitrous oxide is used as part of a general anesthetic.[42]

GABAergic Agonists

Anesthetic agents that are GABA agonist agents have been extensively studied in juvenile animals and all have been implicated in causing an increased level of neuroapoptosis and later neurocognitive deficits. These drugs include barbiturates, benzodiazepines, propofol, and the volatile anesthetics. The neurotoxic injury induced by GABAergic agents generally occurs in different brain locations than the NMDA antagonists, which may explain that in some studies combinations of these two classifications of general anesthetics lead to worse outcomes. One of the theories of the etiology of neurotoxicity of GABAergic agonists is that the GABA receptor in young animals is excitatory rather than inhibitory.[43] Animal studies of young rat pups given sevoflurane will show some epileptiform activity.[43]

Benzodiazepines

High doses of benzodiazepines have induced neuroapoptosis in neonatal mice and rats. A single dose of 5 mg/kg of diazepam will cause neuroapoptosis in young mice but not young rats.[44] This dose was not associated with later learning deficits though. Doubling the dose to 10 mg/kg resulted in neonatal rats exhibiting neuroapoptosis. Similarly, neonatal mice were susceptible to midazolam at a dose of 9 mg/kg, but neonatal rats were not. Clonazepam administered intraperitoneally or subcutaneously has also been implicated in causing neurotoxicity in neonatal rats.

Barbiturates

Pentobarbital in doses of 5–10 mg/kg and phenobarbital in doses of 40/100 mg/kg induce neuroapoptosis in 7-day-old rats.[44] Thiopental, however, even in doses up to 25 mg/kg, did not induce apoptosis.[39] Simultaneous administration of estradiol ameliorates the neurotoxicity of pentobarbital and phenobarbital in rats. The protective effects of estradiol are believed to be due to an increase in the concentration of survival proteins within the cell cytosol.[45]

Propofol

Subanesthetic doses of propofol administered to neonatal rats and mice have been implicated in increased levels of neuroapoptosis.[46] Intraperitoneal propofol doses of 50–60 mg/kg cause increased neuroapoptosis and are associated with later neurocognitive deficits.[46]

Volatile Agents

Volatile anesthetic agents have both GABAergic as well as some NMDA antagonistic properties. However, the GABAergic properties predominate. Neonatal mice are susceptible to the neurotoxic effects of halothane and enflurane after only one-half-hour exposure prenatally. Fetal rats demonstrate learning deficits after a 2-hour prenatal exposure to halothane. In slightly older juvenile rats, prolonged exposure to low doses of halothane is associated with dendritic and synaptic density alterations.

Isoflurane exposure to P7 rats and mice is associated with neuroapoptosis after a 4-hour exposure when given in a concentration of 0.75%. Combinations of midazolam and nitrous oxide with isoflurane lead to a potentiated neurotoxic effect in both rats and guinea pigs.[6]

Sevoflurane even in subclinical doses when given for 2 hours or more has been associated with increased neuroapoptosis in mice pups. Six-hour exposures are associated with abnormal learning and social behaviors.[47]

Mechanisms

Several mechanisms have been postulated to explain anesthetic neurotoxicity in young animals. Understanding the mechanism for neuroapoptosis can aid in the development of ameliorative strategies to protect the developing brain.

Developing cells require external signals to guide their differentiation and synapse formation. General anesthesia can interfere with normal development by interrupting the cells' ability to receive signals as well as the ability of neurons to send signals to other neurons. Cells that are isolated from trophic signaling will upregulate intracellular proteins that can send the cell into a death spiral. In contrast to ischemic cell death, apoptosis cell death is noninflammatory in nature and generally involves single scattered cells rather than groups of cells. Since the cell wall remains intact and intracellular contents are not released into the extracellular fluid, the inflammatory response to cell death is limited. General anesthetics, sedatives, and some anticonvulsants block or alter GABA and NMDA receptors involved in synaptic transmission, putting the neuron at risk for apoptosis. Additional stressors on neurons such as ischemia can also bias a cell toward apoptosis. With rare exceptions, apoptotic cell death is mediated by the caspase enzyme system in the cell cytosol. Staining for activation of the end products of this enzyme system allows for quantification of degree of apoptosis occurring within an organism. Apoptosis can be activated extrinsically by the death receptor pathway or intrinsically by release of proteins from the mitochondria.

Anesthetic drugs can activate the intrinsic pathway by causing the mitochondrial membrane to increase in permeability and release cytochrome C into the cytosol, which then activates the caspase system. There is an intracellular family of regulator proteins known as the Bcl-2 proteins that have two branches—proapoptotic proteins (BAX) and prosurvival proteins (Bcl-2). Activation of the intrinsic system is fairly rapid occurring within 2 hours of exposure. Melatonin has been found to stabilize the mitochondrial membrane, thereby decreasing the release of cytochrome C and thus maintaining the cell in a prosurvival state.[48,49]

NMDA antagonists like ketamine and nitrous oxide are believed to induce cell death by a variety of mechanisms. Antagonism of the NMDA receptor in either a sustained fashion or repetitively causes upregulation of the NR1 subunit of the receptor. These upregulated neurons then require more trophic stimulation to maintain homeostasis. Lack of trophic stimulation leads to an increase in Ca^{2+} influx into the cell and eventually leads to neuronal cell death. Aberrant cell cycle entry has been implicated in cell death in cells exposed to ketamine. Isoflurane and nitrous oxide exposure alters BDNF and akt signaling, leading to activation of both the intrinsic and extrinsic pathways.[21] Isoflurane also has been implicated in activation of the $p75^{NTR}$ receptor, which leads to neuroapoptosis.

Although there are many medications that have demonstrated the ability to block some of the neuroapoptotic pathways in immature anesthetically exposed cells, the clinical relevance of drugs is uncertain. The neurotoxicity of general anesthetics given to young infants has not been proven, and the efficacy and feasibility of administering these neurotoxic blockers to young children remain to be elucidated.

Mitigating Factors

Estradiol

Estradiol given to neonatal rats increases the intracellular levels of phosphorylated extracellular signal regulated kinase and akt. These enzymes are prosurvival enzymes. This hormone does not affect GABA and NMDA neuronal receptors in rats. (The positive effects on immature rats raise the specter that there may be gender-related differences in the neurotoxicity of general anesthetics.)

Melatonin

Melatonin, perhaps by stabilizing mitochondrial membranes, is effective in decreasing the anesthetic-induced neuroapoptosis in the anterior thalamus and cerebral cortex in 7-day-old rat pups.[48,49] It is

plausible that since the intrinsic apoptotic pathway involves release of cytochrome C from mitochondria, stabilization of the mitochondrial membranes might lead to some protection from neuroapoptosis. Upregulation of the prosurvival proteins from the Bcl-X family may be another means by which melatonin is protective.

Xenon

Xenon is similar to nitrous oxide in that both gases are adjunctive general anesthetics, and both are NMDA antagonists. However, unlike nitrous oxide, in rat experiments it decreases isoflurane-induced neuroapoptosis in rat pups but not in mice pups.[50-52]

L-Carnitine

L-carnitine decreases the expression of the proapoptotic proteins in the BAX family and weakly increases the expression of the prosurvival proteins in the Bcl-X (L) family, thereby stabilizing the mitochondrial membranes.[53] Neonatal rats given a combination of nitrous oxide and isoflurane for 6 hours along with L-carnitine were protected from AIDN.[54]

Lithium

Lithium increases the phosphorylation of the extracellular signal regulated protein kinase (ERK) in cells that are exposed to ketamine or propofol. Five-day-old rats were spared AIDN after exposure to these anesthetics when they were pretreated with lithium.[55]

Hypothermia

Moderate hypothermia decreases both normal background neuroapoptosis as well as anesthesia-induced neuroapoptosis.[56] Rat pups that were cooled to 29°C showed no apoptotic response to isoflurane and ketamine exposure. The long-term effects of suppressing normal apoptosis by hypothermia are unknown and in fact may be deleterious.

Dexmedetomidine

The most promising AIDN ameliorating agent is dexmedetomidine. Although it is approved by the Food and Drug Administration (FDA) for sedation in adults, it is being used off label as a sedative in the neonatal and pediatric intensive care units. This medication is an α-2 selective adrenergic agonist with sedative, anxiolytic, and analgesic properties and is used as a general anesthetic adjunct and sedative. Most of the α-2 selective adrenergic receptors are located in the locus ceruleus which, when activated, cause sedation and anxiolysis. Other locations for these receptors include the spinal cord which, when activated, cause analgesia and the autonomic nerves, which, when activated, cause hypotension. The primary action of the α-2 receptors of the heart are chronotropic causing bradycardia, and dexmedetomidine causes a dose-dependent decrease in heart rate. The pharmacodynamic effects of this medication are initial bradycardia with a mild increase in blood pressure followed by bradycardia and hypotension. In addition, there are case reports of sustained severe hypertension in young children given glycopyrrolate to counteract bradycardia.[57] It is not associated with neuroapoptosis in murine studies and may attenuate the apoptosis seen with isoflurane, although in some studies dexmedetomidine is associated with a modest increase in neuroapoptosis.[54]

Narcotics

Opioids are generally considered less neurotoxic than other sedatives. In young rats given narcotics in antinociceptive doses, there is no evidence of apoptosis in the spinal cord.

Local Anesthetics

Local anesthetics have been implicated in both in vitro and in vivo experiments in causing neuroapoptosis. They are associated with apoptotic and necrotic cell death in a dose-dependent manner. A study of rat neuron cells derived from the dorsal ganglion of P7 rat pups revealed that the earliest manifestations of lidocaine neurotoxicity were complete loss of mitochondrial membrane potential, followed by release of cytochrome C into the cytosol at concentration and caspase activation. Another experiment found that many local anesthetics investigated were neurotoxic at concentrations observed intrathecally after spinal anesthesia in humans.[58] The in vitro toxicity of the local anesthetics correlated with their octanol/buffer partition coefficient and thus from a study examining a cell line derived from human neuroblastoma cells their relative clinical potency with the following order of apoptotic potency from high to low toxicity (tetracaine > bupivacaine > prilocaine = mepivacaine = ropivacaine > lidocaine > procaine = articaine).[59] The neuroapoptotic potential of either ketamine or bupivacaine administered intrathecally to P7 rat pups revealed apoptosis in the ketamine but not the bupivacaine-exposed rats.[25]

Clinical Studies

There are several difficulties in extrapolating the results from rat and small mammal studies to the human population. In many of the animal studies, there has been a high mortality of the rat or mice pups while under anesthesia, fortunately a finding not found with human anesthetics. The reasons for this are clear; it is simply impossible to monitor the health of these tiny neonatal animals as carefully as is done in the most premature human infants. Several studies have tried to address this confounder with measuring serum glucoses and venous gases perioperatively.[60] In addition, there is no certainty about when the time of potential vulnerability in humans would occur.

There are other formidable hurdles to adequately studying the issue of anesthetic toxicity in human infants. In general, the need for surgery or radiologic imaging studies in human infants is associated with underlying pathology, so prospective cohort studies or retrospective epidemiologic studies can be confounded by this underlying pathology. In addition, the traumatic effects of surgery such as perioperative fasting, transport, hypothermia, hemodynamic instability, and stress response secondary to surgical stimulus may independently affect neurologic outcomes. The magnitude of the effects of these confounders on eventual neurocognitive outcomes may mask any subtle deleterious effects that general anesthesia may cause in humans. The degree of presurgical morbidity may be one of the reasons that some infants had surgery for patent ductus arteriosus (PDA) and necrotizing enterocolitis rather than medical therapy. In children undergoing inguinal herniorrhaphies, a possible confounder might be a complicated respiratory neonatal course, which has been linked to both a higher incidence of inguinal hernias and poorer neurologic outcomes.[61] These studies can also be affected by informational biases because of their retrospective nature. Prospective cohort studies, which can generally avoid informational biases, are also confounded by surgical and premorbid conditions of the participants. A meta-analysis of 23 clinical reports of patients undergoing neonatal surgery for major noncardiac congenital anomalies revealed lower cognitive scores in a median of 23% of the patients.[62] Randomized controlled trials are very difficult to perform in children who require surgery because for most procedures there are not alternatives to general anesthesia. A single large prospective randomized trial known as the GAS trial compared the effects of general anesthesia with regional anesthesia in very young infants undergoing inguinal herniorrhaphies.[63] A clear limitation of this trial is that the anesthetic exposure duration was limited.

Prenatal Human Exposure to General Anesthesia

There are very few studies examining the prenatal effects of general anesthesia on the neurocognitive outcomes of humans. As of this time, there are no studies looking at the effects of general anesthesia on development in which the general anesthetic was administered well before labor and delivery. A single nonrandomized study from Japan showed that 159 infants exposed to maternal nitrous oxide during the last stages of delivery had statistically different behaviors on postnatal day 5 compared to nonexposed infants.[64] These infants exhibited weaker habituation to sound, stronger muscular habituation, less cuddling, and fewer smiles.

An epidemiologic study based on a birth cohort from Olmstead County in Minnesota found that children exposed to general anesthesia for elective cesarean section deliveries are not more likely to develop learning disabilities than those born of vaginal deliveries.[65] One of the limitations of this study is that it involved two different modes of delivery. A separate study, using this same database, found that there was no impact of neuroaxial labor analgesia on the incidence of childhood learning disabilities.[66]

Neonatal and Young Childhood Human Exposure to General Anesthesia

In the literature are several studies that demonstrate an association between surgery and poor neurodevelopmental outcomes. In premature infants born before 27 weeks' gestation, the Victorian Infant Collaborative Study Group found in a case control study design that infants who underwent surgery for PDA ligation, inguinal herniorrhaphy, gastrointestinal surgery, neurosurgery, and tracheotomy had an increased incident of cerebral palsy, blindness, deafness, and Wechsler Preschool and Primary Scales of Intelligence (WPPSI) < 3 SD below the mean.[67] Several small studies as well as a large study involving almost 3,000 extremely low birth weight infants with a diagnosis of necrotizing enterocolitis found that there was a higher incidence

of cerebral palsy and poor neurocognitive outcomes in those infants who were treated surgically compared with those treated with peritoneal lavage.[68-71] However, the difficulties with adjusting for confounding by indication are illustrated by studies that show that infants undergoing isolated tracheoesophageal fistula repair in the neonatal period do not differ from the general population in terms of intelligence quotient (IQ) measurements.[72,73] Many studies involving infants with serious congenital heart disease have demonstrated an increased incidence of cerebral palsy, speech and language impairment, and motor dysfunction and lower IQs.[74-77] A recently appreciated confounder in studies of cardiac infants involves the relative immaturity of brain development of these infants compared with normal infants.[78] Serial neurocognitive examinations of a prospective cohort of infants born with transposition of the great vessels who were randomized to either circulatory arrest or cardiac bypass during the surgical repair found that the entire group was below population expectations for academic achievement, fine motor function, visuospatial skills, working memory, hypothesis generating and testing, sustained attention, and higher order language skills.[74-76]

Several studies have been published recently specifically examining whether the exposure to general anesthesia in infancy is associated with later learning difficulties. Researchers at the Mayo Clinic in Rochester, Minnesota, published a retrospective cohort study of over 5,000 children, of whom approximately 12% had one or more general anesthetics before the age of 4.[4] This study found that there were significantly more reading, written language, and math learning disabilities in children who had been exposed to two or more general anesthetics but no increase in disabilities in those children who had been exposed to a single anesthetic. The risk of learning disabilities also increased with the cumulative duration of the general anesthesia. In another epidemiologic study, a birth cohort of 5,000 patients was identified from the New York State Medicaid billing codes.[79] Of this group, 383 patients underwent inguinal herniorrhaphy at a young age. After controlling for gender and low birth weight, the authors found nearly a twofold increase in developmental and behavioral issues. A pilot study to test the feasibility of using a validated child behavior checklist in 314 children who had urologic surgery determined that there was more disturbed neurobehavioral development in children who underwent surgery prior to 24 months compared with those who underwent surgery after 24 months of age, although the differences between the two groups were not statistically significant.[80] These studies are provocative, but the data do not reveal whether anesthesia itself may contribute to developmental issues or whether the need for anesthesia is a marker for other unidentified factors that contribute to these.

Another epidemiologic study from the New York State Medicaid dataset examined the developmental behavioral outcomes of 304 children with no risk factors for neurodevelopmental difficulties exposed to anesthesia before age 3 and compared them with a cohort of 10,450 siblings and found a 60% greater incidence of developmental or behavioral problem in children exposed to general anesthesia.[81] A subsequent analysis of both New York and Texas Medicaid databases by the same group reaffirmed an increased rate of mental and developmental delays and attention-deficit disorder in children undoing surgery before 5 years of age. However, the incidence of these disorders was equivalent if the surgery occurred before or after 2 years of age, thereby refuting the practice of delaying surgery to reduce the potential of adverse neurocognitive deficits.[82] A small retrospective study of 53 children who were exposed to general anesthesia before the age of 4 compared with children matched on age, gender, handedness, and socioeconomic status found that the exposed group of children had lower listening comprehension and performance IQ measurements.[83] These decreased measurements were associated with lower gray matter density in the occipital cortex and cerebellum. The duration of anesthesia exposure for the children in this study averaged less than 1 hour.

Separate big data analysis from educational achievement scores in large cohorts (up to 34,000 pediatric patients) from Canada and Sweden divulged a slightly increased odds ratio of decreased education attainment in children exposed to surgery and anesthesia at age greater than 2–4 years.[84–86] Scrutiny of these populations reveals a lower percentage in academic achievement scores for toddlers undergoing ear, nose, and throat surgery.[86] This finding suggests that early derangements in hearing and speech may have an impact on subsequent cognitive domains assessed by school performance.[87]

In contrast to these findings, at least two other large studies have shown no association between receipt of general anesthesia and academic performance. A very large epidemiologic study comparing the academic performance of 2,689 children who had undergone inguinal herniorrhaphy in infancy to a randomly selected, age-matched control group consisting of 5% of the population derived from the Danish Civil Registration System from 1986 to 1990 found that after adjusting for known confounders, there was no statistically significant difference between the exposure and control groups.[88] A similar finding was reported in a Mayo cohort study, which found no increase in learning disabilities in children exposed to a single anesthetic.[4] Bartels et al. from the Netherlands also found no difference in the educational achievements of 1,143 identical twins who were discordant in their exposure to general anesthesia before the age of 3.[89]

In 2007, the GAS trial was initiated and enrolled 722 infants less than 60 weeks postmenstrual age over a period of 6 years. This trial is a randomized controlled equivalence trial comparing general anesthesia with sevoflurane with regional anesthesia with bupivacaine in infants undergoing inguinal herniorrhaphies. The interim 2-year follow-up results have been published and show that there were no differences on the Bayley–III examinations and other neurocognitive tests between the two types of anesthesia.[90] The primary outcome measure—neurocognitive testing at age 5—has not yet been completed. The PANDA trial published results on 105 sibling pairs who were discordant for general anesthesia exposure before the age of 3 years.[91] This small trial found no difference in mean IQ scores between exposed and nonexposed sibling pairs.

Conclusion

The FDA has cautioned health care providers and parents to carefully consider forgoing elective and urgent surgery in children younger than 3 years of age.[92,93] On April 27, 2017, the FDA released a Drug Safety Communication on label changes on common anesthetic and sedative drugs and this issue.[94] The available clinical studies have considerable limitations. Currently the only published prospective randomized controlled trial, the GAS trial, did not find a difference in neurocognitive outcomes in children exposed to general anesthesia in infancy compared with regional anesthesia. However, the outcome measure published was an interim result that needs to be validated by more predictive 5-year neurocognitive results. The results of the retrospective studies are mixed, with approximately half of these studies showing an association with general anesthesia and later neurocognitive impairments. Another obvious limitation of many of these studies is that the duration of anesthesia is limited. Many of these studies have focused on patients undergoing inguinal herniorrhaphies because this type of surgery is common in infancy and in general the patients are healthy. A huge knowledge gap exists in determining whether general anesthesia administered to infants for a period of longer than 2 hours is associated with AIDN. Independent of the concerns about neurotoxicity, general anesthesia is associated with more mortality and complications in the first month of life compared with infancy and more mortality and complications in infancy than in childhood.[3,95] So for the above reasons, the decision to anesthetize a young infant should involve a careful consideration of the risks and benefits of the planned procedure.

References

1. McCann ME, Schouten AN, Dobija N, Munoz C, Stephenson L, Poussaint TY, et al. Infantile postoperative encephalopathy: perioperative factors as a cause for concern. *Pediatrics*. 2014;**133**:e751–7.

2. Centers for Disease Control and Prevention. Update on overall prevalence of major birth defects—Atlanta, Georgia, 1978–2005. *MMWR Morb Mortal Wkly Rep.* 2008;**57**:1–5.

3. Flick RP, Sprung J, Harrison TE, Gleich SJ, Schroeder DR, Hanson AC, et al. Perioperative cardiac arrests in children between 1988 and 2005 at a tertiary referral center: a study of 92,881 patients. *Anesthesiology*. 2007;**106**:226–37; quiz 413–14.

4. Wilder RT, Flick RP, Sprung J, Katusic SK, Barbaresi WJ, Mickelson C, et al. Early exposure to anesthesia and learning disabilities in a population-based birth cohort. *Anesthesiology*. 2009;**110**:796–804.

5. Ing C, Dimaggio C, Whitehouse A, Hegarty MK, Brady J, von Ungern BS, et al. Long-term differences in language and cognitive function after childhood exposure to anesthesia. *Pediatrics*. 2012;**130**(3):e476–85.

6. Jevtovic-Todorovic V, Hartman RE, Izumi Y, Benshoff ND, Dikranian K, Zorumski CF, et al. Early exposure to common anesthetic agents causes widespread

7. Ikonomidou C, Bosch F, Miksa M, Bittigau P, Vockler J, Dikranian K, et al. Blockade of NMDA receptors and apoptotic neurodegeneration in the developing brain. *Science*. 1999;**283**:70–4.

8. Lu Y, Wu X, Dong Y, Xu Z, Zhang Y, Xie Z. Anesthetic sevoflurane causes neurotoxicity differently in neonatal naive and Alzheimer disease transgenic mice. *Anesthesiology*. 2010;**112**:1404–16.

9. Rizzi S, Carter LB, Ori C, Jevtovic-Todorovic V. Clinical anesthesia causes permanent damage to the fetal guinea pig brain. *Brain Pathol*. 2008;**18**:198–210.

10. Brambrink AM, Back SA, Riddle A, Gong X, Moravec MD, Dissen GA, et al. Isoflurane-induced apoptosis of oligodendrocytes in the neonatal primate brain. *Ann Neurol*. 2012;**72**:525–35.

11. Brambrink AM, Evers AS, Avidan MS, Farber NB, Smith DJ, Zhang X, et al. Isoflurane-induced neuroapoptosis in the neonatal rhesus macaque brain. *Anesthesiology*. 2010;**112**:834–41.

12. Olney JW. Fetal alcohol syndrome at the cellular level. *Addict Biol*. 2004;**9**:137–49; discussion 51.

13. Dobbing J, Sands J. Comparative aspects of the brain growth spurt. *Early Hum Dev*. 1979;**3**:79–83.

14. Cande C, Cohen I, Daugas E, Ravagnan L, Larochette N, Zamzami N, et al. Apoptosis-inducing factor (AIF): a novel caspase-independent death effector released from mitochondria. *Biochimie*. 2002;**84**:215–22.

15. Stratmann G, Sall JW, May LD, Bell JS, Magnusson KR, Rau V, et al. Isoflurane differentially affects neurogenesis and long-term neurocognitive function in 60-day-old and 7-day-old rats. *Anesthesiology*. 2009;**110**:834–48.

16. Culley DJ, Cotran EK, Karlsson E, Palanisamy A, Boyd JD, Xie Z, et al. Isoflurane affects the cytoskeleton but not survival, proliferation, or synaptogenic properties of rat astrocytes in vitro. *Br J Anaesth*. 2013;**110**(suppl 1):i19–28.

17. Hofacer RD, Deng M, Ward CG, Joseph B, Hughes EA, Jiang C, et al. Cell-age specific vulnerability of neurons to anesthetic toxicity. *Ann Neurol*. 2013;**73**(6):695–704.

18. Culley DJ, Boyd JD, Palanisamy A, Xie Z, Kojima K, Vacanti CA, et al. Isoflurane decreases self-renewal capacity of rat cultured neural stem cells. *Anesthesiology*. 2011;**115**:754–63.

19. De Roo M, Klauser P, Briner A, Nikonenko I, Mendez P, Dayer A, et al. Anesthetics rapidly promote synaptogenesis during a critical period of brain development. *PLOS ONE*. 2009;**4**:e7043.

20. Briner A, De Roo M, Dayer A, Muller D, Habre W, Vutskits L. Volatile anesthetics rapidly increase

dendritic spine density in the rat medial prefrontal cortex during synaptogenesis. *Anesthesiology.* 2010;**112**:546–56.

21. Lu LX, Yon JH, Carter LB, Jevtovic-Todorovic V. General anesthesia activates BDNF-dependent neuroapoptosis in the developing rat brain. *Apoptosis.* 2006;**11**:1603–15.

22. Creeley CE, Dikranian KT, Dissen GA, Back SA, Olney JW, Brambrink AM. Isoflurane-induced apoptosis of neurons and oligodendrocytes in the fetal rhesus macaque brain. *Anesthesiology.* 2014;**120**:626–38.

23. Sanders RD, Xu J, Shu Y, Fidalgo A, Ma D, Maze M. General anesthetics induce apoptotic neurodegeneration in the neonatal rat spinal cord. *Anesth Analg.* 2008;**106**:1708–11.

24. Walker SM, Westin BD, Deumens R, Grafe M, Yaksh TL. Effects of intrathecal ketamine in the neonatal rat: evaluation of apoptosis and long-term functional outcome. *Anesthesiology.* 2010;**113**:147–59.

25. Yahalom B, Athiraman U, Soriano SG, Zurakowski D, Carpino EA, Corfas G, et al. Spinal anesthesia in infant rats: development of a model and assessment of neurologic outcomes. *Anesthesiology.* 2011;**114**:1325–35.

26. Strunk T, Inder T, Wang X, Burgner D, Mallard C, Levy O. Infection-induced inflammation and cerebral injury in preterm infants. *Lancet Infect Dis.* 2014;**14**:751–62.

27. Tao G, Zhang J, Zhang L, Dong Y, Yu B, Crobsy G, et al. Sevoflurane induces tau phosphorylation and glycogen synthase kinase 3 beta activation in young mice. *Anesthesiology.* 2014;**121**:510–27.

28. Anand KJ, Garg S, Rovnaghi CR, Narsinghani U, Bhutta AT, Hall RW. Ketamine reduces the cell death following inflammatory pain in newborn rat brain. *Pediatr Res.* 2007;**62**:283–90.

29. Paule MG, Li M, Allen RR, Liu F, Zou X, Hotchkiss C, et al. Ketamine anesthesia during the first week of life can cause long-lasting cognitive deficits in rhesus monkeys. *Neurotoxicol Teratol.* 2011;**33**:220–30.

30. Paule MG, Li M, Allen RR, Liu F, Zou X, Hotchkiss C, et al. Ketamine anesthesia during the first week of life can cause long-lasting cognitive deficits in rhesus monkeys. *Neurotoxicol Teratol.* 2011;**33**(2): 220–30.

31. Soriano SG, Anand KJ. Anesthetics and brain toxicity. *Curr Opin Anaesthesiol.* 2005;**18**:293–7.

32. Istaphanous GK, Howard J, Nan X, Hughes EA, McCann JC, McAuliffe JJ, et al. Comparison of the neuroapoptotic properties of equipotent anesthetic concentrations of desflurane, isoflurane, or sevoflurane in neonatal mice. *Anesthesiology.* 2011;**114**:578–87.

33. Massa H, Lacoh CM, Vutskits L. Effects of morphine on the differentiation and survival of developing

pyramidal neurons during the brain growth spurt. *Toxicol Sci.* 2012;**130**:168–79.

34. Sanders RD, Xu J, Shu Y, Januszewski A, Halder S, Fidalgo A, et al. Dexmedetomidine attenuates isoflurane-induced neurocognitive impairment in neonatal rats. *Anesthesiology.* 2009;**110**:1077–85.

35. Shih J, May LD, Gonzalez HE, Lee EW, Alvi RS, Sall JW, et al. Delayed environmental enrichment reverses sevoflurane-induced memory impairment in rats. *Anesthesiology.* 2012;**116**:586–602.

36. Hayashi H, Dikkes P, Soriano SG. Repeated administration of ketamine may lead to neuronal degeneration in the developing rat brain. *Paediatr Anaesth.* 2002;**12**:770–4.

37. Scallet AC, Schmued LC, Slikker W Jr., Grunberg N, Faustino PJ, Davis H, et al. Developmental neurotoxicity of ketamine: morphometric confirmation, exposure parameters, and multiple fluorescent labeling of apoptotic neurons. *Toxicol Sci.* 2004;**81**:364–70.

38. Rudin M, Ben-Abraham R, Gazit V, Tendler Y, Tashlykov V, Katz Y. Single-dose ketamine administration induces apoptosis in neonatal mouse brain. *J Basic Clin Physiol Pharmacol.* 2005;**16**:231–43.

39. Fredriksson A, Ponten E, Gordh T, Eriksson P. Neonatal exposure to a combination of N-methyl-D-aspartate and gamma-aminobutyric acid type A receptor anesthetic agents potentiates apoptotic neurodegeneration and persistent behavioral deficits. *Anesthesiology.* 2007;**107**:427–36.

40. Yon JH, Daniel-Johnson J, Carter LB, Jevtovic-Todorovic V. Anesthesia induces neuronal cell death in the developing rat brain via the intrinsic and extrinsic apoptotic pathways. *Neuroscience.* 2005;**135**:815–27.

41. Haelewyn B, David HN, Rouillon C, Chazalviel L, Lecocq M, Risso JJ, et al. Neuroprotection by nitrous oxide: facts and evidence. *Crit Care Med.* 2008;**36**:2651–9.

42. Chan MT, Wan AC, Gin T, Leslie K, Myles PS. Chronic postsurgical pain after nitrous oxide anesthesia. *Pain.* 2011;**152**:2514–20.

43. Edwards DA, Shah HP, Cao W, Gravenstein N, Seubert CN, Martynyuk AE. Bumetanide alleviates epileptogenic and neurotoxic effects of sevoflurane in neonatal rat brain. *Anesthesiology.* 2010;**112**:567–75.

44. Bittigau P, Sifringer M, Genz K, Reith E, Pospischil D, Govindarajalu S, et al. Antiepileptic drugs and apoptotic neurodegeneration in the developing brain. *Proc Natl Acad Sci USA.* 2002;**99**:15089–94.

45. Asimiadou S, Bittigau P, Felderhoff-Mueser U, Manthey D, Sifringer M, Pesditschek S, et al.

Protection with estradiol in developmental models of apoptotic neurodegeneration. *Ann Neurol.* 2005;58:266–76.

46. Cattano D, Young C, Straiko MM, Olney JW. Subanesthetic doses of propofol induce neuroapoptosis in the infant mouse brain. *Anesth Analg.* 2008;106:1712–14.

47. Zhang X, Xue Z, Sun A. Subclinical concentration of sevoflurane potentiates neuronal apoptosis in the developing C57BL/6 mouse brain. *Neurosci Lett.* 2008;447:109–14.

48. Yon JH, Carter LB, Reiter RJ, Jevtovic-Todorovic V. Melatonin reduces the severity of anesthesia-induced apoptotic neurodegeneration in the developing rat brain. *Neurobiol Dis.* 2006;21:522–30.

49. Xu S, Pi H, Zhang L, Zhang N, Li Y, Zhang H, et al. Melatonin prevents abnormal mitochondrial dynamics resulting from the neurotoxicity of cadmium by blocking calcium-dependent translocation of Drp1 to the mitochondria. *J Pineal Res.* 2016;60:291–302.

50. Cattano D, Williamson P, Fukui K, Avidan M, Evers AS, Olney JW, et al. Potential of xenon to induce or to protect against neuroapoptosis in the developing mouse brain. *Can J Anaesth.* 2008;55:429–36.

51. Ma D, Williamson P, Januszewski A, Nogaro MC, Hossain M, Ong LP, et al. Xenon mitigates isoflurane-induced neuronal apoptosis in the developing rodent brain. *Anesthesiology.* 2007;106:746–53.

52. Shu Y, Patel SM, Pac-Soo C, Fidalgo AR, Wan Y, Maze M, et al. Xenon pretreatment attenuates anesthetic-induced apoptosis in the developing brain in comparison with nitrous oxide and hypoxia. *Anesthesiology.* 2010;113:360–8.

53. Liu F, Rainosek SW, Sadovova N, Fogle CM, Patterson TA, Hanig JP, et al. Protective effect of acetyl-L-carnitine on propofol-induced toxicity in embryonic neural stem cells. *Neurotoxicology.* 2014;42:49–57.

54. Zou X, Sadovova N, Patterson TA, Divine RL, Hotchkiss CE, Ali SF, et al. The effects of L-carnitine on the combination of, inhalation anesthetic-induced developmental, neuronal apoptosis in the rat frontal cortex. *Neuroscience.* 2008;151:1053–65.

55. Straiko MM, Young C, Cattano D, Creeley CE, Wang H, Smith DJ, et al. Lithium protects against anesthesia-induced developmental neuroapoptosis. *Anesthesiology.* 2009;110:862–8.

56. Eberspacher E, Werner C, Engelhard K, Pape M, Gelb A, Hutzler P, et al. The effect of hypothermia on the expression of the apoptosis-regulating protein Bax after incomplete cerebral ischemia and reperfusion in rats. *J Neurosurg Anesthesiol.* 2003;15:200–8.

57. Mason KP, Zgleszewski S, Forman RE, Stark C, DiNardo JA. An exaggerated hypertensive response to glycopyrrolate therapy for bradycardia associated with high-dose dexmedetomidine. *Anesth Analg.* 2009;108:906–8.

58. Johnson ME, Uhl CB, Spittler KH, Wang H, Gores GJ. Mitochondrial injury and caspase activation by the local anesthetic lidocaine. *Anesthesiology.* 2004;101:1184–94.

59. Werdehausen R, Fazeli S, Braun S, Hermanns H, Essmann F, Hollmann MW, et al. Apoptosis induction by different local anaesthetics in a neuroblastoma cell line. *Br J Anaesth.* 2009;103:711–18.

60. Loepke AW, McCann JC, Kurth CD, McAuliffe JJ. The physiologic effects of isoflurane anesthesia in neonatal mice. *Anesth Analg.* 2006;102:75–80.

61. Brooker RW, Keenan WJ. Inguinal hernia: relationship to respiratory disease in prematurity. *J Pediatr Surg.* 2006;41:1818–21.

62. Stolwijk LJ, Lemmers PM, Harmsen M, Groenendaal F, de Vries LS, van der Zee DC, et al. Neurodevelopmental outcomes after neonatal surgery for major noncardiac anomalies. *Pediatrics.* 2016;137:e20151728.

63. Davidson AJ, Disma N, de Graaff JC, Withington DE, Dorris L, Bell G, et al. Neurodevelopmental outcome at 2 years of age after general anaesthesia and awake-regional anaesthesia in infancy (GAS): an international multicentre, randomised controlled trial. *Lancet.* 2016;387:239–50.

64. Eishima K. The effects of obstetric conditions on neonatal behaviour in Japanese infants. *Early Hum Dev.* 1992;28:253–63.

65. Sprung J, Flick RP, Wilder RT, Katusic SK, Pike TL, Dingli M, et al. Anesthesia for cesarean delivery and learning disabilities in a population-based birth cohort. *Anesthesiology.* 2009;111:302–10.

66. Flick RP, Lee K, Hofer RE, Hambel EM, Klein MK, Gunn PW, et al. Neuraxial labor analgesia for vaginal delivery and its effects on childhood learning disabilities. *Anesth Analg.* 2011;112:1424–31.

67. Victorian Infant Collaborative Study Group. Surgery and the tiny baby: sensorineural outcome at 5 years of age. *J Paediatr Child Health.* 1996;32:167–72.

68. Blakely ML, Tyson JE, Lally KP, McDonald S, Stoll BJ, Stevenson DK, et al. Laparotomy versus peritoneal drainage for necrotizing enterocolitis or isolated intestinal perforation in extremely low birth weight infants: outcomes through 18 months adjusted age. *Pediatrics.* 2006;117:e680–7.

69. Hintz SR, Kendrick DE, Stoll BJ, Vohr BR, Fanaroff AA, Donovan EF, et al. Neurodevelopmental and growth outcomes of extremely low birth weight infants after necrotizing enterocolitis. *Pediatrics.* 2005;115:696–703.

70. Walsh MC, Kliegman RM, Hack M. Severity of necrotizing enterocolitis: influence on outcome at 2 years of age. *Pediatrics*. 1989;**84**:808–14.

71. Tobiansky R, Lui K, Roberts S, Veddovi M. Neurodevelopmental outcome in very low birthweight infants with necrotizing enterocolitis requiring surgery. *J Paediatr Child Health*. 1995;**31**:233–6.

72. Lindahl H. Long-term prognosis of successfully operated oesophageal atresia—with aspects on physical and psychological development. *Z Kinderchir*. 1984;**39**:6–10.

73. Bouman NH, Koot HM, Hazebroek FW. Long-term physical, psychological, and social functioning of children with esophageal atresia. *J Pediatr Surg*. 1999;**34**:399–404.

74. Bellinger DC, Rappaport LA, Wypij D, Wernovsky G, Newburger JW. Patterns of developmental dysfunction after surgery during infancy to correct transposition of the great arteries. *J Dev Behav Pediatr*. 1997;**18**:75–83.

75. Bellinger DC, Wypij D, duPlessis AJ, Rappaport LA, Jonas RA, Wernovsky G, et al. Neurodevelopmental status at eight years in children with dextro-transposition of the great arteries: the Boston Circulatory Arrest Trial. *J Thorac Cardiovasc Surg*. 2003;**126**:1385–96.

76. Bellinger DC, Wypij D, Kuban KC, Rappaport LA, Hickey PR, Wernovsky G, et al. Developmental and neurological status of children at 4 years of age after heart surgery with hypothermic circulatory arrest or low-flow cardiopulmonary bypass. *Circulation*. 1999;**100**:526–32.

77. Hovels-Gurich HH, Seghaye MC, Dabritz S, Messmer BJ, von Bernuth G. Cognitive and motor development in preschool and school-aged children after neonatal arterial switch operation. *J Thorac Cardiovasc Surg*. 1997;**114**:578–85.

78. Miller SP, McQuillen PS, Hamrick S, Glidden DV, Charlton N, Karl T, et al. Abnormal brain development in newborns with congenital heart disease. *N Engl J Med*. 2007;**357**:1928–38.

79. DiMaggio CJSL, Kakavouli A, Li G. A retrospective cohort study of the association of anesthesia and hernia repair surgery with behavioral and developmental disorders in young children. *J Neurosurg Anesthesiol*. 2009;**21**(4):286–91.

80. Kalkman CJ, Peelen L, Moons KG, Veenhuizen M, Bruens M, Sinnema G, et al. Behavior and development in children and age at the time of first anesthetic exposure. *Anesthesiology*. 2009;**110**:805–12.

81. Dimaggio C, Sun L, Li G. Early childhood exposure to anesthesia and risk of developmental and behavioral disorders in a sibling birth cohort. *Anesth Analg*. 2011;**113**(5):1143–51.

82. Ing C, Sun M, Olfson M, DiMaggio CJ, Sun LS, Wall MM, et al. Age at exposure to surgery and anesthesia in children and association with mental disorder diagnosis. *Anesth Analg*. 2017;**125**:1988–98.

83. Backeljauw B, Holland SK, Altaye M, Loepke AW. Cognition and brain structure following early childhood surgery with anesthesia. *Pediatrics*. 2015;**136**:e1–12.

84. O'Leary JD, Janus M, Duku E, Wijeysundera DN, To T, Li P, et al. A population-based study evaluating the association between surgery in early life and child development at primary school entry. *Anesthesiology*. 2016;**125**:272–9.

85. Graham MR, Brownell M, Chateau DG, Dragan RD, Burchill C, Fransoo RR. Neurodevelopmental assessment in kindergarten in children exposed to general anesthesia before the age of 4 years: a retrospective matched cohort study. *Anesthesiology*. 2016;**125**:667–77.

86. Glatz P, Sandin RH, Pedersen NL, Bonamy AK, Eriksson LI, Granath F. Association of anesthesia and surgery during childhood with long-term academic performance. *JAMA Pediatr*. 2017;**171**: e163470.

87. Whitton JP, Polley DB. Evaluating the perceptual and pathophysiological consequences of auditory deprivation in early postnatal life: a comparison of basic and clinical studies. *J Assoc Res Otolaryngol*. 2011;**12**:535–47.

88. Hansen TG, Pedersen JK, Henneberg SW, Pedersen DA, Murray JC, Morton NS, et al. Academic performance in adolescence after inguinal hernia repair in infancy: a nationwide cohort study. *Anesthesiology*. 2011;**114**(5):1076–85.

89. Bartels M, Althoff RR, Boomsma DI. Anesthesia and cognitive performance in children: no evidence for a causal relationship. *Twin Res Hum Genet*. 2009;**12**:246–53.

90. Davidson AJ, Disma N, de Graaff JC, Withington DE, Dorris L, Bell G, et al. Neurodevelopmental outcome at 2 years of age after general anaesthesia and awake-regional anaesthesia in infancy (GAS): an international multicentre, randomised controlled trial. *Lancet*. 2016;**387**:239–50.

91. Sun LS, Li G, Miller TL, Salorio C, Byrne MW, Bellinger DC, et al. Association between a single general anesthesia exposure before age 36 months and neurocognitive outcomes in later childhood. *JAMA*. 2016;**315**:2312–20.

92. Rappaport B, Mellon RD, Simone A, Woodcock J. Defining safe use of anesthesia in children. *N Engl J Med*. 2011;**364**:1387–90.

93. Rappaport BA, Suresh S, Hertz S, Evers AS, Orser BA. Anesthetic neurotoxicity—clinical implications of animal models. *N Engl J Med*. 2015;**372**:796–7.

94. US Food and Drug Administration. FDA Drug Safety Communication: FDA approves label changes for use of general anesthetic and sedation drugs in young children. 2017. Available at www.fda.gov/Drugs/Drug Safety/ucm554634.htm.

95. van der Griend BF, Lister NA, McKenzie IM, Martin N, Ragg PG, Sheppard SJ, et al. Postoperative mortality in children after 101,885 anesthetics at a tertiary pediatric hospital. *Anesth Analg*. 2011;**112**:1440–7.

Chapter 20

Perioperative Salt and Water in Pediatric Neurocritical Care

Robert C. Tasker and Frederick Vonberg

Introduction

The overall goal of perioperative care is to prepare the patient for the right surgery, at the right time, under the right circumstances of physiology, all with the best expected outcomes for the child's underlying condition. The prescription of intravenous fluids for children unable to tolerate oral therapy is fundamental in this perioperative period. What we want to know is how much and what type of fluid should we give.

The main aims of this chapter are to cover the essentials of perioperative fluid therapy, the pitfalls in measuring and following electrolyte levels, and the approach to postoperative dysnatremia. We want a patient who is, first, hemodynamically stable, second, receiving intravenous fluids that limits or avoids electrolyte abnormalities, and, third, adequately supplied with glucose for metabolic homeostasis. The first aim requires careful maintenance of intravascular volume. Preoperative fluid restriction may lead to blood pressure instability and even cardiovascular collapse intraoperatively, with problems carrying over into the postoperative phase. Preoperative hyperhydration may lead to abnormalities in salt balance that also carry over into the postoperative period. It is therefore important to know what has happened preoperatively and intraoperatively: the type and volume of fluid given, the estimated blood loss as a proportion of blood volume, as well as fluid inputs and outputs.

Preoperative Intravenous Normal Saline and the Threat to Homeostasis

In common hospital preoperative care, normal saline (NS) is the preferred intravenous fluid for neurosurgery cases since its osmolarity (308 mOsm/L) should minimize the occurrence of hyponatremia (serum sodium concentration $[Na^+] < 135$ mmol/L). In children, we calculate the maintenance fluid required for a child scaled to their weight using the classic Holliday and Segar[1] formula for daily fluids:

100 mL/kg for the first 10 kg in body weight; add 50 mL/kg to the 1,000 mL for the next 10 kg in body weight (i.e., weight 10 to 20 kg); add 20 mL/kg to the 1,500 mL for weight above 20 kg.

The above calculations should be placed in the context of recommended salt (NaCl) intake per day in healthy children. Normal 4- to 8-year-olds require 1.2 g/day (20 mmol/day), but observational studies show that the actual upper limit of intake is ~2.6 g/day (44 mmol/day). Now consider a 20 kg, 6-year-old boy who is placed on 1.5 times fluid maintenance therapy using NS, during the day before surgery, so as to ensure that intravascular volume is optimized for a cerebrovascular procedure. The NaCl intake from NS over 24 hours in this child is 20.2 g/day. Hence, we have taken a child with healthy kidneys and neuroendocrine physiology from a baseline NaCl intake of 2.6 g/day and increased it to 20.2 g/day—an increase from 1 teaspoon to 9 teaspoons of salt per day!

Such an abrupt intervention with preoperative intravenous fluids does result in an expanded arterial volume, which is what was wanted in preparation for surgery, but a foundation has been laid for a subsequent threat to homeostasis. In the proximal tubule, the luminal Na^+ transport system and the basolateral Na^+ pump are removed from membranes of individual proximal tubular cells, so that there is reduced ability to reabsorb filtered Na^+ ions. Of course, the body is aiming to excrete the excess NaCl load. If, however, there is any decrease in the rate of infusion of NS, then the patient will continue to excrete Na^+ because of so-called secondary renal wasting. The potential risk is illustrated by studies in the 1950s to 1990s in healthy adults that looked at transitioning from low to high NaCl intake (0.6 g/day to 20.5 g/day), and the reverse. A change to a high intake leads to a new steady state with high antidiuretic hormone (ADH), low renin, and low aldosterone, which lag behind the acute change in intake by 24–48 hours. When this new steady state of homeostasis is achieved, excess NaCl intake is balanced by increased renal wasting such that serum [Na$^+$] remains stable. Hence, the risk for our patient is that of excess Na$^+$ loss and hyponatremia in the 48 hours after any abrupt decrease in NaCl intake to maintenance levels.

The illustration shows an extreme example with use of 1.5 times maintenance in a preoperative child. When we care for perioperative neurosurgical patients we also need to add to this discussion the intravenous fluids used in the operating room. How long did the procedure take, and how much maintenance fluid was given? It is not unusual for long procedures to necessitate maintenance fluid up to 10 mL/kg/hr. Were any saline boluses given? When more than 60 mL/kg has been used, there is the risk of hyperchloremic metabolic acidosis, which may not be appreciated unless serum chloride concentration ([Cl$^-$]) was measured.

Variations in Sodium and Chloride Measurements

The [Na$^+$] in serum or plasma is quantified by using ion-specific electrode (ISE) technology to measure the activity of Na$^+$ ions in the aqueous (water) phase of plasma. There are two methods that are used for providing clinicians with [Na$^+$] and [Cl$^-$] values: indirect and direct ISE. Indirect ISE technology is used in central laboratory analyzers, and involves presentation of a prediluted serum or plasma sample to the measuring electrode. The measurement assumes that the water content of plasma is constant at 93%. If lipids and/or protein are raised, then the nonwater fraction is >7%, and the diluted sample presented to the ISE contains fewer Na$^+$ ions than would be the case if the sample had a normal proportion of water (93%), i.e., pseudohyponatremia. By similar thinking, if lipid and/or protein are reduced (or diluted by hyperhydration), then the nonwater fraction is <7% and the water fraction is >93%, resulting in falsely high [Na$^+$], i.e., pseudohypernatremia. Direct ISE technology is used in blood gas and other point-of-care analyzers, and requires the presentation of an undiluted sample of whole blood to the measuring electrode. Direct ISE measurements are not affected by changes in lipid and protein concentration because there is no predilution of the sample. What is being reported is the actual [Na$^+$]. Having identified the methods for measuring [Na$^+$] in a particular patient—most likely using indirect ICE technology in the pre- and postoperative periods, and direct ICE technology intraoperatively—the clinician

should consider two issues: (1) the use of population-based reference (normal) intervals in detecting abnormal changes and (2) the significance of changes in consecutive results from an individual.

First, the values of the *reference interval* (RI) are generated and established by your hospital's credentialed laboratory. Sometimes the RI data are stratified according to age and sex. In order to assess how clinicians should interpret changes in measured values, i.e., using the population-based RI versus using the serial values, we need to consider biological variation. The within-person or individual coefficient of variation (CV$_I$) and the between-person coefficient of variation (CV$_G$) for [Na$^+$] are 1% and 1.8%, respectively, and for [Cl$^-$] 1.6% and 2.8%, respectively.[2] The index of individuality is calculated as the ratio of CV$_I$/CV$_G$. A high index (≥ 1.0, or >1.4 for maximum sensitivity) suggests that the population-based RI is appropriate when interpreting an individual's laboratory analyte value. In contrast, a low index (≤ 1.0, or ≤ 0.60 for maximum sensitivity) indicates that under normal circumstances individual results stay within a narrow range compared with the population-based RI. Hence, a low index would suggest that in an individual there is utility in following serial changes in analyte values, and population-based RI would be of limited usefulness.[3,4] Both [Na$^+$] and [Cl$^-$] measurements have a low index of individuality—0.55 and 0.57, respectively.

In view of the above, the second issue of clinical significance of changes in consecutive results from an individual must be considered. The critical significant changes between two results is called the *reference change value* (RCV) and is determined in healthy individuals by the following formula:

$$RCV = k \times \sqrt{2} \times \sqrt{CV_A^2 \times CV_I^2}$$

In this formula CV$_A$ is the laboratory analytical coefficient of variation, and for both [Na$^+$] and [Cl$^-$] it is 0.8%.[2] The value of the constant k is 1.65 for a 1-tailed test and a probability risk α of 95%; k = 1.96 for a 2-tailed test. For example, this formula applied to an analyte result in real time at, say, [Na$^+$] 140 mmol/L gives RCV = 3.5%. This translates into an RCV of 135.3–144.7 mmol/L: a difference in two measurements of [Na$^+$], when starting at a concentration of 140 mmol/L, as large as the upper boundary minus the lower boundary of the 95% confidence interval (CI) could occur at random. If the starting point was

135 mmol/L the 95% CI is 130.3–139.7 mmol/L. When we consider a baseline $[Cl^-]$ 100 mmol/L the RCV is 5% and the 95% CI is 95–105 mmol/L. In clinical practice we are more often concerned with the 1-tailed test; e.g., have we had a significant rise or improvement in $[Na^+]$ from a hyponatremic value of 120 mmol/L since a particular intervention? Based on the above data, with $k = 1.65$, the increase in value in the correction of hyponatremia would have to be to ≥123 mmol/L to be certain of a real change.

Postoperative Dysnatremia

Disorders of Na^+ and water homeostasis are common in postoperative neurosurgical patients. Four main Na^+- and water-handling problems occur, including inappropriate intravenous fluid administration, euvolemic state of ADH excess (i.e., syndrome of ADH excess, SIADH), cerebral salt wasting (CSW), and diabetes insipidus (DI). However, before embarking on detailed analyses of Na^+ and water balance, when an abnormal serum $[Na^+]$ is received from the laboratory, we first need to consider the issues discussed in the first part of this chapter, i.e., the physiological context or priming that has occurred in the pre- and intraoperative periods, and the validity of the measurements themselves. For example, has there been significant use of perioperative radiologic nonionic hyperosmolar contrast medium, which will cause pseudohyponatremia if the measurements come from indirect ICE technology (often reported as "extracellular fluid" $[Na^+]$ rather than "whole blood" $[Na^+]$)? Then, as part of the evaluation, there should be some assessment of cerebrospinal fluid losses (CSF)—for example via CSF drainage.

In the postoperative patient there is a significant risk of hospital-acquired hyponatremia, which approaches 30%.[5] In the pediatric neurosurgical literature there are three recent reports describing the significant scale and impact of this problem.[6–8] In this setting postoperative pain, stress, nausea, vomiting, narcotics, and volume depletion all have the potential to stimulate vasopressin production and induce a state of euvolemic hyponatremia not dissimilar to SIADH—in fact ADH secretion may well be an appropriate survival response. To date, there have been three prospective trials of intravenous fluids in postoperative patients (not specifically neurosurgical patients): two studies in the pediatric intensive care unit,[9,10] and one study in the postoperative ward.[11] Unfortunately, the endpoints in these studies differed

in respect to what and when: either an absolute change in serum $[Na^+]$,[9] or proportion of cases with hyponatremia defined as below 135 mmol/L[9] or below 130 mmol/L;[11] and measurements at 8,[11] 12,[11] or 24 hours.[9–11] (There has also been a recent randomized clinical trial in nonsurgical pediatric patients,[12] and since the findings do not differ from the results in postoperative patients we do not focus on these data.) The general message from the postoperative studies is that isotonic fluids (i.e., NS) prevent postoperative falls in serum $[Na^+]$ and that hypotonic fluids result in falls in $[Na^+]$. In none of the postoperative studies was fluid overload or significant hypernatrema a complication.[9–11] We do not know the current epidemiology of perioperative pediatric neurosurgical intravenous fluid management, but a survey in 2006 of practice in general pediatric surgeons and anesthesiologists using infant and child clinical scenarios showed that significant numbers of clinicians were using hypotonic fluids or fluid restriction.[13] The 2007 Association of Paediatric Anaesthetists of Great Britain and Ireland guideline on perioperative fluid management in children[14] identified the following two gaps in knowledge for postoperative intravenous fluid management:

1. "Consensus was not agreed on what the ideal fluid for postoperative maintenance is. Many felt that Ringer lactate/Hartmann's solution with added dextrose was the most appropriate, but currently this formulation does not exist in the UK. 0.9% sodium chloride with 5% dextrose is the only available isotonic fluid containing dextrose within the UK at present."

2. "Consensus was not agreed on the maintenance fluid rate in the postoperative period. Some would use the full rate as calculated using Holliday and Segar's formula, while others would restrict to 60–70% of full maintenance and additional boluses of isotonic fluid given as required."

Modeling the Effect of Too Much Water versus Too Much Salt

The debate about volume and type of intravenous fluids arises because it is not clear what is maintenance requirement for the postoperative child. We have all seen the edematous child who has received too much free water, or who has received too much Na^+? What is worse?

Figure 20.1 illustrates the arguments for and against volume and concentration by modeling Na^+ and water handling.[15,16] Figure 20.1A shows responses in extracellular (V_e) and intracellular (V_i) volumes in a closed system with two compartments separated by a membrane that permits the movement of water, but is impermeable to Na^+ and potassium (K^+), which are the sole V_e and V_i cations. If the V_i component of the model functions as a perfect osmometer, then the sloping lines represent isopleths, lines of constant overall volume ($V_e + V_i$). The numbers have been normalized to body water, with loss or gain in a percentage for each compartment, relative to the origin (point O), which is steady-state euvolemia. The two vectors represent an accumulated positive balance in the system, either 20 mL/kg of water (vector OW) or 20 mL/kg of

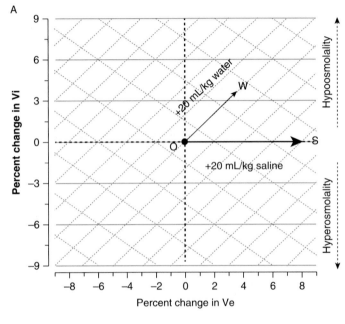

Figure 20.1. (A) Model of fluid shifts due to 20 mL/kg intravenous water or NS (N, saline). (B) Model of fluid shifts due to different tonicities of NS (0.18%, N/5; 0.45%, N/2; and 0.9%, N) and different volumes (i.e., full or two-thirds maintenance).

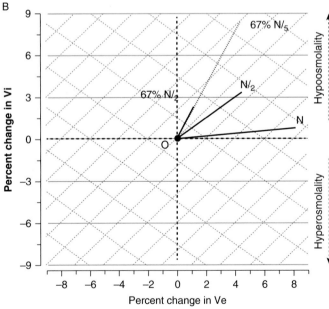

NS (vector OS). In this model, which is applicable between 10 and 30 kg body weight, the effect of gaining 20 mL/kg of saline is an 8% increase in V_e, without any change in V_i or serum osmolarity. The effect of gaining 20 mL/kg of water is an expansion in both V_e and V_i, each by over 3% with an associated fall in serum osmolarity. (The vector SW represents a desalination of 1.5 mmol/kg, and any movement along this same axis above horizontal can be considered as net loss of Na^+ from a particular initial condition.)

The homeostatic challenges are different for the two conditions OW and OS. In the case of gain in NS, the theoretical system must deal with the acute NaCl load, the change in interstitial compliance as V_e increases, and resulting edema. These issues are not trivial. For example, in healthy adults, in the supine position, it takes 2 days to regulate the amount of salt and water provided by an acute saline infusion.[17,18] Experimentally, generalized edema will accelerate after ~15% expansion in V_e, although this response will be different in different tissues as well as being influenced by plasma colloid osmotic pressure.[19–21] In the case of gain in water, the main difference to gain in NS is that the system must defend changes in V_i induced by the hypoosmolality. Is this threat real for the range of values typically seen in postoperative neurosurgical children on maintenance intravenous fluids? In other words, which tissues function as perfect osmometers, like the model?

Experimental studies show that skeletal muscle, which contains the bulk of an organism's water and K^+, is important as a buffer during acute hyponatremia since it serves as a near-perfect osmometer.[22,23] In contrast, within the brain, increases in water content are less than expected, but there are regional differences.[24,25] For example, during acute hyponatremia ([Na^+] reduced from 138 ± 1 to 123 ± 2 mmol/L) the water content of the whole brain and white matter increases, but it is less than expected for perfect osmotic behavior, whereas in the thalamus, water content increases as expected for a perfect osmometer.[23] These data provide the experimental context for interpreting the significance of change in electrolytes summarized in the previous section. It is true that symptomatic hyponatremia with encephalopathy in previously well children has the potential for high neurologic morbidity.[25,26] How likely is this complication in the first 24 hours after an operation and admission to the intensive care unit?

Figure 20.1B uses similar principles to those in Figure 20.1A but, in addition, the model takes account of mass balance for Na^+ and K^+, where the input comes from intravenous fluid and the output in water and electrolytes is considered as solely via urine.[27] The three prospective studies of postoperative and intensive care children provide information about urine tonicity and volume.[9–11] Maintenance fluids were calculated using the Holliday and Segar equation[1] in all three studies. Urine tonicity across the studies is almost fixed: in those receiving NS at full maintenance urine tonicity is ~200 mOsm/L; in those receiving any other prescription urine tonicity is lower, ~160 mOsm/L. Only one study reports urine output,[11] and it appears that irrespective of fluid prescribed mean output over 12 to 24 was ~1.2 mL/kg/hr. These data have been used to generate the four vectors for the 12-hour cumulative fluid and tonicity balance in Figure 20.1B. Starting from the origin (point O), the greatest increase in V_e is seen with full maintenance NS. The likelihood of increased V_i and hypoosmolarity is in the following order: NS, two-thirds restricted half-NS (67% N/2), full maintenance half-NS (100% N/2), and two-thirds one-fifth-NS (67% N/5). The severe derangement occurring with 67% N/5 is nearly three times the theoretical expansion of V_e and hypoosmolality occurring during the other prescriptions. The problem of hypernatremia is not seen in the model, but more complexity in the volume relationships can be added with other variables common in postoperative neurosurgical children, e.g., the sequestration of extracellular water within injured tissues necessitating NS replacement, neuroendocrine stress physiology, and consideration of gains, losses, and urinary desalination.[28–31]

Postoperative Renal Na^+- and Water Handling

The three main renal Na^+- and water-handling problems that occur in such children are euvolemic states of ADH excess (i.e., SIADH), CSW, and DI. Therefore, regular monitoring of intravascular volume, urine output and tonicity, and serum electrolytes is needed during the period of administering intravenous fluids.

Syndrome of Inappropriate ADH Secretion

The risk of postoperative hyponatremia is a major concern since it may go unrecognized until the onset

Table 20.1 Approach to the Diagnosis of Cerebral Salt Wasting in a Patient Who Has a Cerebral Lesion is One of Exclusion; There Must be Excretion of Na^+ and Cl^- Without an Obvious Cause

1. Screening approach to identify potential patients:
   - Hyponatremia with $[Na^+] < 135$ mmol/L
   - Brisk diuresis > 3 mL/kg/hr
   - Elevated urine $[Na^+] > 120$ mmol/L
   - Elevated urine osmolarity > 300 mOsm/L

2. Rule out:
   - A physiologic cause for the excretion of Na^+ and Cl^-:
     An expanded extracellular fluid (ECF) volume from hyperhydration (see text)
     Dietary Na^+ intake >2 mmol/kg/day
     High volumes of isotonic saline (1.5 times maintenance) followed by abrupt decreases in intake (see text)
   - A noncerebral (renal) cause for natriuresis:
     Lack of aldosterone (a stimulator of reabsorption of Na^+)
     Presence of an inhibitor of renal reabsorption of Na^+ such as osmotic agents, high concentration of ligand for calcium-sensing receptor (hyperglycemia, aminoglycoside)
     Renal tubular damage: interstitial nephritis, acute tubular necrosis, obstructive uropathy
     Diuretics
     Adrenocortical insufficiency
     Congenital salt-losing renal tubular disorders: Bartter or Gitelman syndrome
   - Obligatory excretion of Na^+ by the excretion of anions other than Cl^-
   - High-output renal failure
   - Sodium wasting from CSF drainage

3. Possible explanations for salt wasting:
   - Natriuretic agents of cerebral origin
   - Downregulation of renal Na^+ transport by chronic ECF volume expansion
   - Pressure natriuresis from adrenergic agents
   - Suppression of the release of aldosterone

of a seizure.[32] If the cause is perioperative SIADH, and not inadequate NaCl prescription, it has occurred because of free water retention followed at the same time as natriuresis that maintains fluid balance at the expense of serum osmolarity. Because of this risk, many clinicians avoid hypotonic solutions altogether in the perioperative period. It should be noted that Ringer lactate Na^+ content (130 mmol/L) might result in a fall in serum $[Na^+]$. This fluid is often used intraoperatively as it is a balanced solution with a physiologic amount of base, calcium, and K^+, and will limit the hyperchloremic acidosis that occurs with large volumes of Na.

The treatment of SIADH is to reduce free water excess by fluid restriction and diuretics. If a hyponatremic seizure occurs, then 3% hypertonic saline (3%HTS) should be used to correct serum $[Na^+]$; the level to be targeted is that at which the seizure comes under control, often ~130 mmol/L.

Taking 0.6 L/kg body weight as the apparent volume of distribution for Na^+, one should anticipate an immediate increase of 3 to 5 mmol/L in serum sodium concentration with a rapid intravenous bolus of 4 to 6 mL/kg body weight of 3%HTS.[33]

Cerebral Salt Wasting

CSW is a diagnosis of exclusion based on clinical criteria. It appears to be common in children after all types of neurosurgical procedures[6–8,34–36] and it results from excessively high atrial or brain natriuretic peptide levels.[37] The essential features are renal Na^+ and Cl^- wasting in a patient with a *contracted effective arterial blood volume*, where other causes of excess Na^+ excretion have been excluded. Volume contraction is likely to be present when there is a deficit of Na^+ that exceeds 2 mmol/kg.[38] Hyponatremia is a nonspecific clue.

Table 20.1 lists some of the diagnoses that should be excluded before concluding that the patient has CSW. It should be noted that atrial natriuretic peptide level is high in the patient who has been managed with hypervolemic fluid management. In this instance, natriuresis as a response to volume control is part of homeostasis, and not CSW (see initial section on "threat to homeostasis").

As CSW has become more generally recognized as a condition, the syndrome has been diagnosed with increasing frequency. The incidence is apparently of the order of 1–5% of neurosurgical procedures, and it has been reported in association with calvarial remodeling, tumor resection, and hydrocephalus.[6–8,34–36] Hardesty and colleagues[36] reported a 5-year review of postoperative pediatric brain tumor patients they managed. CSW was defined retrospectively as one laboratory measurement of hyponatremia (<135 mmol/L) with brisk diuresis (>3 mL/kg/hr) and elevated urine sodium (>120 mmol/L), when available, or elevated urinary osmolality (>300 mOsm/kg water). The authors did not have any assessment of volume status (see above), but all patients in their institution were treated with NS intra- and postoperatively. However, they found that 5% of all pediatric tumor patients undergoing craniotomy in their center developed CSW, which was more frequently observed than SIADH (3%). The median onset of CSW was on postoperative day 3, lasting a median of 2.5 days. Patients with CSW were more likely to have suffered postoperative stroke, have chiasmatic or hypothalamic tumors, and be younger than patients with normal postoperative sodium concentration. Almost half of the patients with CSW had postoperative hyponatremic seizures (serum [Na$^+$] range 118 to 128 mmol/L). The treatment of CSW involves Na$^+$ administration to match urinary losses and correction of intravascular volume contraction. In some instances, more rapid resolution of hyponatremia after volume expansion has been achieved with fludocortisone.[39]

Diabetes Insipidus

DI results from a deficiency of vasopressin, and it is an expected complication of surgical procedures near the pituitary or hypothalamus. It is most frequently seen in association with craniopharyngioma, where it can be a presenting symptom in 40% of cases.[40] In most patients DI is transient, but approximately 6% develop permanent DI.[41,42] The diagnosis should be suspected when serum sodium rises above 145 mmol/L in association with urine output above 2.5 mL/kg/hr for three consecutive hours, or more than 4 mL/kg/hr in any one hour. The urine osmolarity should be hypotonic (<300 mOsm/L) in the face of increased plasma osmolarity (>300 mOsm/L), in the absence of glycosuria, mannitol use, and renal failure. An important consequence of this condition is severe dehydration and hypovolemia since urine output is driven by lack of vasopressin.

Knowledge of the several patterns of DI that can occur following surgery in the hypothalamic-pituitary area is important. The most common is that associated with local edema as a result of traction or manipulation of the pituitary stalk. This lesion usually results in transient polyuria that begins 2 to 6 hours after surgery and resolves as edema diminishes in 1 to 7 days.[43,44] A "triphasic pattern" has also been described.[41] The initial phase is associated with polyuria in the first postoperative days.[45,46] The second phase is the resumption of normal urinary output or SIADH, probably resulting from the release of previously stored ADH from damaged neurons. Ultimately, transection of the pituitary stalk or destruction of the hypothalamic median eminence will result in permanent DI.[46,47] Frequently, permanent DI, either partial or complete, develops without interphase changes.[43,45]

There are a variety of successful approaches to treating DI. It is useful to have a neuroendocrine assessment preoperatively, with a perioperative care plan, since deficiencies of thyroid and/or adrenocortical hormones can coexist. In the child with known DI, preoperatively, some endocrinologists prefer not to replace vasopressin and to limit total fluid intake to approximately twice-normal maintenance (scaling to body surface area rather than weight, i.e., 3 L/m^2/day), recognizing that this can result in mild hypernatremia and thirst but minimizing the more dangerous risk of water intoxication with vasopressin administration. Others prefer to withhold long-acting desmopressin (DDAVP) in the perioperative period and instead manage DI with intermittent injections of intramuscular vasopressin.[48] Administration of excessive fluids in this setting, as with the perioperative maintenance of DDAVP, can result in hyponatremic seizures.[36,49,50]

Typically, postoperative DI develops 2 to 12 hours after surgery (average, 6 hours following completion of surgery). When DI is recognized, the strategy below should lead to serum [Na$^+$] between 130 and 150 mmol/L. In such patients, new-onset postoperative DI responds to an infusion of aqueous vasopressin (15 units/500 mL). Aqueous vasopressin is used because of its rapid onset of action and brief duration of effect.[51] However, its potential vascular effects (i.e., hypertension) means that close observation in a monitored setting is required. The infusion is started at 0.5 mUnits/kg/hr and titrated upward in 0.5 mUnits/kg/hr increments every 5 to 10 minutes until urine output decreases to <2 mL/kg/hr. The maximum rate should be limited to 10 mUnits/kg/hr.[52] Once a urine output of <2 mL/kg/hr is achieved, the vasopressin infusion is not adjusted downward. Neither is fluid administration adjusted according to urine output. Antidiuresis with vasopressin is essentially an "all-or-none" phenomenon and the aqueous infusion is being used to produce a "functional SIADH" state.[44] This strategy recognizes that renal blood flow remains normal in the normovolemic, but maximally antidiuresed, child. Because urine output is minimal (0.5 mL/kg/hr), other clinical markers of volume status must be followed closely. For example, anuria together with increased heart rate or decreased blood pressure may be evidence of hypovolemia. Vasopressin infusion does not induce acute tubular necrosis, and severe oliguria or anuria is an indication for additional fluid and not for decreasing or discontinuing the infusion. A major caveat when using vasopressin infusion is that management necessitates careful fluid restriction, keeping the total amount of intravenous fluids to two-thirds maintenance. In the presence of full antidiuresis, excessive fluids (oral or intravenous) can lead to intravascular volume overload. In addition, administration of hypotonic fluids (oral or intravenous) can result in dangerous hyponatremia. Again, this complication can be prevented by fluid restriction limited to replacing insensible losses, which is generally considered to be about two-thirds usual maintenance rates.[53]

In children at risk of developing permanent DI, in whom adequate oral intake has been established, intravenous fluids and the vasopressin infusion can be discontinued while permitting free oral intake. Subsequent treatment of DI is withheld until the child demonstrates polyuria. At this time, treatment with DDAVP rather than restarting a vasopressin infusion is recommended. DDAVP is a synthetic vasopressin with duration of action of 12 to 24 hours. It is usually administered intranasally at a dose of 5 to 10 microgram. Oral DDAVP can be used at 10 to 20 times the nasal dose. Antidiuresis generally begins within 1 hour. In children with nasal packing (e.g., transsphenoidal surgery) oral DDAVP is used. In children with known DI, DDAVP treatment can be resumed once an intact thirst mechanism has returned and oral intake without vomiting.

Glucose or No Glucose in Perioperative Intravenous Fluids

Pediatric patients, particularly infants, are at particular risk for perioperative hypoglycemia. Infants, with limited reserves of glycogen and limited gluconeogenesis, require continuous infusions of glucose at 5–6 mg/kg/min in order to maintain serum levels. At the same time, the stress of critical illness and resulting insulin resistance can produce hyperglycemia that, in turn, is associated with neurologic injury and poor outcomes in adults. Hyperglycemia has been linked to poor outcome and it may worsen ischemia, but it remains unclear that the opposite—tight glycemic control—offers significant benefits to children. It is prudent to follow a conservative approach that maintains random serum glucose level in the normal range, below 180 mg/dL. Intraoperatively, the stress response is generally able to maintain normal serum glucose levels without exogenous glucose administration. However, in postoperative infants and small children, particularly if there has been an effective fast of 6 to 12 hours, it is advisable to use glucose-containing fluids to meet baseline demands. NS in 2.5% to 5% dextrose should suffice. In general, older children and adolescents can tolerate 18 to 24 hours of fasting.

References

1. Holliday MA, Segar WE. The maintenance need for water in parenteral fluid therapy. *Pediatrics*. 1957;**19**: 823–32.

2. Larcher DA, Hughes JP, Carroll MD. Biological variation of laboratory analytes based on the 1999–2002 National Health and Nutrition Examination Survey. National Health Statistics Reports no. 21. Hyattsville, MD: National Center for Health Statistics; 2010.

3. Fraser GG. Inherent biological variation and reference values. *Clin Chem Lab Med*. 2004;**42**:758–64.

4. Harris EK. Effects of intra- and interindividual variation on the appropriate use of normal intervals. *Clin Chem*. 1974;**20**:1535–42.

5. Moritz ML, Ayus JC. Water water everywhere: standardizing postoperative fluid therapy with 0.9% normal saline. *Anesth Analg.* 2010;**110**:293–5.

6. Topjian AA, Stuart A, Pabalan AA, et al. Greater fluctuations in serum sodium levels are associated with increased mortality in children with externalized ventriculostomy drains in a PICU. *Pediatr Crit Care Med.* 2014;**15**:846–55.

7. Williams CN, Riva-Cambrin J, Presson AP, et al. Hyponatremia and poor cognitive outcome following pediatric brain tumor surgery. *J Neurosurg Pediatr.* 2015;**15**:480–7.

8. Williams CN, Riva-Cambrin J, Bratton SL. Etiology of postoperative hyponatremia following pediatric intracranial tumor surgery. *J Neurosurg Pediatr.* 2016;**17**:303–9.

9. Yung M, Keeley S. Randomised controlled trial of intravenous maintenance fluids. *J Paediatr Child Health.* 2009;**45**:9–14.

10. Montanana PA, Alapont V, Ocon AP, et al. The use of isotonic fluid as maintenance therapy prevents iatrogenic hyponatremia in pediatrics: a randomised, controlled open study. *Pediatr Crit Care Med.* 2008;**9**: 589–97.

11. Neville KA, Sandeman DJ, Rubinstein A, et al. Prevention of hyponatremia during maintenance intravenous fluid administration: a prospective randomized study of fluid type versus fluid rate. *J Pediatr.* 2010;**156**:313–19.

12. Friedman JN, Beck CE, DeGroot J, et al. Comparison of isotonic and hypotonic intravenous maintenance fluids: a randomized clinical trial. *JAMA Pediatr.* 2015;**169**:445–51.

13. Way C, Dhamrait R, Wade A, et al. Perioperative fluid therapy in children: a survey of current prescribing practice. *Br J Anaesth.* 2006;**97**:371–9.

14. Association of Paediatric Anaesthetists of Great Britain and Ireland. APA consensus guideline on perioperative fluid management in children. 2007. Available at www .apagbi.org.uk/sites/default/files/Perioperative_Fluid_ Management_2007.pdf.

15. Darrow DC, Yannet H. The changes in the distribution of body water accompanying increase and decrease in extracellular electrolyte. *J Clin Invest.* 1935;**14**:266–75.

16. Carpenter RHS. Beyond the Darrow-Jannet diagram: an enhanced plot for body fluid spaces and osmolality. *Lancet.* 1993;**342**:968–70.

17. Crawford B, Ludemann H. The renal response to intravenous injection of sodium chloride solutions in man. *J Clin Invest.* 1951;**30**:1456–62.

18. Drummer C, Gerzer R, Heer M, et al. Effects of an acute saline infusion on fluid and electrolyte metabolism in humans. *Am J Physiol.* 1992;**262**:F744–54.

19. Guyton AC. Interstitial fluid pressure: II. Pressure-volume curves of interstitial space. *Circ Res.* 1965;**16**:452–60.

20. Meyer BJ, Meyer A, Guyton AC. Interstitial fluid pressure: V. Negative pressure in the lungs. *Circ Res.* 1968;**22**:263–71.

21. Guyton AC, Granger HJ, Taylor AE. Interstitial fluid pressure. *Physiol Rev.* 1971;**51**:527–63.

22. Usher-Smith JA, Huang CL, Fraser JA. Control of cell volume in skeletal muscle. *Biol Rev.* 2009;**84**:143–59.

23. Overgaard-Steensen C, Stodkilde-Jorgensen H, Larsson A. Regional differences in osmotic behavior in brain during acute hyponatremia: an in vivo MRI-study of brain and skeletal muscle in pigs. *Am J Physiol Regul Integr Comp Physiol.* 2010; **299**:R521–32.

24. Holliday MA, Kalayci MN, Harrah J. Factors that limit brain volume changes in response to acute and sustained hyper- and hyponatremia. *J Clin Invest.* 1968;**47**:1916–28.

25. Arieff AI, Ayus JC, Fraser CL. Hyponatremia and death or permanent brain damage in healthy children. *Br Med J.* 1992;**304**:1218–22.

26. Moritz ML, Ayus JC. New aspects in the pathogenesis, prevention, and treatment of hyponatremic encephalopathy in children. *Pediatr Nephrol.* 2010;**25**: 1225–38.

27. Carlotti AP, Bohn D, Mallie J-P, et al. Tonicity balance, and not electrolyte-free water calculations, more accurately guides therapy for acute changes in natremia. *Intensive Care Med.* 2001;**27**:921–4.

28. Le Quesne LP, Lewis AAG. Postoperative water and sodium retention. *Lancet.* 1953;**261**:153–8.

29. Shafiee MAS, Bohn D, Hoorn EJ, et al. How to select optimal maintenance intravenous fluid therapy. *Q J Med.* 2003;**96**:601–10.

30. Bailey AG, McNaull PP, Jooste E, et al. Perioperative crystalloid and colloid fluid management in children: where are we and how did we get here? *Anesth Analg.* 2010;**110**:375–90.

31. Steele A, Gowrishankar M, Abrahamson S, et al. Postoperative hyponatremia despite near-isotonic saline infusion: a phenomenon of desalination. *Ann Intern Med.* 1997;**126**:20–5.

32. Hardesty DA, Sanborn MR, Parker WE, et al. Perioperative seizure incidence and risk factors in 223 pediatric brain tumor patients without prior seizures. *J Neurosurg Pediatrics.* 2011;**7**:609–15.

33. Sarnaik A, Meert K, Hackbarth R, et al. Management of hyponatremic seizures in children with hypertonic saline: a safe and effective strategy. *Crit Care Med.* 1991;**19**:758–62.

34. Levine JP, Stelnicki E, Weiner HL, et al. Hyponatremia in the postoperative craniofacial pediatric patient population: a connection to cerebral salt wasting syndrome and management of the disorder. *Plast Reconstr Surg.* 2001;**108**:1501–8.

35. Jimenez R, Casado-Flores J, Nieto M, et al. Cerebral salt wasting syndrome in children with acute central nervous system injury. *Pediatr Neurol.* 2006;**35**:261–3.

36. Hardesty DA, Kilbaugh TJ, Storm PB. Cerebral salt wasting syndrome in post-operative brain tumor patients. *Neurocrit Care.* 2012;**17**:382–7.

37. Singh S, Bohn D, Carlotti AP, et al. Cerebral salt wasting: truths, fallacies, theories, and challenges. *Crit Care Med.* 2002;**30**:2575–9.

38. Hollenberg NK. Set point for sodium homeostasis: surfeit, deficit, and their implications. *Kidney Int.* 1980;**17**:423–9.

39. Papadimitriou DT, Spiteri A, Pagnier A, et al. Mineralocorticoid deficiency in post-operative cerebral salt wasting. *J Pediatr Endocrinol Metab.* 2007;**20**:1145–50.

40. Di RC, Caldarelli M, Tamburrini G, et al. Surgical management of craniopharyngiomas—experience with a pediatric series. *J Pediatr Endocrinol Metab.* 2006;**19**(suppl 1):355–66.

41. Lindsay RC, Seckl JR, Padfield PL. The triple-phase response—problems of water balance after pituitary surgery. *Postgrad Med J.* 1995;**837**:439–41.

42. Hopper N, Albanese A, Ghirardello S, et al. The pre-operative assessment of craniopharyngiomas. *J Pediatr Endocrinol Metab.* 2006;**19**(suppl 1):325–7.

43. Paja M, Lucas T, Garcia-Uria J, et al. Hypothalamic-pituitary dysfunction in children with craniopharyngioma. *Clin Endocrinol.* 1995;**42**:467–73.

44. Hensen J, Henig A, Fahlbusch R, et al. Prevalence, predictors and patterns of postoperative polyuria and hyponatremia in the immediate course after transsphenoidal surgery for pituitary adenomas. *Clin Endocrinol.* 1999;**50**:431–9.

45. Thomas WC Jr. Diabetes insipidus. *J Clin Endocrinol.* 1957;**17**:565–8.

46. Poon WS, Lolin TF, Yeung CP, et al. Water and sodium disorders following surgical excision of pituitary region tumors. *Acta Neurochir.* 1996;**138**:921–7.

47. Davis BB, Bloom ME, Field JB, et al. Hyponatremia in pituitary insufficiency. *Metabolism.* 1969;**18**:821–32.

48. Edate S, Albanese A. Management of electrolyte and fluid disorders after brain surgery for pituitary/suprasellar tumours. *Horm Res Paediatr.* 2015;**83**:293–301.

49. Robson WL, Leung AK. Hyponatremia in children treated with desmopressin. *Arch Pediatr Adolesc Med.* 1998;**152**:930–1.

50. Bhalla P, Eaton FE, Coulter JB, et al. Lesson of the week: hyponatremic seizures and excessive intake of hypotonic fluids in young children. *Br Med J.* 1999;**11**:1554–7.

51. Balestrieri FJ, Chernow B, Rainey TG. Postcraniotomy diabetes insipidus, who's at risk? *Crit Care Med.* 1982;**10**:108–10.

52. Chanson P, Jedynak CP, Dabrowski G, et al. Ultra-low doses of vasopressin in the management of DI. *Crit Care Med.* 1987;**15**:44–6.

53. Wise-Faberowski L, Soriano SG, Ferrari L, et al. Perioperative management of diabetes insipidus in children. *J Neurosurg Anesthesiol.* 2004;**16**:220–5.

Intensive Care Considerations of Pediatric Neurosurgery

Craig D. McClain and Michael L. McManus

Introduction

Pediatric patients who have undergone intracranial and other complicated neurosurgical procedures are often best managed in an intensive care unit (ICU). These patients are at risk of acute changes in hemodynamic, respiratory, and neurologic status postoperatively and will therefore need frequent assessment to ensure a stable recovery. Further, these patients need to be in an environment where diagnostic and therapeutic interventions can be initiated immediately upon recognition of a change in status. Specialized neurocritical care teams have been demonstrated to improve patient outcomes for both adult and pediatric populations in higher volume centers.[1] The transition from operating room to ICU should begin with clear communication of the patient's history, intraoperative course (including relevant events such as airway issues, bleeding, and brain edema), and anticipated postoperative course including potential concerning focal neurologic deficits. Formalized sign-outs can be quite useful for this purpose.

All patients will require an immediate, thorough physiologic and neurologic assessment on arrival to the ICU. These thorough assessments should then be repeated frequently, as changes in the neurologic exam will be sensitive indicators of potential postoperative complications.

Respiratory Support

Most often, the primary plan for patients undergoing neurosurgical procedures will involve an extubated, comfortable, and cooperative patient at the conclusion of the surgery. While this is certainly ideal, not all patients who have undergone neurosurgical procedures meet extubation criteria prior to admission to the ICU. Therefore, clinicians should understand some of the unique considerations in the ventilator management of postoperative neurosurgical patients. In this situation, postoperative mechanical ventilation

aims to support gas exchange while permitting ongoing neurological assessment. These sometimes competing goals present clinicians with challenges. Certain ventilatory modes including triggered modes (i.e., pressure support) offer a method for providing respiratory support without losing the patient's intrinsic drive. This may serve as a marker of neurologic function while also minimizing respiratory muscle deconditioning. Although positive end expiratory pressure (PEEP) is commonly applied to most mechanically ventilated patients, it must be used with caution, especially in smaller children. Even small amounts of PEEP can result in hemodynamic problems.[2] These problems include impairment of venous return, depressed cardiac output, and ultimately impaired cerebral perfusion.[3] In the end, a balance between maintenance of adequate cardiac output and oxygenation must be reached that still allows for adequate cerebral perfusion. PEEP does not seem to increase intracranial pressure (ICP) unless fairly high levels of PEEP are employed. In infants with open fontanelles, there is no association between mean airway and intracranial pressures.

Hemodynamic Support

From a neurocritical care perspective, the primary goal of hemodynamic support is to maintain adequate cerebral perfusion pressure (CPP). Certainly, patients in a critical care setting often have coexisting pathologies that will require a balanced and thoughtful approach to maximizing therapeutic benefit for the patient as a whole. However, this section focuses on hemodynamic goals and support as they relate to the central nervous system (CNS) in critically ill children.

Children of all ages and developmental stages can need neurosurgical procedures that will require a stay in the ICU. In sick neonates, intermittent pressure-passivity of the cerebral circulation is present and can predispose to intracranial hemorrhage. This risk can be exacerbated by significant fluctuations in mean arterial pressure (MAP) and rapid administration of intravenous fluids. However, care must be taken to ensure an adequate CPP. Occasionally this support will require the use of vasopressors and/or inotropes. Even in very low birth weight infants, both dopamine and epinephrine are effective in supporting systemic pressure and restoring cerebral blood flow. Concepts surrounding factors that regulate cerebral perfusion are changing somewhat from classical teaching. It is becoming clearer that the process of cerebral autoregulation is a complicated system that involves much more than simply blood gas tensions and MAP values. Rather, there is synergism and interdependence between these systems as well as a variety of neurogenic mechanisms. Further, it is understood now that cerebral autoregulation does not necessarily maintain a constant perfusion over a range of pressures and that this autoregulation is not controlled solely through the muscles in the pial arterioles. Finally, the autonomic nervous system plays a vital role in modulating cerebral autoregulation and acts as a buffer in surges to perfusion pressure.[4] In fact, recent evidence would suggest that at lower levels of MAP, cerebral autoregulation behaves in a much more pressure-passive manner, whereas at higher levels of blood pressure, autoregulatory mechanisms maintain much tighter control over cerebral blood flow.

Implications for the Neurosurgical Patient

Despite the changing concepts of cerebral autoregulation and its implications on clinical care, we must still have basic guidelines and targets for a given patient.[5] When increased ICP is present, it is generally agreed upon that critical CPP for preschool children (2–6 years) is approximately 50 mmHg, rising to 55–60 mmHg in older children. In neonates and premature babies, the lower limit of pressure autoregulation is approximately 30–35 mmHg, depending on the adjusted postgestational age of the infant. A common rule of thumb for adequate MAP in these infants is to use the gestational age in weeks as a guideline for the lower limit of MAP. Keep in mind, this is not necessarily supported by clear evidence, so individual patients need to be treated accordingly. There are some recent data that would support this idea of much lower limit of mean arterial pressures to provide adequate cerebral blood flow in infants, at least under sevoflurane anesthesia.[6] It must

be mentioned that sevoflurane decreases cerebral metabolic requirement for oxygen ($CMRO_2$), so practitioners should extrapolate with caution.

Fluid Management

Meticulous fluid management is crucial in order to optimize the postoperative outcomes of neurosurgical patients. Pediatric patients are predisposed to a variety of postoperative fluid and electrolyte problems. Factors that contribute to this vary with developmental age but include small size, immature renal function, and other comorbidities. These dispositions are further magnified in neurosurgical patients by the disruption of normal homeostatic controls (see Chapter 20).

Overall, more than 10% of all children experience postoperative hyponatremia, and this percentage is likely higher after neurosurgery.[7–9] The mechanisms for this hyponatremia are varied and often involve the routine administration of hypotonic solutions to children recovering from surgery. In addition, elevated antidiuretic hormone (ADH) levels can result from a variety of factors including surgical stress, manipulation of structures involved in regulation of fluid and serum sodium status, postoperative pain and nausea, and finally fluid shifts and intravascular hypovolemia. Since sudden, unrecognized decreases in serum sodium can provoke seizures, it is prudent to follow serum electrolyte levels closely throughout the perioperative period. For a detailed discussion of perioperative electrolyte disorders and problems with serum sodium regulation, please refer to Chapter 20.

Concerns and Risks

Nonosmotic secretion of ADH increases the risk of hyponatremia after neurosurgical procedures, despite intraoperative fluids that are high in sodium and isotonic—or slightly hypertonic—to plasma (lactated Ringer's, 272 mOsm/L; PlasmaLyte, 295 mOsm/L; normal saline, 308 mOsm/L). Elevated levels of ADH can simply be part of an appropriate stress response to surgical stimulation. Alternatively, there are pathologic conditions of inappropriate ADH secretion that must be considered after many neurosurgical procedures, especially those near the sella turcica. When significant hyponatremia occurs, treatment may include hypertonic saline with free water excesses addressed through fluid restriction and administration of diuretics. It is recommended to avoid hypotonic solutions altogether in the perioperative period.

Management of serum glucose can be challenging as well. Small premature infants, with limited reserves of glycogen and limited gluconeogenesis, require continuous infusions of glucose at 5–6 mg/kg/min in order to maintain serum levels. Such infants are at particular risk for hypoglycemia. The stress of critical illness and resulting insulin resistance can produce hyperglycemia, which, in adults, is associated with poor outcomes. Various strategies to mitigate this phenomenon have been devised. Previously, tight glycemic control has been widely recommended in adults, but recent evidence paints a controversial picture surrounding the concepts of tight or standard glucose control. Hyperglycemia in patients with brain injury has been associated with increased rates of infection, longer ICU stays, and poorer neurologic outcomes. However, the effects of hypoglycemia can be deleterious to patients with brain injury as well. In pediatrics, hyperglycemia has been linked to poor outcome, but it remains unclear that tight glycemic control offers significant benefits to children. There is a growing volume of evidence suggesting that tight control may carry undue risk of hypoglycemia and its deleterious effects.[10] Given the clear evidence that both hyper- and hypoglycemia can be dangerous to patients who have suffered brain injuries, close monitoring of serum glucose should be part of routine neurologic care in the ICU. However, it also remains unclear how to best manage perturbations in glucose homeostasis in these at-risk patients. A conservative approach that maintains random serum glucose levels below 180 mg/dL may be utilized.

Sedation

Pain control and sedation present unique challenges in the pediatric ICU. Ideally, postoperative neurosurgical patients are comfortable, awake, and cooperative with their care. In pediatrics, some level of sedation is often necessary to ensure a safe recovery. This is true for both patients who have been successfully extubated at the conclusion of the neurosurgical procedure as well as those requiring mechanical ventilation. While the ideal sedation regime would include short-acting or reversible agents that can be withdrawn intermittently to permit neurologic assessment while presenting minimal side effects and development of

tolerance, a single agent that fits these criteria and is suitable for children has yet to be developed.

Agents and Their Implications for the Neurosurgical Patient

Propofol

Propofol is a common sedative hypnotic agent that is often used to provide sedation in perioperative and critical care settings. It exerts its effect acting as an agonist at gamma-aminobutyric acid (GABA) receptors. Common side effects of propofol include hypotension, hypoventilation, and apnea. Propofol is metabolized via conjugation in the liver. Small doses of propofol have relatively short clinical effect. This is because propofol is rapidly redistributed from the CNS. Thus, propofol is commonly assumed to be short-acting. The actual half-life is about 1–3 hours. However, continuous infusions of even a few hours will fill the compartments and result in a longer sedation effect. The context-sensitive half-life of propofol infusions is about 40 minutes. It is a potent sedative-hypnotic effect that is extremely useful in adult neurocritical care with limited utility in the pediatric ICU because of its association with the propofol infusion syndrome.[11] This is a fatal syndrome of bradycardia, rhabdomyolysis, metabolic acidosis, and multiple organ failure when propofol is used over extended periods in small children. The mechanism of this disastrous and life-threatening complication remains unclear, although its incidence appears related to both the duration of therapy and the cumulative dose. These difficulties are much less common in adults. If propofol is utilized in pediatric patients, continuous infusions of limited duration are recommended.[12]

Opioids/Benzodiazepines

The mainstay of sedation in the pediatric ICU remains a combination of opioids and benzodiazepine administered via continuous infusion.[13] Titration to a validated sedation score is advised and regular "drug holidays" help ensure that excessive sedation is avoided. Infants and children receiving opioid and/or benzodiazepine infusions for more than 3–5 days are subject to tolerance and experience symptoms of withdrawal when infusions are discontinued. Thus, a plan of discontinuation of sedation regimens should include strategies for weaning and monitoring for withdrawal. Different sedative drugs will have different patterns of weaning. Different classes of sedative drugs will have different signs and symptoms of withdrawal.

Opioids are medications that exert their effect by activating opioid receptors. A complete discussion of the variety of opioid medications useful for analgesia and sedative regimens is beyond the scope of this chapter. However, all opioids produce dose-dependent respiratory depression. Other common side effects include nausea, pruritus, decreased gastric transit time, and constipation. Opioids tend to affect hemodynamics minimally in euvolemic patients, although some individual opioids can have a profound vagolytic effect (e.g., fentanyl, sufentanil). Patients will become more and more tolerant to the effects of opioids over time, thus requiring larger doses to achieve a given clinical effect. When discontinuing sedative regimens that have included opioid medications, a plan must be in place to wean the patient from the induced dependence. This is often done with longer acting opioid medications such as methadone. Patients must be observed for signs of withdrawal during this period.

Benzodiazepine medications such as midazolam, lorazepam, and diazepam are commonly used sedative agents in a critical care setting. These agents can be used as intermittent bolus medications but are most often used as infusions for patients requiring longer term sedation regimens. Benzodiazepines all exert effect by enhancing the activity at GABA receptors. Similar to opioids, benzodiazepines all produce a dose-dependent respiratory depression. Also, in similar fashion, patients can develop a significant tolerance to benzodiazepines, especially after longer term use. These drugs are metabolized through hepatic mechanisms. Thus, with chronic use of benzodiazepines, other medications that also undergo metabolism via various cytochrome p450 pathways may have altered metabolism due to upregulation of hepatic pathways. Finally, much like opioids, weaning strategies must be in place prior to discontinuation of sedative regimens utilizing benzodiazepines. Long-term weans often use longer acting benzodiazepines such as lorazepam.

Dexmedetomidine

Dexmedetomidine is a unique drug that offers tremendous benefit to patients requiring sedation in the ICU following neurosurgical procedures.[14] It has

a completely different mechanism of action than other, classic, sedative agents. It acts by agonizing alpha-2 receptors in the CNS. As such, there is a significant sedative effect exerted with some degree of analgesia. It can be used as a short-acting single-agent sedative in the postoperative period. Apnea has not been described as a problem with dexmedetomidine as respiratory drive is easily maintained, even at relatively high doses when used by itself. There does appear to be some degree of synergism with other sedative/hypnotic drugs including propofol, opioids, and benzodiazepines, so care must be taken when dexmedetomidine is used as part of a multidrug regimen. Pediatric studies are limited, but the drug appears to be safe and effective when used for periods of 24 hours or less. That said, it has been anecdotally reported to be safely used for much longer periods of up to several weeks. Pharmacokinetics of dexmedetomidine in pediatric patients are similar to published adult values. Opioid cross-tolerance makes it a useful agent for treatment of fentanyl or morphine withdrawal. Transient increases in blood pressure can be seen with boluses followed by hypotension and bradycardia as sedation deepens. In our experience, both hypo- and hypertension can occasionally be observed with long-term infusions, and a withdrawal syndrome results when extended infusions are discontinued.

Seizures

Seizures are a common manifestation of neurological illness in pediatrics. In a child with active seizures in the ICU, basic management principles of acutely ill children should be followed with focus on maintenance of oxygenation, ventilation, and hemodynamic stability. Part of this care should include pharmacologic interventions to control the seizure activity. Seizure activity can be seen as an outward manifestation of changes in neurologic disease, and practitioners should be wary of the myriad problems that can precipitate seizure in postoperative neurosurgical patients. In the child with unexplained, altered mental status, nonconvulsive status epilepticus is also an important consideration.[15] Prophylaxis in the perioperative period, particularly for patients having procedures performed in or around the temporal lobes, and aggressive treatment of new seizure activity are well-recognized mainstays of care.

Once the acute problems with seizure activity have been treated, further investigation with laboratory evaluations, neuroimaging, and/or electroencephalography (EEG) may be warranted.

Agents

While phenytoin has been historically the agent used most commonly for prophylaxis, a number of problems with its clinical use have been identified, including the challenge of maintaining therapeutic serum levels through a period of critical illness.[16] More recently, other agents have become more utilized. Namely, levetiracetam has become the agent of choice for prophylaxis in many centers.[17] Advantages include a quite benign side effect profile, no need to monitor serum drug levels, broad spectrum of antiepileptic activity, limited interaction with other drugs, and similar bioavailability from both intravenous and oral dosing. Further, levetiracetam has minimal effect on hemodynamics and level of consciousness, compared to older agents such as phenytoin or phenobarbital.

When levetiracetam cannot be used, a number of alternative agents exist including phenobarbital, carbamazepine, and valproic acid. Though potentially compounding respiratory depression, phenobarbital 20 mg/kg is also an effective first-line antiepileptic drug. For acute treatment of status epilepticus, lorazepam 0.1 mg/kg IV/IM and diazepam 0.5 mg/kg PR are effective. Lorazepam may be repeated after 10 minutes and accompanied by fosphenytoin 20 mg/kg IV or IM if initial doses are ineffective.

Status Epilepticus

Refractory status epilepticus continues to present a significant challenge. Chemically induced coma remains the mainstay of care with antiepileptic drugs titrated to EEG burst suppression. Pentobarbital, midazolam, or phenobarbital may be employed in bolus infusion regimens with adjustment guided by continuous EEG. Mechanical ventilation and invasive monitoring are necessary since therapy often results in hypotension and myocardial depression. In addition, barbiturates have been associated with depression of immune function and increased rate of nosocomial infection. Propofol is also effective in quenching seizures and inducing coma, but the propofol infusion syndrome limits its use in pediatrics. Patients may require hemodynamic support from vasopressors and/or inotropes when being placed in an induced coma.

Intracranial Pressure Monitoring

ICP monitoring is desirable in trauma patients and in neurosurgical patients at risk for brain swelling or sudden expansion of an intracranial bleed or mass lesion (see Chapter 14).[18] Symptoms can be nonspecific in children, and changes in respiratory pattern with intermittent apnea may be its first sign in infancy. Infants have open fontanelles, so it is easy to simply feel if the fontanelle feels full or tense as an indicator of elevated ICP in such patients. Low thresholds are kept for invasive monitoring of unconscious patients since physiologic parameters are less sensitive than mental status changes. As stated, in babies, split sutures and bulging fontanelles provide clinical evidence of increasing ICP, but noninvasive quantitative measures are not reliable. The treatment of increased ICP in infants and children is still largely informed by adult data. A notable exception to this, as discussed above and elsewhere in this book, is that target thresholds for MAP and CPP vary with age. Osmotherapy with 3% (hypertonic) saline (usually 1–3 cm^3/kg initial boluses) is widely used in boluses or infusion to control ICP; it may more rapidly lead to severe hypernatremia in small children than in adults. Other elements of management extrapolated from adult data include avoidance of steroids, the preference of crystalloid over colloid resuscitation fluids, and the reluctance to employ hyperventilation. Regarding the latter, it is particularly important to recognize that small children are subject to inadvertent overventilation and that hyperventilation-associated cerebral ischemia can occur. Careful monitoring of blood gases, minute ventilation, and end-tidal carbon dioxide tensions are therefore recommended. When CPP is low and ICP remains high despite medical management, early decompressive craniectomy may have a better outcome in children than in adults.

Brain Death

Determination of brain death in older children is similar to in adults, but the diagnosis is difficult in infancy.[19] The Uniform Determination of Death Act defines death as "irreversible cessation of circulatory and respiratory function or irreversible cessation of all functions of the entire brain, including the brainstem." Diagnosis requires

- Normothermia
- Normotension
- Normal systemic oxygenation
- Absence of confounding toxins or medications

An apnea test (documenting the absence of respiratory effort despite $pCO_2 > 60$ torr) is conducted last since elevated pCO_2 may exacerbate neurologic injury. To establish irreversibility, age-related observation periods are necessary. For premature newborns and infants under 7 days of age, no such period has been established. For infants 1–8 weeks of age, our institution utilizes two exams and two isoelectric electroencephalograms 48 hours apart. Infants 2–12 months of age require two clinical exams separated by 24 hours. Patients older than 1 year require exams 6–12 hours apart, or 24 hours if the proximate cause of death is hypoxia-ischemia. The exam seeks to establish the complete absence of cortical and brainstem function. Cerebral ^{99}Tc-ECD single photon emission computed tomography (SPECT) scanning is used to document the absence of cerebral perfusion when confounders complicate the clinical diagnosis.

Key Points

- Extubation and initial neurological assessment are ideally accomplished in the operating room.
- Ideally, postoperative neurosurgical patients are comfortable, awake, and cooperative with their care.
- Postoperative mechanical ventilation is directed to support gas exchange while permitting ongoing neurological assessment.
- Hemodynamic goals involve the avoidance of hypotension and maintenance of adequate CPP.
- Sudden, unrecognized decreases in serum sodium can provoke seizures, and can be life-threatening.
- Avoid hypotonic solutions altogether in the perioperative period for neurosurgical patients.
- Seizure prophylaxis in the perioperative period and aggressive treatment of active seizures are well-recognized mainstays of care.
- ICP monitoring is desirable in victims of head trauma and in neurosurgical patients at risk for brain swelling or sudden expansion of an intracranial bleed or mass lesion.

- In babies, split sutures and bulging fontanelles provide clinical evidence of increasing ICP, but noninvasive quantitative measures are not reliable.
- The Uniform Determination of Death Act defines death as "irreversible cessation of circulatory and respiratory function or irreversible cessation of all functions of the entire brain, including the brainstem."

References

1. Bell MJ, Carpenter J, Au AK, Keating RF, Myseros JS, Yaun A, et al. Development of a pediatric neurocritical care service. *Neurocrit Care.* 2009;**10**(1):4–10.

2. Caricato A, Conti G, Della Corte F, Mancino A, Santilli F, Sandroni C, et al. Effects of PEEP on the intracranial system of patients with head injury and subarachnoid hemorrhage: the role of respiratory system compliance. *J Trauma.* 2005;**58**(3):571–6.

3. Nemer SN, Caldeira JB, Santos RG, Guimarães BL, Garcia JM, Prado D, et al. Effects of positive end-expiratory pressure on brain tissue oxygen pressure of severe traumatic brain injury patients with acute respiratory distress syndrome: a pilot study. *J Crit Care.* 2015;**30**(6):1263–16.

4. Willie CK, Tzeng YC, Fisher JA, Ainslie PN. Integrative regulation of human brain blood flow. *J Physiol.* 2014;**592**(5):841–59.

5. Strandgaard S, Paulson OB. Cerebral autoregulation. *Stroke.* 1984;**15**(3):413–16.

6. Rhondali O, André C, Pouyau A, Mahr A, Juhel S, De Queiroz M, et al. Sevoflurane anesthesia and brain perfusion. *Paediatr Anaesth.* 2015;**25**(2):180–5.

7. Judd BA, Haycock GB, Dalton N, Chantler C. Hyponatraemia in premature babies and following surgery in older children. *Acta Paediatr Scand.* 1987;**76**(3):385–93.

8. Bohn D. The problem of acute hyponatremia in hospitalized children: the solution is in the solution. *Pediatr Crit Care Med.* 2008;**9**(6):658–9.

9. Eulmesekian PG, Pérez A, Minces PG, Bohn D. Hospital-acquired hyponatremia in postoperative pediatric patients: prospective observational study. *Pediatr Crit Care Med.* 2010;**11**(4):479–83.

10. Jauch-Chara K, Oltmanns KM. Glycemic control after brain injury: boon and bane for the brain. *Neuroscience.* 2014;**283**:202–9.

11. Bray RJ. Propofol-infusion syndrome in children. *Lancet.* 1999;**353**(9169):2074–5.

12. Koriyama H, Duff JP, Guerra GG, Chan AW. Is propofol a friend or a foe of the pediatric intensivist? Description of propofol use in a PICU. *Pediatr Crit Care Med*. 2014;**15**(2):e66–71.

13. Zalieckas J, Weldon C. Sedation and analgesia in the ICU. *Semin Pediatr Surg*. 2015;**24**(1):37–46.

14. Plambech MZ, Afshari A. Dexmedetomidine in the pediatric population: a review. *Minerva Anestesiol*. 2015;**81**(3):320–32.

15. Abend NS, Dlugos DJ. Nonconvulsive status epilepticus in a pediatric intensive care unit. *Pediatr Neurol*. 2007;**37**(3):165–70.

16. Wolf GK, McClain CD, Zurakowski D, Dodson B, McManus ML. Total phenytoin concentrations do not accurately predict free phenytoin concentrations in critically ill children. *Pediatr Crit Care Med*. 2006;**7**(5):434–9; quiz 440.

17. Abend NS, Monk HM, Licht DJ, Dlugos DJ. Intravenous levetiracetam in critically ill children with status epilepticus or acute repetitive seizures. *Pediatr Crit Care Med*. 2009;**10**(4):505–10.

18. Huang SJ, Hong WC, Han YY, Chen YS, Wen CS, Tsai YS, et al. Clinical outcome of severe head injury using three different ICP and CPP protocol-driven therapies. *J Clin Neurosci*. 2006;**13**(8):818–22.

19. Mathur M, Petersen L, Stadtler M, Rose C, Ejike JC, Petersen F, et al. Variability in pediatric brain death determination and documentation in Southern California. *Pediatrics*. 2008;**121**(5):988–93.

Index

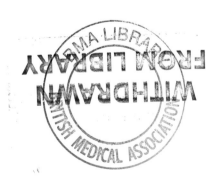